Study Guide

Maternity Nursing

8th Edition

Deitra Leonard Lowdermilk, RNC, PhD, FAAN
Shannon E. Perry, RN, CNS, PhD, FAAN
Kitty Cashion, RN, BC, MSN

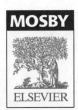

MOSBY

ELSEVIER

MOSBY
ELSEVIER

3251 Riverport Lane
St. Louis, Missouri 63043

STUDY GUIDE FOR MATERNITY NURSING, 8th EDITION　　　　ISBN: 978-0-323-08571-7

ISBN: 978-0-323-08571-7

Executive Editor: Robin Carter
Managing Editor: Laurie K. Gower
Publishing Services Manager: Deborah L. Vogel
Project Manager: John W. Gabbert
Cover Designer: Maggie Reid

Printed in the United States of America

Last digit is the print number:　9　8　7　6　5

Working together to grow
libraries in developing countries

www.elsevier.com | www.bookaid.org | www.sabre.org

ELSEVIER　BOOK AID International　Sabre Foundation

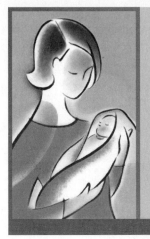

Introduction

This study guide is designed to help students effectively use the textbook, *Maternity Nursing,* 8th Edition. In addition to reviewing content of the text, this study guide encourages students to think critically in applying their knowledge.

Chapter Review Activities focus on recall and application of critical concepts and essential terminology. These activities are specifically designed to help you identify the important content of the chapter and test your level of knowledge and understanding after reading the chapter. Completion of each of the activities will provide you with an excellent resource to use when you are reviewing important content prior to course examinations. The knowledge that you attain by completing the activities will help you develop the theoretical foundation you need to answer the Critical Thinking Exercises that follow, to successfully pass course examinations and the NCLEX-RN® examination, and to manage the care of your patients in the clinical setting. Answers or answer guidelines for the activities are provided in the Answer Key at the end of this study guide.

Critical Thinking Exercises focus primarily on the application of critical chapter content. Typical patient care situations are presented, and you are required to apply concepts found in the chapter to solve problems, make decisions concerning care management, and provide responses to a patient's questions and concerns. These exercises may be completed on your own or with members of your study group. Completing the Critical Thinking Exercises will help you prepare for clinical experiences, course examinations, and the NCLEX-RN® examination, all of which focus on problem solving and application of nursing knowledge. Guidelines for completing the exercises, as well as specific chapter sections, boxes, or tables where the content for the answer can be found, are provided in the Answer Key at the end of this study guide.

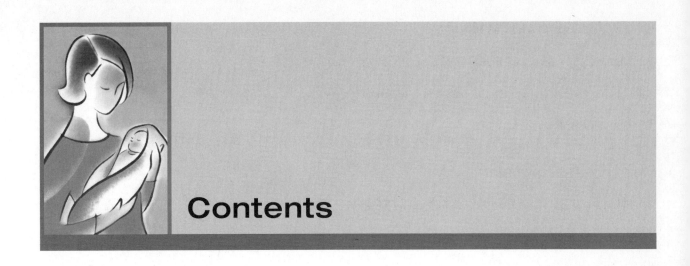

Contents

1 21st Century Maternity Nursing: Culturally Competent, Family and Community Focused, *1*

UNIT ONE: REPRODUCTIVE YEARS

2 Assessment and Health Promotion, *9*

3 Common Concerns, *25*

4 Contraception, Abortion, and Infertility, *37*

UNIT TWO: PREGNANCY

5 Genetics, Conception, and Fetal Development, *47*

6 Anatomy and Physiology of Pregnancy, *55*

7 Nursing Care of the Family during Pregnancy, *65*

8 Maternal and Fetal Nutrition, *77*

UNIT THREE: CHILDBIRTH

9 Labor and Birth Processes, *85*

10 Management of Discomfort, *91*

11 Fetal Assessment during Labor, *99*

12 Nursing Care of the Family during Labor and Birth, *107*

UNIT FOUR: POSTPARTUM PERIOD

13 Maternal Physiologic Changes, *117*

14 Nursing Care of the Family during the Fourth Trimester, *121*

15 Transition to Parenthood, *129*

UNIT FIVE: THE NEWBORN

16 Physiologic and Behavioral Adaptations of the Newborn, *137*

17 Assessment and Care of the Newborn and Family, *145*

18 Newborn Nutrition and Feeding, *155*

UNIT SIX: COMPLICATIONS OF CHILDBEARING

19 Assessment of High Risk Pregnancy, *167*

20 Pregnancy at Risk: Preexisting Conditions, *175*

21 Pregnancy at Risk: Gestational Conditions, *187*

22 Labor and Birth at Risk, *205*

23 Postpartum Complications, *219*

24 The Newborn at Risk, *231*

Answer Key, *247*

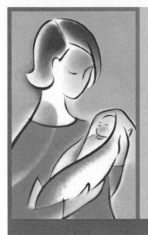

21st Century Maternity Nursing: Culturally Competent, Family and Community Focused

CHAPTER 1

CHAPTER REVIEW ACTIVITIES

MATCHING: Match the definition in Column I with the appropriate descriptive term in Column II.

COLUMN I

_____ 1. Number of births in 1 year per 1000 women

_____ 2. Infant who is born before completing 38 weeks of gestation

_____ 3. Number of women who die as a result of births and complications of pregnancy, childbirth, and the puerperium (the first 42 days after termination of the pregnancy) per 100,000 live births

_____ 4. Number of stillbirths and number of neonatal infant deaths per 1000 live births

_____ 5. Number of births per 1000 women between the ages of 15 and 44 (inclusive), calculated annually

_____ 6. Infant whose weight at birth is less than 2500 g (5 lb, 8 oz)

_____ 7. Number of deaths during the first year of life per 1000 live births

_____ 8. Number of deaths of infants younger than 28 days of age per 1000 live births

_____ 9. Miss S. lives with her 2-year-old adopted Romanian daughter, Anna.

_____ 10. Sara and Jim are married and live with their son, David, and Jim's mother, Jean.

_____ 11. Jane and Tom are a married couple living with their new baby boy, Alex.

_____ 12. Sue and Rose are a lesbian couple living with Sue's adopted daughter, Elise, whom they are raising together.

_____ 13. This family consists of Roy, his second wife Tara, and Roy's two daughters by a previous marriage.

_____ 14. Denise and Mike have been divorced for 3 years. They share custody of their four children.

COLUMN II

A. Fertility rate
B. Infant mortality rate
C. Birth rate
D. Maternal mortality rate
E. Neonatal mortality rate
F. Perinatal mortality rate
G. Low-birth-weight
H. Preterm infant
I. Binuclear family
J. Single-parent family
K. Homosexual family
L. Nuclear family
M. Extended family
N. Reconstituted (blended) family

FILL IN THE BLANKS: Insert the term that corresponds to each of the following.

15. _____ is a specialty area of nursing practice that focuses on the care of childbearing women and their families through all stages of pregnancy and childbirth, as well as the first 4 weeks after birth.

16. _____ is a practice that is based on findings obtained through research and clinical trials.

17. _____ is an umbrella term for the use of communication technologies and electronic information to provide or support health care when the participants are separated by distance.

18. Mrs. M., a newly delivered Mexican-American woman, tells the nurse not to include certain foods on her meal tray because her mother told her to avoid those foods while breastfeeding. The nurse tells her that she doesn't have to avoid any foods and should eat whatever she desires. _____

19. Ms. P., an immigrant from Vietnam, has lived in the United States for 1 year. She tells you that she enjoys the comfort of wearing blue jeans and sneakers on casual occasions such as shopping, even though she never would have done so in Vietnam. _____

20. A family of Cambodian boat people immigrated to the United States and have been living in Denver for over 5 years. The parents express concern about their children, ages 10, 13, and 16, stating, "The children act so differently now. They are less respectful to us and want to eat only American food and go to rock concerts. It's hard to believe they are our children." _____

21. The nurse is preparing a healthy diet plan for Mrs. O, who is Polish-American. In doing so, she takes the time to identify and include the Polish foods that are favorites of Mrs. O. _____

22. A central concern of nurses is to plan and provide care that reflects and respects the values, beliefs, and practices to which the patient and family adhere as part of a particular social group. _____

23. _____ is a set of guidelines that an individual inherits as a member of a particular society that tells people how to view the world and how to relate to other people, supernatural forces, and the natural environment.

24. _____ is a nursing practice approach that focuses on the way that people of different cultures perceive life events and the health care system.

Family Theory

25. _____ are interaction and communication processes that allow family members to perform essential activities by working cooperatively with each other and assuming appropriate social roles. Family members use _____ to determine roles and role responsibilities. _____ are set up by a family between itself and society. A family sets up _____ through which it interacts with society and ensures that its members receive their share of resources.

26. _____ is a family theory that is based on a science of wholeness characterized by interaction among the components of the family and between the family and the environment. The family is viewed as a whole that is different from the sum of the individual members.

27. _____ is a family theory that focuses on the family as it moves in time and through transitions. Each family member progresses through phases of growth, from dependence through active independence to interdependence. The family structure and function also vary over time.

28. _____ is a family theory that is concerned with the ways families react to stressful events and suggests factors that promote adaptation to these events. Stress must be studied within the _____ and _____ contexts in which the family is living.

29. Analyzing individual census tracts helps identify subpopulations, or _____, with differing needs.

30. _____ are groups of people who are at higher risk of developing physical, mental, or social health problems or who are more likely to have worse outcomes resulting from these health problems than the population as a whole. Women who are _____, _____, _____, or _____ are often considered vulnerable.

MULTIPLE CHOICE: Circle the one correct option and state the rationale for the option chosen.

31. A family with open boundaries:
    A. Uses available support systems to meet its needs.
    B. Is more prone to crises related to increased exposure to stressors.
    C. Discourages family members from setting up channels.
    D. Strives to maintain family stability by avoiding outside influences.

32. Which one of the following nursing actions is most likely to reduce a patient's anxiety and enhance the patient's personal security as it relates to the concept of personal space needs?
    A. Touching the patient before and during procedures
    B. Providing explanations when performing tasks
    C. Making eye contact as much as possible
    D. Reducing the need for the patient to make decisions

33. A Native-American woman gave birth to a baby girl 12 hours ago. The nurse notes that the woman keeps her baby in the bassinet except for feeding and states that she will wait until she gets home to begin breastfeeding. The nurse recognizes this behavior as a reflection of:
    A. Embarrassment.
    B. Delayed attachment.
    C. Disappointment that the baby is a girl.
    D. Her belief that babies should not be fed colostrum.

34. A Hispanic woman has just given birth to a baby boy. The nurse caring for the woman should recognize that the woman will likely:
    A. Have a meal of refried beans brought from home.
    B. Request that a fan be placed in the room to cool her body.
    C. Remain on bed rest for 3 days after birth.
    D. Request to take a shower as soon as possible.

TRUE OR FALSE: Circle T if true or F if false for each of the following statements. Correct the false statements.

T   F   35. Currently the highest birth rates are for women between 25 and 29 years of age.

T   F   36. Births to unmarried women are frequently related to less favorable outcomes because there are typically a large number of adolescents in this group.

T   F   37. One fourth of all births in the United States are to unmarried women.

T   F   38. The infant mortality rate can be reduced by shifting the emphasis from high technology to improved access to preventive health care services, especially for low-income families.

T   F   39. The greatest risk for giving birth to a low-birth-weight infant occurs among Hispanic women.

T   F   40. The U.S. ranking of 26th for infant mortality among industrialized nations relates to the high rate of low birth weight infants born in the United States compared with other countries.

T   F   41. The maternal mortality rate is a common indicator of the adequacy of prenatal care and the health of the nation as a whole.

T   F   42. The most significant barrier to accessible prenatal care is the inability to pay.

T   F   43. The incidence of high risk pregnancies has been decreasing steadily.

T   F   44. The two most frequently reported maternal medical risk factors are hypertension associated with pregnancy and diabetes.

T   F   45. Cultural beliefs and practices related to childbearing and parenting for a subculture must be assessed for each woman and family representing that subculture because variations in beliefs and practices are possible.

T   F   46. Women from Southeast Asia often vocalize while experiencing the pain and discomfort associated with the childbirth process.

T   F   47. African-American women seek prenatal care early because they view pregnancy as a time when women require medical care and supervision.

T   F   48. Hispanic women appreciate the opportunity to shower or bathe as soon as possible after birth.

T   F   49. The nurse should recognize that a Vietnamese woman might not wish to breastfeed until her milk comes in; she believes newborns should not be fed colostrum because it is dirty.

T   F   50. European-American women typically prefer a technology-dominated childbirth approach rather than a natural approach.

T   F   51. Native-American women often use herbal preparations to promote uterine contractions during labor and stop bleeding in the postpartum period.

T   F   52. Hispanic-American women often desire and expect reduced activity or even bed rest for as long as 3 days after birth.

T   F   53. Women make up one-third of the homeless people in America.

T   F   54. Migrant women are more likely than others to receive early prenatal care.

T   F   55. Over time, health disparities decline for the migrant population.

T   F   56. The perinatal continuum of care starts with family planning and preconception care and ends when the infant is 1 year of age.

57. *IDENTIFY* the factors that contribute to infant mortality in the United States.

58. *STATE* three changes that have occurred in the health care of women and their infants. *DESCRIBE* how each change has affected the quality of health care.

59. *LIST* the most common barriers to early and ongoing prenatal care in the United States.

60. *DISCUSS* the importance of using family theory as a basis for managing the care of pregnant women and their families.

61. *DISCUSS* why the nurse should take each of the following "products of culture" into consideration when providing care within a cultural context:

A. Communication
B. Space
C. Time
D. Family roles

62. Nurses must avoid making stereotypical assumptions when caring for patients from specific sociocultural or religious groups. *IDENTIFY* the factors that influence the degree to which a woman and her family adhere to the traditional beliefs and practices related to childbearing and parenting of their subculture.

63. A committee of experts from many community health-related organizations has identified a set of indicators that can be used to assess the health and well-being of a community.

A. *LIST* the indicators of health status outcome.

B. *LIST* the indicators of risk factors.

64. *CITE* the social and health problems faced by migrant laborers and their families.

65. *STATE* three characteristics of refugees that can significantly increase the difficulties they experience.

CRITICAL THINKING EXERCISES

1. *SUPPORT* the accuracy of the following statement: An emphasis on high-technology medical care and lifesaving techniques will not reduce the rate of preterm and low-birth-rate-weight infants in the United States.

2. *PROPOSE* three changes in health care and its delivery that you believe can improve the health status and well-being of mothers and their infants and reduce the rate of infant and maternal mortality. *SUPPORT* your answer by using the content presented in Chapter 1 and your own experiences with the health care system.

3. Self-management approaches in health care management are appealing to women who want to assume responsibility for their own level of wellness and become active partners with their health care providers. *DISCUSS* the care measures that you as a nurse would implement when providing maternal health care to enhance a pregnant woman's responsibility for herself and partnership with you.

4. *IMAGINE* that you are a nurse working in a clinic that provides prenatal services to a multicultural community predominated by Hispanic, African-American, and Asian families. *DESCRIBE* how you would adapt care measures to reflect the cultural beliefs and practices of pregnant women and their families from each of the following cultural groups.

Hispanic

African-American

Asian

5. Pamela is a 20-year-old Native-American woman. She is 3 months pregnant and has come to the prenatal clinic on the reservation where she lives for her first visit to obtain some prenatal vitamins, which her friends at work told her are important.

A. *STATE* the questions the nurse should ask to determine Pamela's cultural expectations about childbearing.

B. *DESCRIBE* the communication approach you would consider when interviewing Pamela.

C. *IDENTIFY* the Native-American beliefs and practices regarding childbearing that might influence Pamela's approach to her pregnancy and birth.

6. A nurse has been providing care to a Hispanic family. This family recently experienced the birth of twin girls at 38 weeks of gestation. It is the first birth experience for both parents and the first grandchildren for the extended family. Both newborns are healthy and living at home.

A. *OUTLINE* how the nurse should accomplish the goal of providing health care to this family within a cultural context.

B. *DESCRIBE* the cultural beliefs and practices that this family, as a Hispanic family, might use as guidelines to provide care to their twin girls.

7. The nurse-midwife at a prenatal clinic has been assigned to care for a refugee couple from Bosnia who has recently emigrated to the United States. The woman has just been diagnosed as 2 months pregnant. Neither she nor her husband speaks English. Outline the process this nurse should use when working with a translator to facilitate communication with this couple, thereby enhancing care management.

8. As a nurse working in home care, it is helpful for the nurse to become familiar with the neighborhood and resources with which her or his patients interact.

A. *DESCRIBE* the walking survey of a community.

B. *DISCUSS* how the nurse could use the findings from this survey to provide health care to patients who reside in the assessed community.

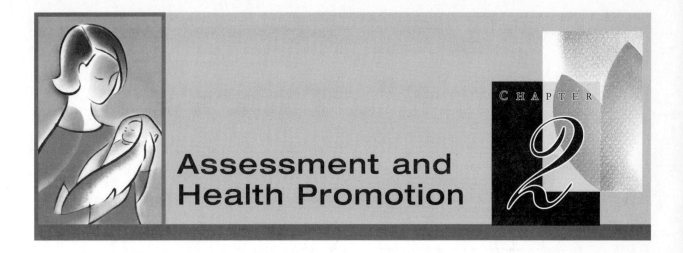

Assessment and Health Promotion

CHAPTER 2

CHAPTER REVIEW ACTIVITIES

1. Preconception care has become an integral component of perinatal health care.

   A. *DESCRIBE* the concept of preconception care, including its importance in achieving the goal of a healthy and positive pregnancy outcome for the parents, newborn, and family.

   B. *LIST* the purposes of preconception care and counseling.

   C. *STATE* the components of preconception care.

   D. *IDENTIFY* the individuals who should participate in this type of health care service.

2. *IDENTIFY* the most common reasons why women seek health care.

TRUE OR FALSE: Circle T for true or F for false for each of the following statements. Correct the false statements.

T F 3. Preconception care and counseling is a health care service designed primarily for women of childbearing age who have chronic health problems.

T F 4. During the climacteric women should continue to use birth control because pregnancy can still occur.

T F 5. Women tend to use primary care services more often and more effectively than men.

T F 6. Women older than 35 years of age are at risk for age-related conditions such as chronic diseases that can adversely affect pregnancy.

T F 7. Smoking increases the risk for osteoporosis after menopause.

T F 8. Women are more likely than men to abuse drugs.

T F 9. Maternal cocaine use is the leading cause of fetal mental retardation in the United States.

T F 10. Birth defects have been related to moderate-to-high caffeine intake.

T F 11. The choice of contraceptive influences a woman's risk for contracting a sexually transmitted infection.

T F 12. Human papillomavirus (HPV) is the most common cause of cervical cancer.

T F 13. Many female sexual abuse and assault victims experience posttraumatic stress disorder.

T F 14. Race, religion, social background, age, and educational level are very significant factors in identifying and differentiating women at risk for abuse.

T F 15. The key feature for establishing rape is the absence of consent; threat or coercion implies the lack of consent.

T F 16. It is recommended that a woman be tested by a Papanicolaou (Pap) test for the first time at the age of 18 years, or when the woman becomes sexually active.

T F 17. Clinical breast examination by a health care provider is recommended every year for women after the age of 30.

T F 18. The best time for women experiencing menstrual periods to perform a breast self-examination is several days after the end of each period or when the breasts are not tender or swollen.

T F 19. The American Cancer Society recommends an annual mammogram, beginning at age 38.

T F 20. Women should be encouraged to drink at least four to six glasses of water daily.

T F 21. Anorexia nervosa is the most common eating disorder.

T F 22. Swimming improves cardiovascular fitness and helps prevent osteoporosis.

T F 23. Kegel exercises help strengthen abdominal and pelvic muscles.

T F 24. Pregnancy is possible at any time after menarche occurs.

T F 25. Variations in the length of the follicular phase account for almost all variations in the length of menstrual cycles.

T F 26. Implantation of a fertilized ovum usually occurs about 14 days after ovulation.

T F 27. Mittelschmerz refers to the stretchable quality of cervical mucus that occurs in response to estrogen secretion before ovulation.

T F 28. Men and women are very different in terms of their physiologic response to sexual excitement and orgasm.

T F 29. For many women modesty, fear, and anxiety can make the health history interview and physical examination an ordeal.

T F 30. Vulvar (genital) self-examination should be performed by all women who are either sexually active or 18 years of age or older at least once a month, between menstrual periods.

31. *LIST* the components that should be included in well-woman health care.

32. *DISCUSS* three barriers to seeking health care that women face. *IDENTIFY* one nursing intervention that can be used to help a woman overcome each barrier.

33. *STATE* the impact on the maternal-fetal unit of using each of the following illicit drugs while pregnant:

Cocaine

Heroin

Marijuana

34. *DESCRIBE* the concept of "cycle of violence."

FILL IN THE BLANKS: Insert the term that corresponds to each of the following.

Health Promotion

35. _____, _____, _____, and _____ or _____ are all terms applied to a pattern of assaultive and coercive behaviors that includes _____, _____, and _____ attacks and _____ coercion inflicted by a male partner in a marriage or another heterosexual significant intimate relationship. _____ is often a time when violence begins or escalates.

36. _____ is an act of violence rather than a sexual act, and in its strictest sense it is the _____ of the female _____ or _____ without the woman's consent. _____ is a term used to describe an act of force with a much broader definition, which includes unwanted or uncomfortable _____, _____, _____, _____, _____, or other _____ acts.

37. A nurse is teaching a group of male and female adolescents about sexually transmitted infections (STIs). One of the students asks the nurse about the effects that these infections can have. *LIST* the possible consequences of STIs that the nurse might describe.

38. A nurse involved in the health care of women must be alert for factors in a woman's health history that have been associated with an increased risk for specific reproductive tract malignancies. *IDENTIFY* the factors that increase a woman's risk for each of the following gynecologic cancers.

| **Cervical** | **Endometrial** | **Ovarian** |

39. Imagine that you are a nurse working in a women's health clinic. Recognizing that more and more women are involved in violent relationships, you include assessment for clues that indicate whether your patients are in such relationships. *CITE* the characteristics of women in battering relationships for which you would be alert during the assessment process.

FILL IN THE BLANKS: Insert the term that corresponds to each of the following.

Female Reproductive Tract and Breasts

40. _____ Fatty pad that lies over the anterior surface of the symphysis pubis

41. _____ Two rounded folds of fatty tissue covered with skin that extend downward and backward from the mons pubis (their purpose is to protect the inner vulvar structures)

42. _____ Two flat reddish folds composed of connective tissue and smooth muscle that are supplied with extremely sensitive nerve endings

43. _____ Hoodlike covering of the clitoris

44. _____ Fold of tissue under the clitoris

45. _____ Thin flat tissue formed by the joining of the labia minora, found underneath the vaginal opening at the midline

46. _____ Small structure composed of erectile tissue with numerous sensory nerve endings that increases in size during sexual arousal

47. _____ Almond-shaped area enclosed by the labia minora that contains openings to the urethra, Skene's glands, vagina, and Bartholin's gland

48. _____ Skin-covered muscular area between the fourchette and the anus that covers the pelvic structures

49. _____ Fibromuscular collapsible tubular structure that extends from the vulva to the uterus and lies between the bladder and rectum (its mucosal lining is arranged in transverse folds called _____; _____ and _____ glands secrete mucus for its lubrication)

50. _____ Anterior, posterior, and lateral pockets that surround the cervix

51. _____ Muscular pelvic organ located between the bladder and the rectum just above the vagina (_____ is a deep pouch, or recess, posterior to the cervix formed by the posterior ligament)

52. _____ Upper triangular portion of the uterus

53. _____ Also known as the lower uterine segment, the short constricted portion that separates the corpus of the uterus from the cervix

54. _____ Dome-shaped top of the uterus

55. _____ Highly vascular lining of the uterus

56. _____ Layer of the uterus composed of smooth muscles that extend in three different directions

57. _____ Passageways between the ovaries and the uterus, attached at each side of the dome-shaped top of the uterus

58. _____ Almond-shaped organs located on each side of the uterus (their two functions are _____ and the production of the hormones _____, _____, and _____)

59. _____ Lower cylindric portion of the uterus composed of fibrous connective tissue and elastic tissue. The _____ canal connects the uterine cavity to the vagina; the opening between the uterus and this canal is the _____; the opening between the canal and the vagina is the _____. The _____ junction is the location in the cervix where the squamous and columnar epithelia meet. This is the most common site for neoplastic changes; therefore cells from this site are scraped for the _____ smear.

60. _____ Paired mammary glands

61. _____ Segment of mammary tissue that extends into the axilla

62. _____ Mammary papilla

63. _____ Pigmented section of the breast that surrounds the nipple

64. _____ Sebaceous glands that cause the areola to appear rough

65. _____ Breast structures lined with epithelial cells that secrete colostrum and milk

66. _____ Milk reservoirs

67. A nurse working in the field of women's health must have knowledge of the female reproductive system, including the internal and external structures, the interrelationship of these structures, and their normal characteristics. *LABEL* each of the following illustrations as indicated. *DESCRIBE,* on a separate sheet of paper, the normal characteristics and functions of each structure (use the figures in Chapter 4 and those found in a physical assessment or anatomy textbook to assist you with the labels and descriptions).

A. **External female genitalia**

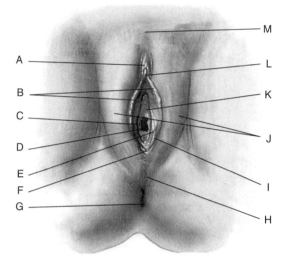

B. **Perineal body with surrounding tissues and organs**

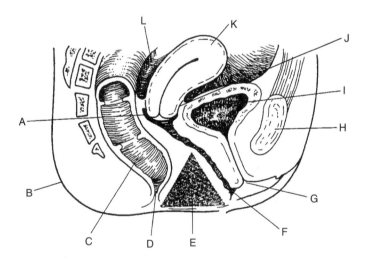

C. Cross section of uterus, adnexa, and upper vagina

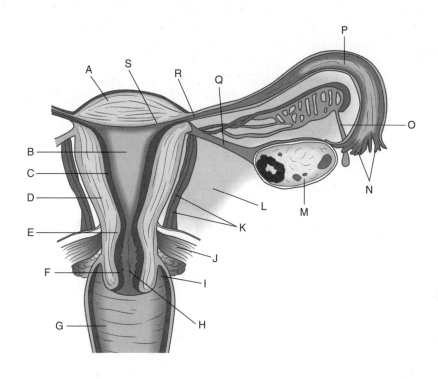

D. Female breast

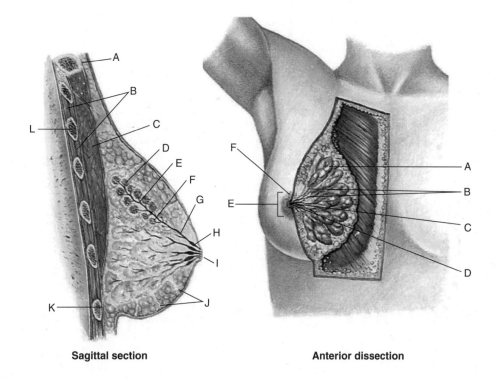

Sagittal section

Anterior dissection

E. **Female pelvis**

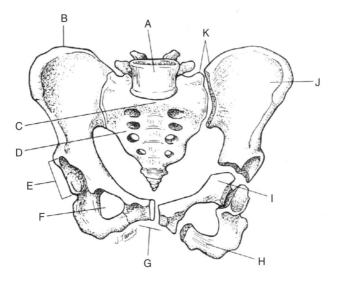

68. The diagram below illustrates the cyclic changes that occur during the menstrual cycle of a woman of childbearing age.

A. *LABEL* the diagram as indicated in terms of hormones, phases and cycles, and specific ovarian structures.

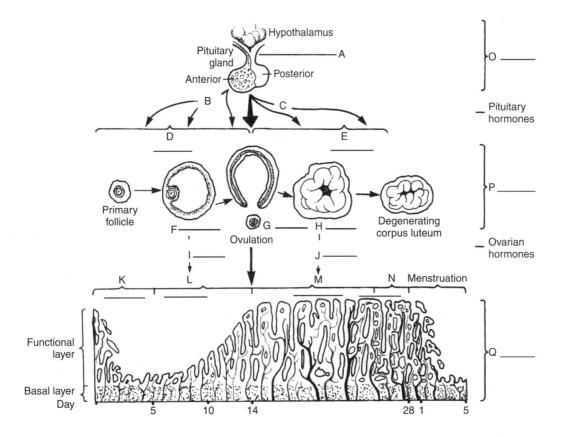

B. Hormones play an important role in the regulation of the menstrual cycle. *DESCRIBE* how each of the following hormones influences the changes and events that occur during the cycle:

Gonadotropin-releasing hormone

Follicle-stimulating hormone

Luteinizing hormone

Estrogen

Progesterone

Prostaglandins

69. *DESCRIBE* each of the following components of the pelvic examination:

External inspection and palpation

Internal examination

Bimanual palpation

Rectovaginal palpation

70. It is essential that guidelines for laboratory and diagnostic procedures be followed exactly to ensure the accuracy of the results obtained. *OUTLINE* the guidelines that should be followed when performing a Pap test in terms of each of the following.

Patient preparation and instruction

Timing during examination when the specimen is obtained

Sites for specimen collection

Handling of specimens

Frequency of performance

71. Sara, a 20-year-old woman, tells the nurse that she performs a breast self-examination (BSE) on a regular basis. The nurse evaluates Sara's understanding of BSE and her ability to perform the technique correctly. The nurse's findings are documented below. *INDICATE* with a "+" the findings that reflect accurate knowledge and correct technique, and use a "−" for the findings that require further instruction and demonstration. *STATE* the nursing instruction for the findings that require further teaching and demonstration.

A. Performs examination every 1 to 2 months _____

B. Performs BSE about 4 days after menstruation begins _____

C. Begins BSE by standing in front of a mirror with her arms in at least two positions—at rest at her sides and above her head—and observing characteristics of her breasts _____

D. Observes the size of her breasts, the direction of her nipples, the appearance of her skin, and any dimples or lumps anywhere when looking at her breasts in the mirror _____

E. Lies down on her bed and puts a pillow under the shoulder of the breast she is going to palpate; places the arm on that side under her head _____

F. Uses the tips of her four fingers to palpate her breast _____

G. Begins to palpate at her nipple and then moves in a circular pattern around her entire breast _____

H. Squeezes her nipple between her thumb and forefinger to check for discharge _____

I. Palpates her breasts and up into her axilla while taking a shower _____

MULTIPLE CHOICE: Circle the one correct option and state the rationale for the option chosen.

72. Which of the following is most accurate regarding persons who should participate in preconception counseling?

A. All women and their partners as they make decisions about their reproductive future

B. All women during their childbearing years

C. Sexually active women who do not use birth control

D. Women with chronic illnesses such as diabetes who are planning to get pregnant

73. A newly married 25-year-old woman has been smoking since she was a teenager. She has come to the women's health clinic for a checkup before she begins trying to get pregnant. The woman demonstrates a need for further instruction about the effects of smoking on reproduction and health when she states:

A. "Smoking can interfere with my ability to get pregnant."

B. "My husband also needs to stop smoking because second-hand smoke can have an adverse effect on my pregnancy and the development of the baby."

C. "Smoking can make my pregnancy last longer than it should."

D. "Smoking can reduce the amount of calcium in my bones."

74. A nurse has instructed a female patient regarding self-examination of the external genitalia. Which of the statements made by the patient require further instruction?

A. "I will perform this examination at least once a month, especially if I change sexual partners or am sexually active."

B. "I will become familiar with how my genitalia look and feel so I will be able to detect changes."

C. "I will use the examination to determine when I should get medications at the pharmacy for yeast infections."

D. "I will wash my hands thoroughly before and after I examine myself."

75. To enhance the accuracy of the Pap test, the nurse should instruct the patient to:

A. Take a tub bath the morning of the test.

B. Stop taking her birth control pill for 2 days before the test.

C. Avoid intercourse for 24 hours before the test.

D. Douche with a specially prepared antiseptic solution the night before the test.

76. When assessing women, it is important for the nurse to keep in mind the possibility that they are victims of violence. The nurse should:

A. Use an abuse assessment screen during the assessment of every woman.

B. Recognize that abuse rarely occurs during pregnancy.

C. Assess a woman's legs and back as the most commonly injured areas.

D. Notify the police immediately if abuse is suspected.

1. Alice and her husband, George, have just gotten married. At her annual gynecologic checkup, Alice tells the nurse practitioner that she and her husband plan to get pregnant in about 1 year. *DESCRIBE* the process that the nurse should follow in providing Alice and George with preconception care and counseling.

2. Joyce, a 30-year-old woman, arrives at the women's health clinic and is assigned to a nurse practitioner for care. The nurse notes that Joyce is very nervous and seems embarrassed when she tells the nurse that this is the first time she has ever come for "female care." *DESCRIBE* how the nurse should approach Joyce to ensure quality care that meets Joyce's needs and reduces her level of anxiety and embarrassment.

3. Laura is a 28-year-old pregnant woman at 8 weeks of gestation. This is her first pregnancy. During the health history interview, she reveals that she smokes at least one pack of cigarettes each day. When discussing this practice with the nurse, Laura states, "My friends smoked when they were pregnant, and their babies are okay. In fact, two of them had pregnancies that were a little shorter than expected, and they had nice small babies." *DESCRIBE* how the nurse should respond to Laura's comments.

4. As a nurse working at a women's health clinic, you have been assigned to design a health promotion and illness prevention class for a group of young adult women.

   A. *OUTLINE* the content that you would include in the class and the teaching methodologies that you would use when discussing each of the following topics.

   Nutrition

   Exercise

Health risk prevention

    B. During the class one of the women asks what safer sex means and who needs to use it. *DESCRIBE* how you would respond to her question.

    C. Another woman expresses concern about the increase in violence against women. She states, "One of my friends was raped, and a colleague at work was beaten by her boyfriend." *DISCUSS* how you would respond to this woman's concern and what you would tell the group about measures they could use to protect themselves from violence and injury.

5. Mary comes to the women's health clinic for her annual gynecologic checkup. During the health history interview, she tells the nurse, "I have just about reached the end of my rope." Mary cites family and work pressures as the cause.

    A. *IDENTIFY* the physical and emotional effects that Mary might experience as a result of her high level of stress.

    B. *DESCRIBE* the stress management techniques that the nurse could recommend to Mary to help her reduce her level of stress and cope with it in a healthy manner.

6. As a nurse working in a women's health clinic, you have been assigned to interview a new female patient to obtain her health history.

   A. *WRITE* a series of questions that you would ask to obtain data related to her reproductive and sexual health and practices.

   B. *LIST* several examples of communication variations that can occur even when the nurse and the patient speak the same language.

7. Breast and vulva (genitalia) self-examination are important assessment techniques to teach a woman. *OUTLINE* the procedure you would use to teach each technique to one of your patients. *INCLUDE* the teaching methodologies you would use to enhance learning.

Breast self-examination

Vulvar (genital) self-examination

8. Lu is a 25-year-old exchange student from China who has been living in the United States for 3 months. This is the first time she has been away from home. She comes to the university women's health clinic for a checkup and to obtain birth control. *DESCRIBE* how the nurse assigned to Lu might approach and communicate with her in a culturally sensitive manner.

9. Nurses working in women's health care must be aware of the growing problem of violence against women. All women should be screened when being assessed during health care for the possibility of abuse.

   A. *DESCRIBE* how you as a nurse would adjust the environment where the health history interview and physical examination take place to elicit a woman's confidence and trust.

   B. *IDENTIFY* indicators of possible abuse that you would look for before the appointment and then during the health history interview and physical examination.

   C. *STATE* the questions that you would ask to screen for abuse.

   D. *DISCUSS* the approach that you would take if abuse is confirmed during the assessment.

10. As a student, you might be assigned to assist a health care provider during the performance of a pelvic examination for one of your patients.

   A. *DESCRIBE* how you would do the following:

   Prepare your patient for the examination

   Support your patient during the examination

Assist your patient after the examination

B. *DESCRIBE* how you would assist the health care provider who is performing the examination.

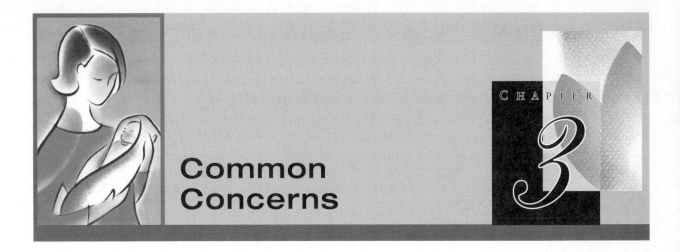

Common Concerns

CHAPTER REVIEW ACTIVITIES

FILL IN THE BLANKS: Insert the term that corresponds to each of the following.

Menstrual Disorders

1. _____ refers to the absence or cessation of menstrual flow.

2. _____ or painful menstruation is one of the most common gynecologic problems for women of all ages.

3. _____ dysmenorrhea is a type of painful menstruation that occurs because of a physiologic alteration in some women.

4. Both _____ and _____ are necessary for primary dysmenorrhea to occur.

5. _____ is a type of painful menstruation that is acquired after age 25 and associated with pelvic pathology. Pain often begins _____.

6. _____ is the appearance of physical and psychologic symptoms that begin in the luteal phase of the menstrual cycle. A diagnosis is only made if the following criteria are met: _____, _____, _____, _____, and _____.

7. _____ is a menstrual disorder characterized by the presence and growth of endometrial tissue outside the uterus. This tissue responds to hormonal stimulation by growing during the _____ and _____ phases of the menstrual cycle and bleeds during or immediately after _____, resulting in a(n) _____ response with subsequent _____ and _____ to adjacent organs.

8. The major symptoms of endometriosis are _____, _____ and _____. Many women also experience bowel symptoms such as _____, _____, and _____.

9. _____ is the term used to describe infrequent menstrual periods. One of the most common causes of scanty menstrual flow is the use of _____.

10. _____ refers to bleeding between menstrual periods.

11. _____ is excessive or profuse menstrual bleeding.

12. _____ is excessive bleeding with no demonstrable, organic cause. It is most commonly caused by _____ when there is no surge of _____ or if insufficient _____ is produced by the _____ to support the endometrium so it begins to involute and shed. This most often occurs when the menstrual cycle is just becoming established at _____ or when it draws to a close at _____.

TRUE OR FALSE: Circle T if true or F if false for each of the following statements. Correct the false statements.

T F 13. A pregnancy test is recommended as an initial step when a woman experiences amenorrhea.

T F 14. The pain associated with primary dysmenorrhea usually occurs at the onset of menstruation.

T F 15. The exact cause of premenstrual syndrome (PMS) is unknown.

T F 16. When a woman is experiencing primary dysmenorrhea, she should avoid exercise.

T F 17. Oral contraceptives are the first-line medications for the treatment of primary dysmenorrhea.

T F 18. Endometriosis is a menstrual disorder primarily affecting Caucasian women during their late teens to early twenties.

T F 19. Synarel (nafarelin) is a gonadotropic-releasing hormone agonist administered at a dose of 200 mcg twice daily by nasal spray to treat endometriosis.

T F 20. The only definitive cure for endometriosis is a total abdominal hysterectomy with a bilateral salpingo-oophorectomy.

T F 21. Aspirin can be used to reduce the size of myomas (fibroids) before a myomectomy.

T F 22. Sexually transmitted infections (STIs) are among the most common health problems in the United States today.

T F 23. The majority of women contracting chlamydia are over 30 years of age.

T F 24. Human papillomavirus (HPV) is the most common STI contracted by American women today.

T F 25. The VDRL and rapid plasma reagin tests are used as screening tests for syphilis.

T F 26. New human immunodeficiency virus (HIV) infections occur more often in African-American women than in other groups of women in the United States.

T F 27. Once HIV enters the body, seroconversion to HIV positivity usually occurs within 2 to 4 weeks.

T F 28. Presence of HIV antibody in infants younger than 18 months of age is not diagnostic of HIV infection.

T F 29. Standard Precautions are to be used once patients have been diagnosed with a blood-borne infection.

T F 30. Fibroadenoma is a rare benign condition of the breast most commonly seen in middle-age women.

T F 31. One in ten American women develop breast cancer in their lifetime.

T F 32. The most important predictor for breast cancer is age.

T F 33. It is estimated that most breast lumps detected by women are malignant.

34. *COMPLETE* the following table related to sexually transmitted infections and vaginal infections.

Infection	Clinical Manifestations	Screening/Diagnosis	Management
Chlamydia trachomatis			
Gonorrhea			
Syphilis			
Genital herpes simplex virus			
Human papillomavirus			
Bacterial vaginosis			
Candidiasis			
Trichomoniasis			

FILL IN THE BLANKS: Insert the pelvic inflammatory disease term that corresponds to each of the following.

35. Pelvic inflammatory disease (PID) is an infectious process that most commonly involves the _____, _____ and, more rarely, the _____ and _____ surfaces.

36. _____ is estimated to cause _____ of all cases of PID. Most PID results from the ascending spread of microorganisms from the _____ and _____ to the _____. This spread most frequently happens at the end of or just after _____, following reception of a(n) _____. PID may also develop after a(n) _____, _____, or _____.

37. Women who have had PID are at increased risk for _____, _____, and _____. Other problems associated with PID include _____, _____, _____, and _____.

38. Signs and symptoms of PID include _____ and one or more of the following: _____, _____, _____, _____, _____, and _____.

39. The most important nursing intervention related to PID is _____ by _____ and _____.

40. *IDENTIFY* factors that place women at risk for contracting a hepatitis B infection.

41. Women are the fastest growing population of individuals with HIV infection.

   A. *STATE* the mode of transmission for HIV infection.

   B. *LIST* the signs and symptoms that might occur during seroconversion to HIV positivity.

   C. *IDENTIFY* the behaviors that place a woman at risk for HIV infection.

D. *OUTLINE* the care management approach for women who test positive for HIV.

42. *STATE* two specific precautions for each of the following.

Standard Precautions

Precautions for invasive procedures

43. *LIST* the probable risk factors for breast cancer.

MULTIPLE CHOICE: Circle the one correct option and state the rationale for the option chosen.

44. Women experiencing primary dysmenorrhea should be advised to avoid which of the following foods?
    A. Red meats
    B. Asparagus
    C. Cranberry juice
    D. Whole-grain cereals

45. The nurse counseling a 30-year-old woman regarding effective measures to use to relieve symptoms associated with PMS might suggest that she:
    A. Decrease her intake of fruits, especially peaches and watermelon.
    B. Reduce exercise during the luteal phase of the menstrual cycle when symptoms are at their peak.
    C. Take a vitamin supplement containing vitamin B_6 twice a day.
    D. Avoid tobacco, alcohol, and caffeine.

46. A 28-year-old woman has been diagnosed with endometriosis. She has been placed on a course of treatment with danazol (Danocrine). The woman exhibits understanding of this treatment when she says:
    A. "Because this medication stops ovulation, I do not need to use birth control."
    B. "I will need to take this medication until I reach menopause."
    C. "I can experience decreased breast size, oily skin, and facial hair growth as a result of taking this medication."
    D. "I will need to spray this medication into my nose twice a day."

47. Dysfunctional uterine bleeding is most likely to occur when women:
    A. Experience ovulatory cycles.
    B. Weigh less than their expected body weight.
    C. Are experiencing signs of the onset of perimenopause.
    D. Secrete high levels of prostaglandin.

48. Infections of the female midreproductive tract such as chlamydia are dangerous primarily because these infections:
    A. Are asymptomatic.
    B. Cause infertility.
    C. Lead to PID.
    D. Are difficult to treat effectively.

49. A finding associated with HPV infection includes which of the following?
    A. White curdlike adherent discharge
    B. Soft papillary swelling occurring singly or in clusters
    C. Vesicles progressing to pustules and then to ulcers
    D. Yellow-to-green frothy malodorous discharge

50. A recommended medication effective in the treatment of vulvovaginal candidiasis is which of the following?
    A. Metronidazole
    B. Clotrimazole
    C. Penicillin
    D. Acyclovir

51. When providing a woman recovering from primary herpes with information regarding the recurrence of herpes infection of the genital tract, the nurse tells her that:
    A. Fever and flulike symptoms precede a recurrent infection.
    B. Little can be done to control the recurrence of infection.
    C. Transmission of the virus is only possible when lesions are open and draining.
    D. Itching and tingling often occur before the appearance of vesicles.

52. When assessing a woman with a diagnosis of fibroadenoma, a characteristic the nurse would expect to find is:
    A. Bilateral tender lumps behind the nipple.
    B. Milky discharge from one or both nipples.
    C. Soft and nonmovable lumps.
    D. Small, well-delineated lump in the upper outer quadrant of one breast.

CRITICAL THINKING EXERCISES

1. Maria is a 16-year-old gymnast who has been training vigorously for a placement on the U.S. Olympic team. She has been experiencing amenorrhea, and the development of her secondary sexual characteristics has been limited. Maria expresses concern because her nonathletic friends have all been menstruating for at least 1 year and have well-developed breasts. After a health assessment, Maria was diagnosed with hypogonadotropic amenorrhea.

    A. *STATE* the risk factors for this disorder that Maria most likely exhibited during the assessment process.

B. *STATE* one nursing diagnosis reflective of Maria's concern.

C. *WRITE* two expected outcomes for a plan of care for Maria.

D. *OUTLINE* a typical care management plan for Maria that addresses the issues associated with hypogonadotropic amenorrhea.

2. Mary, a 17-year-old who experienced menarche at age 16, comes to the women's health clinic for a routine checkup. She complains to the nurse that her last few periods have been very painful. "I have missed a few days of school because of it. What can I do to reduce the pain I feel during my periods?" Physical examination and testing reveal normal structure and function of Mary's reproductive system. A medical diagnosis of primary dysmenorrhea is made.

A. *STATE* the priority nursing diagnosis appropriate for Mary.

B. *IDENTIFY* appropriate relief measures for primary dysmenorrhea that the nurse might suggest to Mary.

3. Susan experiences physical and psychologic signs and symptoms associated with PMS during every ovulatory menstrual cycle.

A. *LIST* the signs and symptoms most likely described by Susan that led to the diagnosis of PMS.

B. *IDENTIFY* one nursing diagnosis that might be appropriate for Susan when she is experiencing the signs and symptoms of PMS.

C. *DESCRIBE* the approach the nurse would use in helping Susan deal with this menstrual disorder.

4. Lisa is a 26-year-old who has recently been diagnosed with endometriosis.

A. *LIST* the signs and symptoms that Lisa most likely exhibited that led to this medical diagnosis.

B. Lisa asks the nurse, "What is happening to my body as a result of this disease?" *DESCRIBE* the nurse's response.

C. Lisa asks about her treatment options. "Are there medications that I can take to make me feel better?" *DESCRIBE* the actions, effects, and potential side effects for each of the following pharmacologic approaches to treatment.

Oral contraceptive pills

Gonadotropin-releasing hormone agonists

Androgenic synthetic steroids

D. *IDENTIFY* support measures that the nurse can suggest to help Lisa cope with the effects of endometriosis.

5. Suzanne has just been diagnosed with severe acute PID as a result of a chlamydia infection. Intravenous antibiotics will be used as the primary medical treatment, followed by oral antibiotics.

A. *OUTLINE* a nursing management plan for Suzanne in terms of each of the following.

Position/activity

Comfort measures

Support measures

Health education

B. *LIST* the recommendations for Suzanne's self-care during the recovery phase.

6. Gloria has tested positive for hepatitis B. *DESCRIBE* the measures that the nurse should teach Gloria to implement in an effort to decrease the chance of transmission of the virus to others in Gloria's life.

7. Sonya is concerned that she has been exposed to HIV and has come to the women's health clinic for testing.

   A. While taking the health history, the nurse questions Sonya about behaviors that might have placed her at risk for HIV transmission. *CITE* the behaviors that the nurse would be looking for.

   B. *EXPLAIN* the testing procedure that is most likely to be followed to determine Sonya's HIV status.

   C. *OUTLINE* the counseling protocol that should guide the nurse when caring for Sonya before and after the test.

   D. Sonya's test result is negative. *DISCUSS* the instructions that the nurse should give Sonya regarding guidelines that she should follow to reduce her risk for the transmission of HIV with future sexual partners.

8. Julia, a 20-year-old woman, has just been diagnosed with a primary herpes simplex virus 2 (HSV-2) infection. In addition to the typical systemic symptoms, Julia exhibits multiple painful genital lesions.

    A. Relief of pain and healing without the development of a secondary infection are two expected outcomes for care. *IDENTIFY* several measures that the nurse can suggest to Julia in an effort to help her achieve the expected outcomes of care.

    B. Julia asks the nurse if there is anything she can do so this infection does not return. *DISCUSS* what the nurse should tell Julia about the recurrence of HSV-2 infection and the influence of self-care measures.

9. Molly, a 50-year-old woman, found a lump in her left breast during breast self-examination. She comes to the women's health clinic for help.

    A. *DESCRIBE* the diagnostic protocol that should be followed to determine the origin of the lump that Molly found in her breast.

    B. Molly's lump is diagnosed as cancerous, and she elects to have a simple mastectomy based on the information provided by her health care providers and after consulting with her husband. *DESCRIBE* the nursing care management for each of the following phases of Molly's treatment.

    Preoperative phase

    Immediate postoperative phase

C. Molly will be discharged within 48 hours after her surgery. *OUTLINE* the instructions that the nurse should give Molly to prepare her for self-care at home.

D. *DISCUSS* support measures that the nurse should use to address the concerns that Molly and her husband will most likely experience and express.

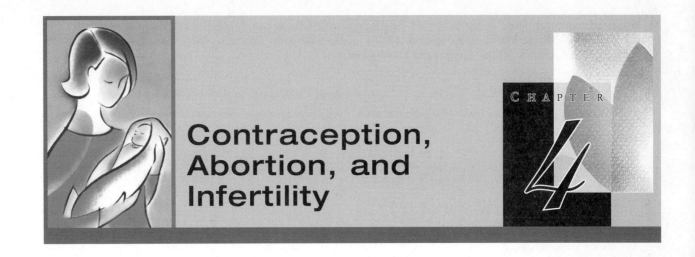

Contraception, Abortion, and Infertility

CHAPTER 4

CHAPTER REVIEW ACTIVITIES

TRUE OR FALSE: Circle T if true or F if false for each of the following statements about contraception and abortion. Correct the false statements.

T   F   1. Contraception failure rate refers to the percentage of contraceptive users who are expected to experience an accidental pregnancy during the first year of use, even when they use the method consistently and correctly.

T   F   2. The fertile period extends from 4 days before to 3 to 4 days after ovulation.

T   F   3. When preparing to use the rhythm method of periodic abstinence, a woman needs to accurately record the lengths of the previous two menstrual cycles.

T   F   4. Nonoxinol 9 offers some protection against the transmission of sexually transmitted infections such as gonorrhea and chlamydia.

T   F   5. Implanon provides contraceptive effectiveness for at least 3 years.

T   F   6. Implanon completely suppresses ovulation.

T   F   7. The most common side effect of Implanon is irregular menstrual bleeding.

T   F   8. Use of a diaphragm can increase the risk for toxic shock snydrome.

T   F   9. Women using combined estrogen and progestin as oral contraception should expect heavier menstrual bleeding.

T   F   10. Following a vasectomy, another form of birth control should be used until the sperm count is zero for at least two consecutive semen analyses.

T   F   11. A vasectomy reduces the volume of ejaculate.

T   F   12. Most women having abortions are Caucasian, younger than 24 years old, and unmarried.

T   F   13. Mifepristone (RU 486) can be taken up to 9 weeks after the last menstrual period to terminate a pregnancy.

T   F   14. Dilation and evacuation can be performed to terminate a pregnancy up to 26 weeks of gestation.

15. *STATE* the characteristics of the ideal contraceptive.

16. Informed consent is a vital component when helping a woman choose a contraceptive method that is right for her. The acronym **"BRAIDED"** is useful in ensuring that all elements of an informed consent have been met and documented. *INDICATE* the action represented by each letter.

B

R

A

I

D

E

D

17. June's religious and cultural beliefs prohibit her from using any artificial method of birth control. She is interested in learning about periodic abstinence or natural family planning as a method of contraception.

    FILL IN THE BLANKS in each of the following statements concerning this method.

    A. Women with _____ have the greatest risk for failure using the periodic abstinence method.
    B. Using the calendar method, June and her husband would abstain from day _____ to day _____ of her menstrual cycle because her shortest cycle was 23 days and her longest cycle was 33 days.
    C. The Billings method, also called the _____ method, requires June to recognize and interpret the cyclic changes in the characteristics of her _____ such as _____ and _____.
    D. The symptothermal method combines _____ and _____ methods, with awareness of cycle- or phase-related symptoms such as _____, _____, _____, _____ or _____, and _____.
    E. The urine predictor test for ovulation detects the sudden surge of _____ in the urine that occurs approximately _____ to _____ hours before ovulation.

18. Alice and Bob use nonprescription chemical and mechanical contraceptive barriers. *LABEL* each of the following actions with C if correct or I if incorrect. *INDICATE* how the action should be changed for those actions labeled I.

    A. _____ When using a spermicide, Alice inserts it deeply into her vagina so that it contacts her cervix.
    B. _____ Alice reapplies the spermicide before each act of intercourse.
    C. _____ Alice douches within 2 hours of intercourse because she finds that the spermicidal foam is sticky and uncomfortable.
    D. _____ Bob applies a condom over his erect penis, leaving an empty space at the tip.

E. _____ Bob often lubricates the outside of the condom with Vaseline, a petroleum-based lubricant.

F. _____ Bob uses the same condom if he and Alice repeat intercourse.

19. Joyce has chosen the diaphragm as her method of contraception. *LABEL* each of the following actions with C if correct or I if incorrect. *INDICATE* how the action should be changed for those actions labeled I.

A. _____ Joyce came to be refitted for her diaphragm after healing was complete following the vaginal birth of her son.

B. _____ Joyce applies a spermicide only to the rim of the diaphragm just before insertion.

C. _____ Joyce empties her bladder before inserting the diaphragm.

D. _____ Joyce inserts the diaphragm about 3 to 4 hours before intercourse to increase spontaneity.

E. _____ Joyce applies more spermicide for each act of intercourse.

F. _____ Joyce removes the diaphragm within 1 hour of intercourse.

G. _____ Joyce washes the diaphragm with warm water and an antiseptic-type soap, dries it, and then applies baby powder after its removal.

H. _____ Joyce always uses the diaphragm during her menstrual periods.

20. *CITE* four factors that might contribute to a woman's decision to seek an induced abortion.

TRUE OR FALSE: Circle T if true or F if false for each of the following infertility statements. Correct the false statements.

T   F   21. Infertility implies subfertility, a prolonged time to conceive.

T   F   22. A female factor is responsible for infertility in approximately 40% to 55% of infertile couples.

T   F   23. Unexplained factors and causes related to both partners account for 5% to 10% of infertility cases.

T   F   24. Hysterosalpingography is used to determine tubal patency.

T   F   25. An endometrial biopsy is typically performed late in the menstrual cycle about 2 to 3 days before menstruation is expected to begin.

T   F   26. An increase in scrotal temperature, through use of hot tubs and saunas, may adversely affect spermatogenesis.

T   F   27. The use of condoms during genital intercourse for 2 to 3 months reduces female antibody production in most women who have elevated antisperm antibody titers.

28. Mary and Jim have come for their first visit to the fertility clinic. You must instruct them on the interrelated structures, functions, and processes essential for conception, emphasizing that they are a biologic unit of reproduction.

A. *IDENTIFY* and *DESCRIBE* each component required for normal fertility.

B. *SUPPORT* this statement: Assessment of infertility must involve both partners.

29. With some forms of infertility, pharmacologic measures might be effective. *INDICATE* classification, mode of action, contraindications, administration, side effects, and nursing implications, including content for health teaching, for each of the following medications. *USE* a drug manual to assist you in gathering this information.

Clomiphene citrate (Clomid, Serophene)

Purified FSH (Metrodin)

Human chorionic gonadotropin (Profasi)

Human menopausal gonadotropins (Pergonal)

30. Alternative reproductive technologies are being developed and perfected, creating a variety of ethical, legal, financial, and psychosocial concerns.

A. *DEFINE* each of the following reproductive alternatives.

In vitro fertilization−embryo transfer

Gamete intrafallopian transfer

Zygote intrafallopian transfer)

Therapeutic donor insemination

Gestational carrier (embryo host)

B. *DISCUSS* the religious and cultural concerns engendered by these alternative technologies.

MULTIPLE CHOICE: Circle the one correct option and state the rationale for the option chosen.

31. A single young adult woman receives instructions from the nurse regarding the use of an oral contraceptive. The woman demonstrates a need for further instruction if she:
    A. Stops asking her sexual partners to use condoms with spermicide.
    B. Enrolls in a smoking cessation program.
    C. Takes a pill every morning.
    D. Uses a barrier method of birth control if she misses two or more pills.

32. Oral contraception in the form of a combination of low-dose estrogen and progesterone:
    A. Reduces the pH of cervical mucus, thereby destroying sperm.
    B. Protects against iron deficiency anemia by reducing blood loss with menses.
    C. Prevents the transmission of sexually transmitted infections.
    D. Is 90% effective in preventing pregnancy when used correctly.

33. A woman must assess herself for signs that ovulation is occurring. Which of the following is a sign associated with ovulation?
    A. Reduction in level of luteinizing hormone in the urine 12 to 24 hours before ovulation
    B. Spinnbarkeit
    C. Drop in basal body temperature following ovulation
    D. Increase in amount and thickness of cervical mucus

34. An infertile woman may be given danazol (Danocrine) to:
    A. Stimulate her pituitary gland.
    B. Treat endometriosis.
    C. Induce ovulation.
    D. Help her to relax before intercourse.

1. Kathy has come to Planned Parenthood for information on birth control methods and assistance with making her choice. *DISCUSS* the approach that the nurse should use to help Kathy make an informed decision in choosing contraception that is right for her.

2. June plans to use a combination estrogen-progestin oral contraceptive.

   A. *DESCRIBE* the mode of action for this type of contraception.

   B. *LIST* the advantages of using oral contraception.

   C. *IDENTIFY* the factors that, if present in June's health history, constitute a contraindication to the use of oral contraception with estrogen and progesterone.

   D. Using the acronym **"ACHES,"** *IDENTIFY* the signs and symptoms that would require June to stop taking the pill and notify her health care provider.

      A

      C

      H

E

S

E. *SPECIFY* the instructions that you would give June about taking the pill to ensure maximum effectiveness.

3. Beth has decided to try the cervical cap. *DESCRIBE* the principles that should guide Beth's use of this method to maximize effectiveness and minimize or prevent complications.

4. Anita has just had a copper T-380A intrauterine device inserted. *SPECIFY* the instructions that you would give to Anita before she leaves the women's health clinic after the insertion.

5. Judy (6-4-1-1-3) and Allen, both age 36, are contemplating sterilization now that their family is complete. They are seeking counseling regarding this decision.

   A. *DESCRIBE* the approach that a nurse should use in helping Judy and Allen make the right decision for them.

   B. They decide that Allen will have a vasectomy. *DISCUSS* the preoperative and postoperative care and instructions required by Allen.

6. Anne and her husband, Ian, will be using the symptothermal method of natural family planning.

   A. *LIST* the assessment components of this method.

   B. *OUTLINE* the teaching plan that you would use to ensure that Anne and Ian do the following accurately:

   Measure basal body temperature

   Evaluate cervical mucus characteristics

7. Mark and his wife, Mary, are undergoing testing for impaired fertility.

   A. *LIST* the components of the assessment for both Mark and Mary.

   Assessment for the man

   Assessment for the woman

   B. Mark must provide a specimen of semen for analysis. *DESCRIBE* the procedure that he should follow to ensure accuracy of the test.

C. *STATE* the semen characteristics that will be assessed and the values expected for each.

D. *DESCRIBE* nursing support measures that should be used when working with Mark and Mary.

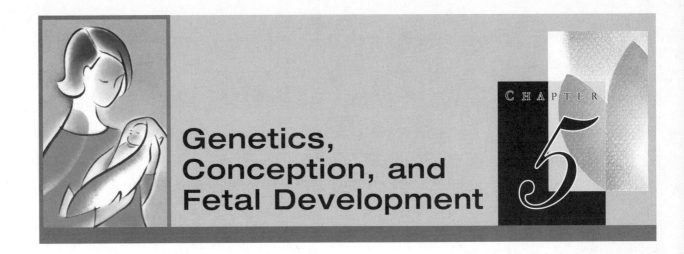

Genetics, Conception, and Fetal Development

CHAPTER 5

CHAPTER REVIEW ACTIVITIES

FILL IN THE BLANKS: Insert the term that corresponds to each of the following.

Process of Conception and Implantation

1. At ovulation, the _____ is released from the ruptured _____. The _____ of the uterine tube capture(s) the ovum and propel(s) it through the uterine tube toward the uterus. Ova are fertile for about _____ hours after ovulation.

2. Following ejaculation, _____ reach the site of fertilization in an average of _____ hours and remain viable in a woman's reproductive system for _____ days. With the process of _____, the protective coating from the sperm heads is removed, allowing enzymes to escape. Fertilization occurs in the _____ of the uterine tube. Once penetrated by a sperm, the membrane surrounding the ovum becomes impenetrable through a process termed the _____.

3. With the fusion of the male and female _____, the _____ number of chromosomes is restored. The new cell is called a(n) _____. Within _____ days a 16-cell ball called the _____ is formed. A cavity develops within this ball of cells, creating the _____, which is ____ _____ into the endometrium _____ days after conception. The endometrium is now called the _____. Fingerlike projections called _____ develop from the _____. These projections tap into maternal blood vessels in the decidua _____.

4. Each of the following structures plays a critical role in fetal growth and development. *LIST* the functions of each of the following structures.

   Yolk sac

   Amniotic membranes and fluid

Umbilical cord

Placenta

5. Fetal circulation differs from neonatal circulation. *DESCRIBE* the location and purpose for each of the following fetal circulatory structures.

Ductus venosus

Ductus arteriosus

Foramen ovale

TRUE OR FALSE: Circle T if true or F if false for each of the following statements. Correct the false statements.

T   F   6. All normal human somatic cells contain 46 chromosomes.

T   F   7. Hemophilia and color blindness are examples of sex chromosome abnormalities caused by nondisjunction during gametogenesis.

T   F   8. Neural tube defects and cleft lip and palate result from a combination of genetic and environmental factors.

T   F   9. For a recessive trait to be expressed in their offspring, both parents must contribute the abnormal gene.

T   F   10. In autosomal dominant inheritance, if one parent is affected by the disorder, there is a 100% chance of passing the abnormal gene to an offspring during each pregnancy.

T   F   11. Cystic fibrosis and phenylketonuria, both inborn errors of metabolism, follow the autosomal dominant inheritance pattern.

T   F   12. The stage of the fetus lasts from 9 weeks of gestation until the end of pregnancy.

T   F   13. The umbilical cord is composed of two veins, one artery, and Wharton's jelly.

T   F   14. Human chorionic gonadotropin, which is produced by the placenta, reaches its peak serum level at 24 weeks of gestation.

T   F   15. The corpus luteum produces estrogen and progesterone to maintain the pregnancy until the placenta is mature enough to take over as an endocrine gland.

T   F   16. The placenta functions as an effective barrier to substances such as viruses and drugs, thereby protecting the fetus from their potentially harmful effects.

T   F   17. Oligohydramnios is associated with fetal renal abnormalities.

T   F   18. Meconium, fetal waste products in the intestine, can be passed into the amniotic fluid if fetal hypoxia occurs.

T   F   19. If a couple gives birth to a child with an autosomal dominant disorder, there is a 50% reduction in risk that the next pregnancy will result in an affected child.

T   F   20. Fetal viability is first reached at 30 weeks of gestation.

T   F   21. The limitations on survival outside the uterus are based on central nervous system function and oxygenation capability of the lungs.

T   F   22. The occurrence of multifetal pregnancies with three or more fetuses has steadily decreased as a result of increased exposure to teratogens.

23. Genetic counseling is rapidly becoming an important health care service for families during the childbearing years.

    A. *DISCUSS* each of the following steps in the process of genetic counseling.

      Estimation of risk

      Interpretation of risk

    B. *DESCRIBE* the role of the nurse in genetic counseling.

    C. *CITE* several ethical considerations related to genetics and genetic counseling.

24. *COMPLETE* the following table by naming the three primary germ layers and identify the tissues or organs that develop from each layer.

Primary Germ Layer	Tissue/Organ Formation

25. Suzanne, a primigravida, has come for her first prenatal visit. *IDENTIFY* the questions that the nurse should ask during the health history interview to determine whether factors are present that might place Suzanne at risk for giving birth to a baby with a congenital or inheritable disorder.

26. *EXPLAIN* each of the following types of inheritance and give an example of each.

Unifactorial inheritance

Multifactorial inheritance

X-linked inheritance

MULTIPLE CHOICE: Circle the one correct option and state the rationale for the option chosen.

27. On the basis of genetic testing of a newborn, a diagnosis of dwarfism has been made. The parents ask the nurse whether this could happen to future children. Because this is an example of autosomal dominant inheritance, the nurse tells the parents:
    A. "For each pregnancy there is a 50:50 chance that the child will be affected by dwarfism."
    B. "This will not happen again because the dwarfism was caused by the harmful genetic effects of the infection you had during pregnancy."
    C. "For each pregnancy there is a 25% chance that the child will be a carrier of the defective gene but unaffected by the disorder."
    D. "Because you already have had an affected child, there is a decreased chance for this to happen in future pregnancies."

28. A female carries the gene for hemophilia on one of her X chromosomes. Now that she is pregnant, she asks the nurse how this might affect her baby. The nurse should tell her:
    A. "A female baby has a 50% chance of also being a carrier."
    B. "A male baby can be a carrier or have hemophilia."
    C. "Female babies are never affected by this disorder."
    D. "Hemophilia is always expressed if a male inherits the defective gene."

29. A pregnant woman carries a single gene for cystic fibrosis. The father of her baby does not carry this gene. Which of the following is true concerning the genetic pattern of cystic fibrosis as it applies to this family?
    A. The pregnant woman has cystic fibrosis herself.
    B. There is a 50% chance that her baby will have the disorder.
    C. There is a 25% chance that her baby will be a carrier.
    D. The baby will not have cystic fibrosis but may be a carrier for this disorder.

30. When teaching a class of pregnant women about fetal development, the nurse includes which of the following:
    A. "The gender of your baby is determined by the 9th week of pregnancy."
    B. "The baby's heart begins to pump blood during the 10th week of pregnancy."
    C. "The baby's heartbeat will be audible using a special ultrasound stethoscope as early as the 18th week of pregnancy."
    D. "You should be able to start feeling your baby move between weeks 16 and 20 of your pregnancy."

CRITICAL THINKING EXERCISES

1. Imagine that you are a nurse-midwife working in partnership with an obstetrician. *FORMULATE* a response to each of the following concerns or questions directed to you from some of your prenatal patients.

    A. June (2 months pregnant), Mary (5 months pregnant), and Alice (7 months pregnant) ask for a description of their fetuses at the present time.

June	Mary	Alice

B. Jessica states that a friend told her that babies born after about 35 weeks have a better chance to survive because they can breathe more easily. She asks whether this is true.

C. Susan, who is 6 months pregnant, states that she read in a magazine that a fetus can actually hear and see. She believes that this is totally unbelievable!

D. Alexa is 2 months pregnant. She asks how the gender of her baby was determined and whether a sonogram might indicate if she were having a boy or a girl.

E. Karen is pregnant for the first time. She reveals that she has a history of twins in her family. She wants to know what causes twin pregnancies to occur and the difference between identical and fraternal twins.

2. Mr. and Mrs. G. are newly married and planning for pregnancy. They express to the nurse their concern that Mrs. G. has a history of Tay-Sachs disease in her family. Mr. G. has never investigated his family history.

A. *DESCRIBE* the process that the nurse should follow in assisting Mr. and Mrs. G. to determine their genetic risk.

B. Both Mr. and Mrs. G. are found to be carriers of the disorder. *DESCRIBE* the chance that they have for giving birth to a child who is normal, a carrier, or affected by the disorder.

C. *DISCUSS* the decision-making process that should be followed with couples such as Mr. and Mrs. G. who might give birth to a child with a genetic disorder.

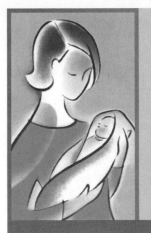

Anatomy and Physiology of Pregnancy

CHAPTER 6

CHAPTER REVIEW ACTIVITIES

FILL IN THE BLANKS: Insert the term that corresponds to each of the following.

1. _____ Pregnancy
2. _____ Number of pregnancies in which the fetus(es) has (have) reached viability, not the number of fetuses (e.g., twins) born (whether the fetus is born alive or is stillborn—i.e., the fetus who shows no signs of life at birth, after viability is reached, has no effect on this numeric designation)
3. _____ Woman who is pregnant
4. _____ Woman who has never been pregnant
5. _____ Woman who has not completed a pregnancy with a fetus (or fetuses) who has (have) reached the stage of fetal viability
6. _____ Woman who is pregnant for the first time
7. _____ Woman who has completed one pregnancy with a fetus or fetuses who have reached the stage of fetal viability
8. _____ Woman who has had two or more pregnancies
9. _____ Woman who has completed two or more pregnancies to the stage of fetal viability
10. _____ Capacity to live outside the uterus, about 22 to 24 weeks since the last menstrual period, or a fetal weight more than 500 g
11. _____ Term referring to a pregnancy that has reached 20 weeks of gestation but before completion of 37 weeks of gestation
12. _____ Term used to describe a pregnancy from the beginning of the 38th week of gestation to the end of the 42nd week of gestation
13. _____ Two terms used to describe a pregnancy that goes beyond 42 weeks of gestation
14. _____ Substance whose presence in urine or serum results in a positive pregnancy test result

MATCHING: Match the assessment finding in Column I with the appropriate descriptive term in Column II.

COLUMN I

_____ 15. Menstrual bleeding no longer occurring

_____ 16. Fundal height decreased, fetal head in pelvic inlet

_____ 17. Cervix and vagina violet-blue in color

_____ 18. Swelling of ankles and feet at the end of the day

_____ 19. Cervical tip softened

_____ 20. Increased hair growth on face and abdomen

_____ 21. Fetal head rebounding with gentle upward tapping through vagina

_____ 22. White mucoid vaginal discharge with faint musty odor

_____ 23. Enlarged sebaceous glands in areola on both breasts

_____ 24. Plug of mucus filling endocervical canal

_____ 25. Pink stretch marks on breasts and abdomen

_____ 26. Thick, creamy fluid expressed from nipples

_____ 27. Cheeks, nose, and forehead blotchy, hyperpigmented

_____ 28. Pigmented line extending up abdominal midline

_____ 29. Varicosities around anus

_____ 30. Heartburn experienced after supper

_____ 31. Lumbosacral curve increased

_____ 32. Paresthesia and pain in right hand radiating to elbow

_____ 33. Spotting following cervical palpation or intercourse

_____ 34. Hematocrit decreased from 40% to 36%

_____ 35. Vascular spiders on neck and thorax

_____ 36. Palms pinkish red, mottled

_____ 37. Abdominal wall muscles separated

COLUMN II

A. Colostrum

B. Operculum

C. Amenorrhea

D. Telangiectasis (angioma)

E. Pyrosis

F. Friability

G. Striae gravidarum

H. Physiologic anemia

I. Linea nigra

J. Ballottement

K. Chadwick sign

L. Diastasis recti abdominis

M. Lordosis

N. Leukorrhea

O. Chloasma (mask of pregnancy)

P. Lightening

Q. Hemorrhoids

R. Palmar erythema

S. Goodell sign

T. Physiologic edema

U. Hirsutism

V. Montgomery tubercles

W. Carpal tunnel syndrome

38. *COMPLETE* the following table related to the three categories of signs and symptoms of pregnancy by filling in the blanks and listing the appropriate signs and symptoms for each category.

_____, changes felt by the woman	_____, changes observed by an examiner	_____, signs attributed only to the presence of the fetus

39. *DESCRIBE* the obstetric history for each of the following women, using the four- and five-digit systems.

    A. Alice is pregnant. Her first pregnancy resulted in a stillbirth at 36 weeks of gestation, and her second pregnancy resulted in the birth of her daughter at 42 weeks of gestation.

        Four-digit

        Five-digit

    B. Angela is 6 weeks pregnant. Her previous pregnancies resulted in the live birth of a daughter at 40 weeks of gestation, the live birth of a son at 38 weeks of gestation, and a miscarriage at 10 weeks of gestation.

        Four-digit

        Five-digit

    C. Constance is experiencing her fourth pregnancy. Her first pregnancy ended in a miscarriage at 12 weeks, the second resulted in the live birth of twin boys at 32 weeks, and the third resulted in the live birth of a daughter at 39 weeks.

        Four-digit

        Five-digit

TRUE OR FALSE: Circle T if true or F if false for each of the following statements. Correct the false statements.

T   F   40. Pregnancy tests are based on the presence of human chorionic gonadotropin in a pregnant woman's urine or serum.

T   F   41. Most home pregnancy tests are based on enzyme-linked immunosorbent assay technology.

T   F   42. Drugs such as diuretics can contribute to a false-positive pregnancy test result.

T   F   43. Fetal movements palpated by an examiner are an example of a positive sign of pregnancy.

T F 44. The uterine fundus should be above the level of the symphysis pubis by the eighth week of gestation.

T F 45. Evaluating abnormal Papanicolaou tests during pregnancy can be complicated.

T F 46. During pregnancy the pH of vaginal secretions decreases.

T F 47. Lactation does not occur during pregnancy as a result of the inhibiting effect of high prolactin levels.

T F 48. Physiologic anemia is diagnosed in a pregnant woman when the hemoglobin value falls to 10 g/dl or less or if the hematocrit value falls to 35% or less.

T F 49. A woman is at greater risk for the development of thrombosis during pregnancy and the postpartum period as a result of increases in certain clotting factors and depression of fibrinolytic activity.

T F 50. Pregnancy is a state of respiratory alkalosis compensated by a mild metabolic acidosis.

T F 51. A supine position with head elevated is the best maternal position to increase renal perfusion.

T F 52. A proteinuria value of 1 is acceptable during pregnancy.

T F 53. Carpal tunnel syndrome occurs during the third trimester of pregnancy as a result of edema that compresses the median nerve beneath the carpal ligament in the wrist.

T F 54. Increased triglyceride levels as a result of higher estrogen levels might account for the development of gallstones during pregnancy.

55. When assessing the pregnant woman, the nurse should keep in mind that baseline vital sign values change as she progresses through her pregnancy. *DESCRIBE* how each of the following changes during pregnancy.

Blood pressure (BP)

Heart rate and patterns

Respiratory rate and patterns

Body temperature

56. *CALCULATE* the mean arterial pressure for each of the following BP readings.

120/76

114/64

110/80

150/90

57. *SPECIFY* the changes that occur in the following laboratory test results as a result of expected physiologic adaptations to pregnancy.

Complete blood count: hematocrit, hemoglobin, white blood cell count

Clotting activity

Acid-base balance values

Blood glucose level

Urinalysis

58. *DESCRIBE* the expected adaptations in elimination that occur during pregnancy. *INCLUDE* in your answer the basis for the changes that occur.

Renal   **Bowel**

59. *EXPLAIN* how and why the levels of each of the following substances change during pregnancy.

   A. **Parathyroid hormone**

B. **Insulin**

C. **Estrogen**

D. **Progesterone**

E. **Thyroid hormones**

F. **Human chorionic gonadotropin (hCG)**

G. **Prolactin**

MULTIPLE CHOICE: Circle the one correct option and state the rationale for the option chosen.

60. A pregnant woman at 10 weeks of gestation exhibits the following signs of pregnancy during a routine prenatal checkup. Which one is categorized as a probable sign of pregnancy?
   A. hCG in the urine
   B. Breast tenderness
   C. Morning sickness
   D. Fetal heart sounds

61. A pregnant woman with four children reports the following obstetric history: a stillbirth at 32 weeks of gestation, triplets (two sons and a daughter) born by cesarean section at 30 weeks of gestation, a miscarriage at 8 weeks of gestation, and a daughter born vaginally at 39 weeks of gestation. Which of the following accurately expresses this woman's current obstetric history using the five-digit system?
   A. 5-1-4-1-4
   B. 4-1-3-1-4
   C. 5-2-2-0-3
   D. 5-1-2-1-4

62. An essential component of prenatal health assessment of pregnant women is the determination of vital signs. An expected change in vital signs as a result of pregnancy would be:
   A. Increase in systolic BP by 30 mm Hg or more after assuming a supine position.
   B. Increase in diastolic BP by 5 to 10 mm Hg beginning in the first trimester.
   C. Increased awareness of the need to breathe as pregnancy progresses.
   D. Gradual decrease in baseline pulse rate of approximately 20 beats/min.

63. A woman exhibits understanding of instructions for performing a home pregnancy test to maximize accuracy if she:
   A. Uses urine collected at the end of the day, just before going to bed.
   B. Avoids using Tylenol or aspirin for a headache for about 1 week before performing the test.
   C. Performs the test on the day after she misses her first menstrual period.
   D. Records the day of her last normal menstrual period and her usual cycle length.

64. During an examination of a pregnant woman, the nurse notes that her cervix is soft on its tip. The nurse would document this finding as:
   A. Friability.
   B. Goodell's sign.
   C. Chadwick's sign.
   D. Hegar's sign.

CRITICAL THINKING EXERCISES

1. *DESCRIBE* your response to each of the following patient concerns and questions.

   A. Tina is 14 weeks pregnant. She calls the prenatal clinic to report that she noticed slight painless spotting this morning. She reveals that she did have intercourse with her partner the night before.

B. Lisa suspects that she is pregnant because her menstrual period is already 3 weeks late. She asks her friend, who is a nurse, how to use the pregnancy test she just bought so she obtains the best results.

C. Joan is 3 months pregnant. She tells you that she's worried because a friend told her that vaginal and bladder infections are more common during pregnancy. She wants to know if this could be true and, if so, why.

D. Tammy, who is 20 weeks pregnant, tells you that she has noted some "problems" with her breasts. There are "little pimples" near her nipples, and her breasts feel "lumpy and bumpy" and "leak a little" when she does a breast self-examination.

E. Tamara is concerned because she read in a book about pregnancy that a pregnant woman's position could affect her circulation and especially affect the baby. She asks what positions are good for her circulation now that she is pregnant.

F. Beth, a pregnant woman, calls to tell you that she had a nosebleed this morning and has noticed occasional feelings of fullness in her ears. She asks if these are anything to worry about.

G. Karen is 7 months pregnant and works as a full-time secretary. She asks you if she should take a "water pill" that a friend gave her because she has noticed that her ankles "swell up" at the end of the day.

H. Jan is in her third trimester of pregnancy. She tells you that her posture seems to have changed and that she occasionally experiences low back pain.

I. Monica, who is 36 weeks pregnant with her first baby, calls the clinic, stating that she knows that the baby is coming because she felt some uterine contractions before getting out of bed in the morning. Monica confirms that they seem to have decreased in intensity and frequency since she got out of bed and walked around.

J. Nina is a primigravida who is at 32 weeks of gestation. When she comes for a prenatal visit, she reports that she has been experiencing occasional periods of shortness of breath during the day and sometimes has to use an extra pillow to sleep comfortably. Nina expresses concern that she is developing a breathing problem.

2. Accurate BP readings are critical if significant changes in the cardiovascular system are to be detected as a woman adapts to pregnancy during the prenatal period. *WRITE* a protocol for BP assessment that can be used by nurses working in a prenatal clinic to ensure accuracy of the results obtained during BP assessment.

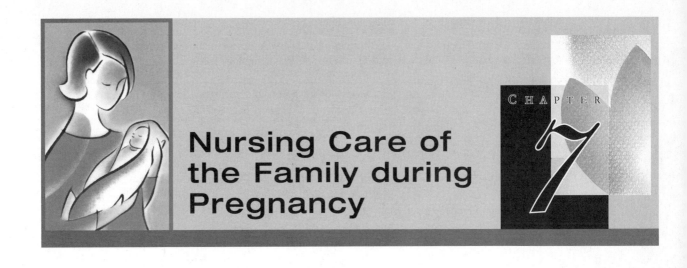

Nursing Care of the Family during Pregnancy

CHAPTER 7

CHAPTER REVIEW ACTIVITIES

FILL IN THE BLANKS: Insert the term that corresponds to each of the following.

Nursing Care

1. Pregnancy can be diagnosed by assessing a woman for the presence of specific signs and symptoms associated with pregnancy. _____ indicators of pregnancy can be caused by conditions other than gestation and are not reliable for diagnosis. _____ indicators of pregnancy are those observed by the health care provider. _____ indicators of pregnancy verify that a woman is pregnant.

2. _____ rule is used to determine the _____ by subtracting _____ from and adding _____ to the first day of the _____. Pregnancy is divided into three 3-month periods called _____.

3. _____ can occur when a woman is placed in the lithotomy position because of the compression of the vena cava and aorta by the weight of the abdominal contents, including the uterus. Signs and symptoms indicating that this has occurred include _____, _____, _____, _____, _____, _____, and _____.

4. A variety of assessment methods are used to evaluate the progress of pregnancy. _____ is measured beginning in the second trimester as one indicator of the progress of fetal growth. The _____ test determines whether nipples are everted or inverted by placing the thumb and forefinger on the areola and pressing inward gently.

5. The health status of the fetus is assessed by evaluating _____, the _____, and abnormal _____. The fetal _____ is estimated after determining the duration of pregnancy and the estimated date of birth (EDB).

6. Maternal adaptation during pregnancy includes mastery of certain _____ tasks that include _____, _____, _____, and _____.

7. As a pregnant woman establishes a relationship with her fetus, she progresses through three phases. In phase 1 she accepts the _____ and needs to be able to state _____. In phase 2 the woman accepts the _____ and as a(n) _____. She can now say _____. Finally, in phase 3 the woman prepares realistically for the _____ and _____. She expresses the thought _____.

8. _____ refers to rapid and unpredictable changes in mood. Having conflicting feelings simultaneously regarding the pregnancy is termed _____.

9. The _____ phase is the early period of paternal adaptation during which the father accepts the biologic fact of pregnancy. During the _____ phase, the father adjusts to the reality of the pregnancy. The father becomes actively involved in the pregnancy and the relationship with his child during the _____ phase. The _____ syndrome refers to the phenomenon of men experiencing pregnancy-like symptoms.

10. The _____ is a tool used by parents to communicate the childbirth options that they have chosen to their health care providers.

11. Certain cultural practices are expected by women of all cultures to ensure a good outcome to their pregnancy. Cultural _____ are directives that tell a woman what to do during pregnancy. Cultural _____ are directives that tell a woman what not to do during pregnancy; they establish _____.

12. Quadruple screening is used to detect _____, _____, and _____. It is done ideally between _____ and _____ weeks of gestation and measures levels of _____, _____, _____, and _____.

13. Target body parts for battering during pregnancy include the _____, _____, _____, and _____. _____ is common.

14. *CALCULATE* the EDB for each of the following pregnant women using Nägele's rule.

   A. Denise's last menses began on May 5, 2010, and ended on May 10, 2010.

   B. Anna had intercourse on February 21, 2010. She has not had a menstrual period since the one that began on January 14, 2010, and ended 5 days later.

   C. Charlene's last period began on July 4, 2010, and ended on July 10, 2010. Charlene noted that her basal body temperature began to rise on July 28, 2010.

15. Cultural beliefs and practices are important influencing factors during the prenatal period.

   A. *DESCRIBE* how cultural beliefs can affect a woman's participation in prenatal care as it is defined by the Western biomedical model of care.

B. *IDENTIFY* one **prescription** and one **proscription** for each of the following areas.

Emotional response

Clothing

Physical activity and rest

Sexual activity

Diet

16. *COMPLETE* the following table by identifying data to be collected for each component of maternal assessment during the initial and follow-up visits during pregnancy.

Component	Initial Visit	Follow-up Visits
Interview and history		
Physical examination		
Laboratory and diagnostic testing		

17. Marie asks the nurse what can be done during a prenatal visit to "make sure that my baby is healthy, growing, and doing well." *IDENTIFY* and *DESCRIBE* what the nurse might tell Marie about the components of fetal assessment that are used during prenatal visits to determine the health status of her baby.

18. Nurses responsible for the care management of pregnant women must be alert for warning signs of potential complications that women might develop as pregnancy progresses from trimester to trimester.

    A. *LIST* the warning signs of potential complications for each trimester of pregnancy. *INDICATE* possible causes for each sign listed.

    First Trimester   **Second and Third Trimesters**

    B. *DESCRIBE* the approach a nurse should take when discussing these warning signs and potential complications with a pregnant woman and her family.

TRUE OR FALSE: Circle T if true or F if false for each of the following statements. Correct the false statements.

T   F   19. Women should consider avoiding weight-bearing exercises such as jogging and running during pregnancy.

T   F   20. The use of a condom is necessary during pregnancy if the woman is at risk for a sexually transmitted infection.

T   F   21. Intercourse is safe during a normal pregnancy as long as it is not uncomfortable.

T   F   22. Exposure to secondhand smoke is associated with growth restriction and an increase in perinatal and infant morbidity and mortality.

T   F   23. It is not necessary to screen pregnant women for human immunodeficiency virus because there is no effective measure to reduce transmission to the fetus.

T   F   24. A woman should be scheduled for prenatal visits once a month until the 36th week of pregnancy.

T   F   25. A 1-hour glucose tolerance test is performed on all pregnant women at 28 weeks of gestation to screen for the presence of gestational diabetes.

T   F   26. During the second and third trimesters (weeks 18 to 30), the height of the fundus in inches is approximately the same as the weeks of gestation if the woman's bladder is full.

T   F   27. Quickening usually occurs between weeks 16 and 20 of gestation.

T   F   28. A woman should avoid tub bathing and should shower instead once she reaches the midpoint of her pregnancy.

T   F   29. The side-lying position promotes uterine perfusion and fetoplacental oxygenation.

T   F   30. Once the uterus enlarges, the pregnant woman should use only the lap belt and avoid using a shoulder harness while she is in a motor vehicle.

T F 31. A woman with inverted nipples should perform nipple rolling and tugging exercises during the third trimester to break adhesions.

T F 32. Hepatitis B vaccination is contraindicated during pregnancy.

T F 33. All pregnant women should be taught to recognize signs and symptoms of preterm labor.

T F 34. Breast shells can be used by women with inverted or flat nipples to help the nipples evert or become erect, thereby facilitating latch-on of the newborn once breastfeeding begins after birth.

T F 35. Women who are positive for hepatitis B should not breastfeed.

T F 36. Women often react to the confirmation of pregnancy with mixed feelings or ambivalence.

T F 37. Emotional lability (mood swings) might be related to profound hormonal changes that are part of the maternal response to pregnancy.

T F 38. Children typically respond to their mother's pregnancy in terms of their age and dependency needs.

T F 39. The reaction of a mother to her daughter's pregnancy can influence her daughter's self-confidence about her pregnancy.

40. *CREATE* a protocol for fundal measurement that facilitates accuracy.

41. *IDENTIFY* four factors that can be used to estimate the gestational age of the fetus.

42. Prevention of injury is an important goal for nurses as they teach pregnant women about how to care for themselves during pregnancy.

   A. *DESCRIBE* three principles of body mechanics that pregnant women should be taught to prevent injury.

   B. *IDENTIFY* five safety guidelines that you would include in a pamphlet titled Safety During Pregnancy that is to be distributed to pregnant women during their prenatal visit. INCLUDE the rationale for each guideline identified.

43. During the third trimester parents often make a decision concerning the method that they will use to feed their new-born. *LIST* the contraindications for breastfeeding.

MULTIPLE CHOICE: Circle the one correct option and state the rationale for the option chosen.

44. A nurse is assessing a pregnant woman during a prenatal visit. Several presumptive indicators of pregnancy are documented. Which one of the following is a presumptive indicator?
   A. Uterine enlargement
   B. Quickening
   C. Ballottement
   D. Palpation of fetal movement by the nurse

45. A woman's last menstrual period began on September 10, 2010, and ended on September 15, 2010. Using Nägele's rule, the EDB would be:
   A. June 17, 2011.
   B. June 22, 2011.
   C. August 17, 2011.
   D. December 3, 2011.

46. A woman at 30 weeks of gestation assumes a supine position for a fundal measurement and Leopold maneuvers. She begins to complain about feeling dizzy and nauseous. Her skin feels damp and cool. The nurse's first action would be to:
   A. Assess the woman's respiratory rate and effort.
   B. Provide the woman with an emesis basin.
   C. Elevate the woman's legs 20 degrees from her hips.
   D. Turn the woman on her side.

47. The nurse evaluates a pregnant woman's knowledge about prevention of urinary tract infections at the prenatal visit following a class on infection prevention that the woman attended. The nurse recognizes that the woman needs further instruction when she tells the nurse about which one of the following measures she now uses to prevent urinary tract infections:
   A. "I drink about 1 quart of fluid a day."
   B. "I have stopped using bubble baths and bath oils."
   C. "I have started wearing panty hose and underpants with a cotton crotch."
   D. "I drink cranberry juice instead of orange juice and have yogurt for lunch."

CRITICAL THINKING EXERCISES

1. A health history interview of the pregnant woman by the nurse is included as part of the initial prenatal visit.

   A. *STATE* the purpose of the health history interview.

B. *LIST* the components that should be included in the prenatal health history.

C. *WRITE* two questions for each component identified. Questions should be clear, concise, and understandable. Most of the questions should be open-ended to elicit the most complete response from the patient.

2. *IMAGINE* that you are a nurse working in a prenatal clinic. You have been assigned to be the primary nurse for Martha, an 18-year-old, who has come to the clinic for confirmation of pregnancy. She tells you that she knows she is pregnant because she has already missed three periods and a home pregnancy test she used last week was positive. Martha states that she has had very little contact with the health care system and the only reason she came today is because her boyfriend insisted that she "make sure" that she is really pregnant. *DESCRIBE* the approach you would take regarding data collection and nursing interventions appropriate for this woman.

3. Terry is a primigravida in her first trimester of pregnancy. She is accompanied by her husband, Tim, to her second prenatal visit. *ANSWER* each of the following questions asked by Terry and Tim.

A. "At the last visit I was told that my EDB is December 25! Can I really count on my baby being born on Christmas Day?"

B. "Before I became pregnant, my friend told me that I should be doing Kegel exercises. I was too embarrassed to ask her about them. What are they, and is it safe for me to do them while I am pregnant?"

C. "What effect will pregnancy have on our sex life? We're willing to abstain during pregnancy if we have to to keep our baby safe."

D. "This morning sickness I'm experiencing is driving me crazy. I become nauseous in the morning and again late in the afternoon. Occasionally I vomit or have the dry heaves. Will this last for my entire pregnancy? Is there anything I can do to feel better?"

4. Tara is 2 months pregnant. She tells the nurse at the prenatal clinic that she is used to being active and exercises every day. Now that she is pregnant, she wonders if she should reduce or stop her exercise routine. *DISCUSS* the nurse's response to Tara.

5. *WRITE* one nursing diagnosis for each of the following situations. *STATE* one expected outcome, and *LIST* appropriate nursing measures for the nursing diagnoses that you identified.

A. Beth is 6 weeks pregnant. During the health history interview she tells you that she has limited her intake of fluids and tries to hold her urine as long as she can because "I just hate having to go to the bathroom so frequently."

Nursing Diagnosis   **Expected Outcome**   **Nursing Measures**

B. Doris, who is 23 weeks pregnant, tells you that she is beginning to experience more frequent lower back pain. You note that, when she walked into the examining room, her posture exhibited a moderate degree of lordosis and neck flexion. She was wearing shoes with 2-inch narrow heels.

Nursing Diagnosis   **Expected Outcome**   **Nursing Measures**

C. Lisa, a primigravida at 32 weeks of gestation, comes for a prenatal visit accompanied by her partner, the father of the baby. They both express anxiety about the impending birth of the baby and how they will handle the experience of labor. Lisa is especially concerned about how she will survive the pain, and her partner is primarily concerned about how he can help Lisa cope with labor and make sure that she and the baby are safe.

Nursing Diagnosis	**Expected Outcome**	**Nursing Measures**

6. While a nurse is measuring a pregnant woman's fundus, the woman becomes pale and diaphoretic. The woman, who is at 23 weeks of gestation, states that she feels dizzy and lightheaded.

   A. *STATE* the most likely explanation for the assessment findings exhibited by this woman.

   B. *DESCRIBE* the nurse's immediate action.

7. Kelly is a primigravida in her third trimester of pregnancy. *ANSWER* each of the following questions that Kelly asks during a prenatal visit.

   A. "My husband and I have decided to breastfeed our baby, but friends told me that it is very difficult if my nipples do not come out. Is there any way I can tell now if my nipples are okay for breastfeeding?"

   B. "My ankles are swollen by the time I get home from work late in the afternoon." (Kelly teaches second grade.) "I've been trying to drink about 3 liters of fluid every day. Should I reduce the amount of liquid I'm drinking or ask my doctor for a water pill?"

C. "I woke up last night with a terrible cramp in my leg. It finally went away, but my husband and I just did not know what to do. What if this happens again tonight?"

8. Marge, a pregnant woman (2-0-0-1-0) beginning her third trimester, expresses concern about preterm birth. "I already had one miscarriage, and my sister's baby died after being born too early."

   A. *INDICATE* what the nurse can teach Marge about the signs of preterm labor. (See Chapter 22.)

   B. *DESCRIBE* the actions Marge should take if she experiences signs of preterm labor. (See Chapter 22.)

9. Carol is 4 months pregnant and beginning to "show." She asks the nurse what reactions she should expect from her 13-year-old daughter and 3-year-old son. *DESCRIBE* the nurse's response.

10. Your neighbor, Jane, is in her second month of pregnancy. Knowing that you are a nurse, her husband, Tom, confides in you that he just can't figure Jane out. "One minute she's happy, and the next minute she's crying for no reason at all! I don't know how I'll be able to cope with this for 7 more months." *DISCUSS* how you would respond to his concern.

11. Tony and Andrea are hoping to deliver their second baby at home. They have been receiving prenatal care from a certified nurse-midwife who has experience with home birth. Their 5-year-old son and both sets of grandparents will be present for the birth. *DISCUSS* the preparation measures that you would recommend to Tony and Andrea to ensure a safe and positive experience for everyone.

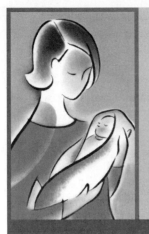

Maternal and Fetal Nutrition

CHAPTER 8

CHAPTER REVIEW ACTIVITIES

FILL IN THE BLANKS: Insert the term that corresponds to each of the following.

Nutrition

1. A(n) _____ before conception is the best way to ensure that adequate nutrients are available for the developing fetus. _____ intake is of particular concern to prevent _____ defects.

2. Maternal malnutrition can impair fetal growth and development, resulting in _____. Poor weight gain early in pregnancy increases the risk for giving birth to a(n) _____ infant, whereas inadequate gain during the last half of pregnancy increases the risk for _____ birth.

3. When individualizing the recommended daily intake of nutrients during pregnancy and lactation, nurses need to consider variations in a pregnant woman's situation, including _____, _____, _____, _____, and _____. _____ needs are met by carbohydrates, fats, and protein in the diet and should be increased during the second and third trimesters by _____ and _____ respectively above prepregnancy needs.

4. Women at greatest risk for inadequate protein intake include _____, _____, and _____.

5. Poor iron intake and absorption can lead to the development of _____ during pregnancy. If iron deficiency anemia is present, doses of _____ are recommended.

6. _____ is the inability to digest milk sugar because of the absence of the lactase enzyme in the small intestine.

7. _____ is the practice of consuming nonfood substances such as _____, _____, or _____ or excessive amounts of foodstuffs low in nutritional value such as _____, _____, _____, or _____. A(n) _____ is the urge to consume specific types of foods such as ice cream, pickles, and pizza.

8. Assessment of nutritional status begins with a diet history, which should include _____, _____, _____, and _____. Physical examination includes _____ measurements such as _____ and _____. Calculation of the _____ is a method of evaluating the appropriateness of weight for height and is used to guide a woman's weight gain during pregnancy.

9. Vegetarian diets can vary in terms of the foods allowed. Basic to all vegetarian diets are _____, _____, _____, _____, _____, and _____. A(n) _____ diet includes fish, poultry, eggs, and dairy products but does not allow beef or pork. _____ consume dairy products and plant products. _____ or _____ consume only plant products.

10. _____ or heartburn is caused by reflux from the stomach into the esophagus.

11. *COMPLETE* the following table by stating the importance of each of the following nutrients for healthy maternal adaptation to pregnancy and optimum fetal growth and development. *INDICATE* the major food sources for each nutrient.

Nutrient	Importance for Pregnancy	Common Food Sources
Protein		
Iron		
Calcium and phosphorus		
Zinc		
Fat-soluble vitamins (A, E, D)		
Water-soluble vitamins (folate, B_6, B_{12}, C)		

12. When assessing pregnant women, it is critical that nurses be alert for factors that might place women at nutritional risk so early intervention can be implemented. *STATE* five of the indicators or risk factors of which the nurse should be aware.

13. At her first prenatal visit Marie, a 20-year-old primigravida, reports that she has been a strict vegetarian for the past 3 years. *IDENTIFY* two major guidelines that the nurse should follow when planning menus with Marie.

14. Evaluation of nutritional status is an essential part of a thorough physical assessment of pregnant women. *CITE* four signs of good nutrition and four signs of inadequate nutrition for which the nurse should watch during the assessment of a pregnant woman.

15. *IDENTIFY* three nursing measures appropriate for each of the following nursing diagnoses:

   A. Imbalanced nutrition: less than body requirements related to inadequate intake associated with moderate nausea and vomiting (morning sickness)

   B. Constipation related to decreased intestinal motility associated with increased progesterone levels during pregnancy

16. *DETERMINE* the approximate body mass index (BMI) for each of the following pregnant women and *INDICATE* the recommended weight gain and pattern for each woman based on her calculated BMI.

Woman	BMI	Weight gain

June: 157.5 cm, 54.5 kg

Alice: 165 cm, 93 kg

Ann: 162.5 cm, 43 kg

TRUE OR FALSE: Circle T if true or F if false for each of the following statements. Correct the false statements.

T F 17. Good maternal nutrition before and during pregnancy is an important measure to reduce the risk for giving birth to a low-birth-weight infant.

T F 18. A series of 24-hour diet recalls is the best way to determine the appropriateness of a woman's kilocalorie intake.

T F 19. Women capable of becoming pregnant should consume approximately 800 mcg of folic acid daily.

T F 20. A woman whose BMI is 28 (overweight) should gain approximately 0.3 kg/week during the second and third trimesters of pregnancy.

T F 21. Adolescents are at increased nutritional risk because their growth requirements compete with those of the fetus for nutrients.

T F 22. A caloric increase of 600 kcal/day is recommended for pregnant women beginning in the first trimester.

T F 23. Ketonuria has been associated with preterm labor.

T F 24. Pregnant women should avoid caffeine because research has indicated that caffeine can adversely affect uterine perfusion.

T F 25. Women should begin taking an iron supplement at the onset of pregnancy.

T F 26. If moderate peripheral edema occurs during pregnancy, the woman's sodium intake should be reduced.

T F 27. Excessive intake of fat-soluble vitamins such as vitamin A during pregnancy can result in congenital malformations of the fetus.

T F 28. Development of neural tube defects appears to be more common in the fetuses of pregnant women whose diet is low in vitamin B_6.

T F 29. Dehydration can stimulate the onset of premature labor.

T F 30. Lactating women need to consume at least 2500 kcal/day.

T F 31. Lactating women should be informed that loss of the weight gained during pregnancy begins after they stop breastfeeding.

T F 32. The most common nutrition-related laboratory tests for a pregnant woman are hematocrit and hemoglobin measurements.

33. Joanne is going to breastfeed her infant until she returns to work in 6 months. *STATE* three guidelines that the nurse should teach Joanne to follow to ensure adequate nutrition during lactation.

34. Addie asks why her nutrient needs increase during pregnancy. *STATE* four factors that the nurse should explain to Addie as reasons why her nutrient needs increase during pregnancy.

MULTIPLE CHOICE: Circle the one correct option and state the rationale for the option chosen.

35. A nurse teaching a pregnant woman about the importance of iron in her diet tells her to avoid consuming which of the following foods at the same time as her iron supplement because it decreases iron absorption.
   A. Tomatoes
   B. Strawberries
   C. Meat
   D. Eggs

36. A 25-year-old pregnant woman is at 10 weeks of gestation. Her BMI is calculated to be 24. Which one of the following is recommended in terms of weight gain during pregnancy?
   A. Total weight gain of 18 kg
   B. First-trimester weight gain of 1 to 2.5 kg
   C. Weight gain of 0.4 kg/week for 40 weeks
   D. Weight gain of 3 kg/month during the second and third trimesters

37. A pregnant woman at 6 weeks of gestation tells her nurse-midwife that she has been experiencing nausea with occasional vomiting every day. The nurse could recommend which of the following as an effective relief measure?
   A. Eat starchy foods such as buttered popcorn or peanut butter with crackers in the morning before getting out of bed.
   B. Avoid eating before going to bed at night.
   C. Alter eating patterns to small meals every 2 to 3 hours.
   D. Skip a meal if nausea is experienced.

38. A woman demonstrates an understanding of the importance of increasing her intake of foods high in folic acid when she includes which of the following foods in her diet?
   A. Seafood
   B. Legumes
   C. Green leafy vegetables
   D. Cheese

39. A 30-year-old woman at 16 weeks of gestation comes for a routine prenatal visit. Her 24-hour dietary recall is evaluated by the nurse. Which of the following entries indicates that this woman needs further instruction regarding nutrient needs during pregnancy?

A. Six servings from the meat, poultry, fish, dry beans, eggs, and nuts group

B. Total intake is 300 kcal above her calculated prepregnancy needs

C. Daily iron supplement taken at bedtime with a glass of orange juice

D. Four servings from the milk, yogurt, and cheese group

CRITICAL THINKING EXERCISES

1. Nutrition and weight gain are important areas of consideration for nurses who care for pregnant women. In addition, weight gain is often a source of stress and body image alteration for the pregnant woman. *DISCUSS* the approach that you would use in each of the following situations.

   A. Kelly (5' 8" and 130 pounds) complains to you that her physician recommended a weight gain of approximately 25 to 35 pounds during her pregnancy. She states, "Babies only weigh about 7 pounds when they are born! Why do I have to gain much more than that?"

   B. Kate (5' 4" and 125 pounds) has just found out that she is pregnant. She states, "I am so glad to be pregnant. I love to eat, and now I can start eating for two. It will be great not to have to watch the scale or what I eat."

   C. June tells you that she does not have to worry about her nutrient intake during her pregnancy. "I take plenty of vitamins—everything from A to Z!"

   D. Erin is 7 months pregnant. She asks you what she can do to relieve the heartburn she experiences after meals, especially dinner.

E. Sara (BMI 28.7) is 1 month pregnant. She asks you for dietary guidance, including a weight reduction diet, because she does not want to gain too much weight during this pregnancy.

F. Beth is 2 months pregnant. She states, "I have cut down on my water intake. I do get a little thirsty, but it is worth it because I do not have to urinate so often."

G. Hedy is 2 months pregnant and has come for her second prenatal visit. During a discussion about nutrition needs during pregnancy, she states, "I know I will not get enough calcium because I get sick when I drink milk."

H. Lara is 36 weeks pregnant. She states that she would like to breastfeed her baby but is concerned about getting back into shape and losing weight after the baby is born. "My friends told me that I will lose weight more slowly because I will not be able to start on a weight reduction diet as long as I am breastfeeding."

2. Yvonne's hemoglobin is 13 g/dl, and her hematocrit is 37% at the onset of her pregnancy. She asks the nurse if she will have to take iron during her pregnancy if she tries to follow a good diet. "My friend took iron when she was pregnant, and it made her sick to her stomach." *DISCUSS* the appropriate response by the nurse.

3. Gloria is an 18-year-old Native-American woman (5' 6" and 98 pounds) who has just been diagnosed as 8 weeks pregnant. In her discussions with you at her first prenatal visit, she expresses a lack of knowledge regarding the nutritional requirements of pregnancy and an interest in learning about what to eat because she wants to have a healthy baby.

A. *OUTLINE* the approach that you would use to help Gloria learn about and meet the nutritional requirements of her pregnancy.

B. *PLAN* a 1-day menu that incorporates Gloria's nutritional needs and reflects the traditions of her culture.

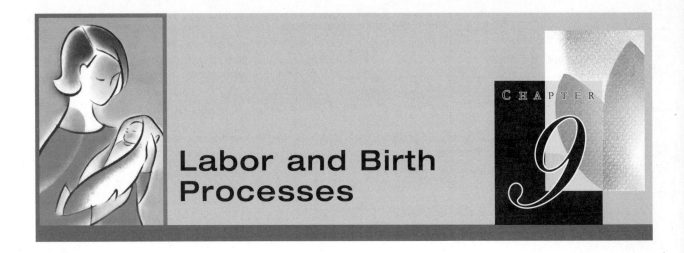

Labor and Birth Processes

CHAPTER REVIEW ACTIVITIES

FILL IN THE BLANKS: Insert the term that corresponds to each of the following.

Labor and Birth

1. Fontanels are _____ that are located where _____ in the fetal or neonatal skull intersect.

2. Molding is the slight _____ of the _____ of the fetal skull that occurs during childbirth.

3. Fetal presentation refers to the _____ that enters the pelvic _____ first. The three main types are _____ (head first), _____ (buttocks or feet first), and _____.

4. The presenting part is the part of the fetal body _____ during a(n) _____ examination. The three most common parts are _____, _____, and _____.

5. The vertex presentation occurs when the fetal head is completely _____, making the _____ the fetal part first felt by the examining finger.

6. Fetal lie is the relationship of the _____ to the _____. There are two types—longitudinal (vertical), when the _____, and transverse (horizontal), when the _____.

7. Fetal attitude is the relationship of the _____. The most common type is one of general _____.

8. The biparietal diameter is the largest _____ diameter of the fetal skull. The suboccipitobregmatic diameter is the smallest _____ diameter of the fetal skull to enter the maternal pelvis when the fetal head is in complete _____.

9. Fetal position refers to the relationship of the fetal _____ to the four _____ of the maternal _____.

10. Engagement occurs when the _____ diameter of the presenting part has passed through the maternal _____ into the _____, reaching the level of the _____ or station _____.

11. Station is the relationship of the _____ of the fetus to an imaginary line drawn between the maternal _____. It is measured in _____ above or below the _____, thereby serving as a method of determining the progress of fetal _____.

12. Effacement refers to the _____ and _____ of the _____ during the _____ stage of labor. Degree of effacement is expressed in _____ from _____ to _____.

13. Dilation is the _____ or _____ of the _____ and the _____, which occurs once labor has begun. Degree of progress is expressed in _____ from less than _____ to full dilation or _____.

14. Lightening or "_____" occurs when the fetal _____ descends into the _____ approximately _____ before term in the primigravida and at the _____ in the multiparous woman.

15. Bloody show is _____, representing the passage of the _____ as the cervix _____ in preparation for labor.

16. The mechanism of labor is the fetal _____ necessary in the human birth process to facilitate passage through the _____. The seven _____ of labor in a vertex presentation are _____, _____, _____, _____, _____, _____, and finally birth by _____.

17. Mary is a primigravida at 34 weeks of gestation. She asks you how she will know when labor is getting closer. *IDENTIFY* the signs that indicate that she is experiencing prodromal labor (period immediately preceding the onset of true labor).

18. *STATE* the five factors (the five P's) that affect the process of labor and birth. *INCLUDE* the manner in which each factor affects the progress of childbirth in your description.

19. *LIST* the events that occur during each of the four stages of labor.

20. *LABEL* the following illustrations of the fetal skull and the maternal pelvis with the appropriate landmarks and diameters.

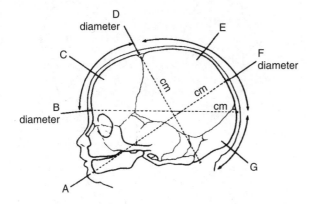

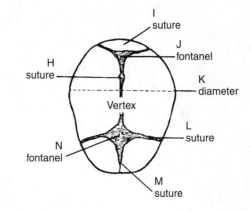

Fetal Skull

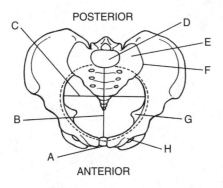

Pelvic Brim from Above

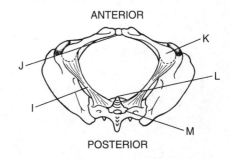

Pelvic Outlet from Above

Maternal Pelvis

21. *INDICATE* the presentation, presenting part, position, lie, and attitude of the fetus for each of the following illustrations.

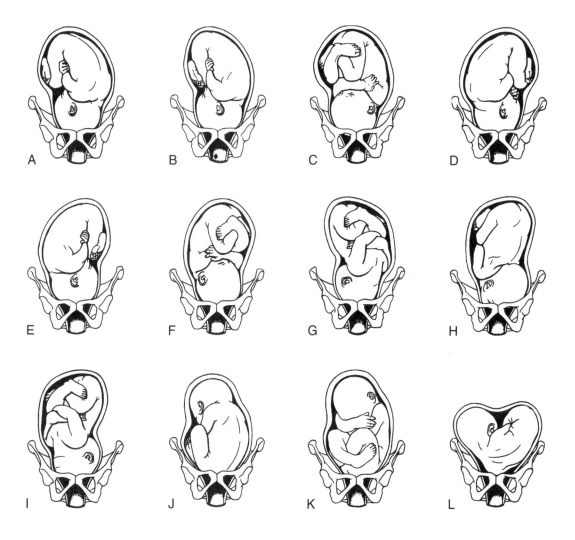

22. *STATE* the three factors that affect fetal circulation.

TRUE OR FALSE: Circle T if true or F if false for each of the following statements. Correct the false statements.

T   F   23. The most common fetal attitude is one of full extension of body parts.

T   F   24. A longitudinal lie results in either a cephalic or a breech presentation.

T   F   25. Fetal position is unlikely to change once labor begins.

T   F   26. A woman must have a gynecoid pelvis to experience a spontaneous vaginal birth.

T   F   27. Effacement usually precedes dilation for a nulliparous woman but progresses simultaneously with dilation for the multiparous woman.

T   F   28. Women with a history of sexually transmitted infections might experience slowed or ineffective progress of dilation as a result of cervical scarring.

T   F   29. The hands-and-knees position is most helpful when the fetal position is anterior.

T   F   30. Women often experience decreased dyspnea after lightening occurs.

T   F   31. The expected range of the fetal heart rate of a full-term fetus is 100 to 140 beats/min.

T   F   32. An increase in fetal P_{O_2} and arterial pH and a decrease in P_{CO_2} prepare the fetus for initiating respirations immediately after its birth.

T   F   33. Because systolic blood pressure increases during a first-stage contraction by approximately 10 mm Hg, assessment of maternal blood pressure *between* contractions provides more accurate data.

T   F   34. The maternal white blood cell count increases in response to physical or emotional stress, tissue trauma, and increased activity level associated with childbirth.

T   F   35. During labor a woman should be encouraged to do toe-pointing leg exercises to reduce the incidence of leg cramps.

T   F   36. Endogenous endorphins secreted during labor raise a woman's pain threshold.

MULTIPLE CHOICE: Circle the one correct option and state the rationale for the option chosen.

37. A vaginal examination during labor reveals the following information about the fetus: RMT, −2. An accurate interpretation of the data would be:
    A. Attitude: flexed.
    B. Station: above the ischial spines.
    C. Presenting part: vertex.
    D. Lie: Transverse.

38. Changes occur as a woman progresses through labor. Which of the following maternal adaptations are expected during labor?
    A. Increase in both systolic and diastolic blood pressure during uterine contractions in the first stage of labor
    B. Decrease in white blood cell count to below 14,000/mm^3
    C. Slight increase in temperature, pulse, and respiration findings
    D. Increase in gastric motility leading to vomiting, especially during the latent and active phases of the first stage of labor

39. Duration of labor varies from woman to woman and is often influenced by a woman's obstetric history, including parity. An expected duration for a nulliparous woman's stages of labor would be:
    A. First stage of labor: up to 20 hours for full dilation to be achieved.
    B. Second stage of labor: average of 20 minutes or less.
    C. Third stage of labor: 45 to 60 minutes.
    D. Fourth stage of labor: 6 to 8 hours.

40. When instructing a group of primigravid women about the onset of labor, the nurse tells them to be alert for:
    A. Urinary retention.
    B. Weight gain of 2 kg.
    C. Quickening.
    D. Energy surge.

CRITICAL THINKING EXERCISES

1. As part of their care of the laboring woman, nurses perform vaginal examinations and interpret the results. *STATE* the meaning of each of the following vaginal examination findings.

Exam I	Exam II	Exam III	Exam IV
ROP	RMA	LST	OA
−1	0	+1	+3
50%	25%	75%	100%
3 cm	2 cm	6 cm	10 cm

2. Brooke is a primigravida at 36 weeks of gestation. During a prenatal visit at 34 weeks of gestation, she asks you the following questions regarding her approaching labor. *DESCRIBE* how you would respond.

   A. "What causes labor to start?"

   B. "Are there things that I should watch for that would tell me my labor is getting closer to starting?"

   C. "How long can I expect my labor to last once it starts?"

   D. "My friend just had a baby, and she told me that the nurses kept helping her change her position and even encouraged her to walk! Isn't that dangerous for the baby and painful for the mom?"

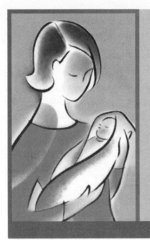

Management of Discomfort

CHAPTER REVIEW ACTIVITIES

FILL IN THE BLANKS: Insert the term that corresponds to each of the following.

Childbirth Pain

1. _____ pain originates in the body organs during labor and birth. This type of pain results from _____ changes and uterine _____. It is located over the _____ of the abdomen and radiates to the _____ area of the back and down the _____.

2. _____ pain is well localized. During labor and birth this type of pain is experienced as _____ discomfort that results from stretching and distention of _____ to allow passage of the fetus and from traction on the _____ and _____ supports during contractions.

3. _____ pain is felt in areas of the body other than the area of pain origin. Pain originating in the abdominal viscera is felt in the _____, _____, _____, _____, _____, and _____.

4. The _____ theory of pain is based on the principle that pain sensations travel along sensory nerve pathways to the brain but only a limited number of sensations or messages can travel through these nerve pathways at one time. Pain relief techniques based on this theory include _____ or _____, _____, _____, and concentration on _____ and _____ techniques.

5. _____ are endogenous opioids secreted by the pituitary gland that act on the central and peripheral nervous systems to reduce pain.

Nonpharmacologic Techniques for Management of Discomfort

6. Three major childbirth preparation methods taught in the United States are _____, _____, and _____.

7. Breathing techniques provide _____, thereby reducing the _____ and helping the woman maintain control throughout contractions. _____ breathing is breathing at approximately _____ the woman's normal breathing rate. It is usually the first technique used in early labor.

8. As contractions increase in frequency and intensity, chest breathing is used, with breathing becoming more _____ in depth and increasing to about _____ the normal breathing rate.

9. A(n) _____ should begin and end each breathing technique and contraction.

10. A breathing technique using a pattern of breaths and puffs in a ratio of 4:1, 6:1, or 8:1 is used to enhance concentration during the _____ phase of the first stage of labor. An undesirable effect of this type of breathing might be _____ or rapid, deep respirations, which can result in _____, as exhibited by the symptoms of _____, _____, _____, or _____. It can be overcome by having the woman _____. This enables the woman to rebreathe _____ and replace the _____ ions.

11. _____, or light stroking of the abdomen or other body part in rhythm with breathing during contractions and _____, or steady pressure against the lower back especially during back labor, are two examples of nonpharmacologic methods to relieve discomfort that are based on the _____ theory of pain.

12. *DESCRIBE* the factors that could influence the nursing diagnosis of acute pain related to the processes involved in labor and birth, identified for a woman in labor.

13. *EXPLAIN* the theoretic basis of techniques such as massage, stroking, music, and imagery to reduce the sensation of pain during childbirth.

MATCHING: Match the description in Column I with the appropriate pharmacologic pain relief measure in Column II.

COLUMN I

_____ 14. Abolition of pain perception by interrupting nerve impulses going to the brain (loss of sensation, partial or complete, and sometimes loss of consciousness occurs)

_____ 15. Method to repair a tear in the dura mater around the spinal cord as a result of spinal anesthesia

_____ 16. Single-injection subarachnoid anesthesia useful for pain control during birth but not for labor

_____ 17. Systemic analgesic that provides analgesia without significant maternal or neonatal respiratory depression

_____ 18. Used for rapid perineal anesthesia for performing and repairing an episiotomy

_____ 19. Medication such as a barbiturate that can be used to relieve anxiety and induce sleep in prodromal or early latent labor

_____ 20. Analgesic potentiators such as tranquilizers

_____ 21. Drug that reverses effects of opioids including neonatal narcosis (central nervous system depression of the newborn)

_____ 22. Medications such as opioid agonists that are administered intramuscularly or intravenously for pain relief during labor

_____ 23. Alleviation of pain sensation or raising of the pain threshold without loss of consciousness

_____ 24. Relief from pain of uterine contractions and birth by injecting a local anesthetic and/or opioid agonist such as fentanyl into the peridural space

_____ 25. Anesthetic that eliminates pain in the lower vagina, vulva, and perineum, making it useful for episiotomy, birth, and forceps- or vacuum-assisted birth

COLUMN II

A. Opioid agonist-antagonist
B. Anesthesia
C. Analgesia
D. Ataractics
E. Epidural block
F. Epidural blood patch causing
G. Local infiltration anesthesia
H. Spinal block/anesthesia
I. Opioid antagonist
J. Pudendal block
K. Systemic analgesia
L. Sedative

26. *COMPLETE* the following table by listing the effects, criteria and timing for use, and nursing management for each of the following commonly used nerve block anesthetics.

Anesthetic	Effects	Criteria and Timing	Management
Local infiltration			
Pudenal block			
Spinal block/anethesia			
Epidural block			

27. Systemic analgesics cross the placenta and affect the fetus.

    A. *LIST* three factors that influence the effect that systemic analgesics have on the fetus.

    B. *DESCRIBE* the fetal effects of systemic analgesics.

28. *COMPLETE* the following table by giving one example for each of the following medication classifications, stating guidelines for its administration, and explaining why it is used during the childbirth process.

Medication	Guidelines for Administration	Purpose of Administration
Opioid agonist analgesic		
Opioid agonist-antagonist analgesic		
Analgesic potentiator		
Opioid antagonist		

TRUE OR FALSE: Circle T if true or F if false for each of the following statements. Correct the false statements.

T F 29. Somatic pain occurs as a result of perineal stretching and pressure exerted by the presenting part on the pelvic organs and structures.

T F 30. A woman's perception of her birth experience as "good" or "bad" is influenced by the degree to which she believes she has met her personal goals related to coping with pain effectively.

T F 31. Water therapy can be used even if the laboring woman's membranes are ruptured.

T F 32. Water therapy can worsen the pain associated with "back labor".

T F 33. Barbituates given without an analgesic when a laboring woman is experiencing pain can magnify pain perception because the woman's normal coping mechanisms may be blunted.

T F 34. Intramuscular administration of analgesics during labor offers a more predictable onset of pain relief.

T F 35. Naloxone (Narcan) is contraindicated if a woman has an opioid dependency because it may cause symptoms of withdrawal.

T F 36. Before initiating her epidural anesthesia, a woman should be adequately hydrated using an intravenous (IV) solution of 5% glucose in water.

T F 37. Epidural anesthesia is useful as a pain relief measure for both labor and birth.

T F 38. Keeping the woman in a flat position for at least 8 hours after birth is the most effective way to prevent headaches following a spinal block.

T F 39. The woman can be assisted into a sitting position for the induction of both spinal anesthesia and lumbar epidural blocks.

T F 40. Maternal hypotension is a major adverse reaction to both spinal anesthesia and epidural blocks.

41. *EXPLAIN* why the IV route is preferred to the intramuscular route for the administration of systemic analgesics during labor.

MULTIPLE CHOICE: Circle the one correct option and state the rationale for the option chosen.

42. The use of ataractics can potentiate the action of analgesics. An ataractic that the nurse might expect to give to a laboring woman would be:
    A. Naloxone (Narcan).
    B. Hydroxyzine (Vistaril).
    C. Butorphanol tartrate (Stadol).
    D. Fentanyl (Sublimaze).

43. The doctor has ordered meperidine (Demerol) 25 mg IV q2-3h prn for pain associated with labor. In fulfilling this order, the nurse should know that:
    A. The onset of the effect of this analgesic after IV administration is approximately 10 minutes.
    B. The dosage of the analgesic is too high for IV administration, necessitating a new order.
    C. Respiratory depression of the woman or fetus is not a concern with this analgesic.
    D. The newborn should be observed for respiratory depression if birth occurs within 4 hours after administration.

44. An anesthesiologist is preparing to begin a continuous epidural block using a combination of local anesthetic and narcotic analgesic as a pain relief measure for a laboring woman. A nursing measure related to this type of nerve block would be to:
    A. Assist the woman into a modified Sims or upright position with her back curved.
    B. Keep the woman in a semirecumbent position after administration to ensure equal distribution of the pharmacologic agents.
    C. Assess the woman for headaches, especially after birth.
    D. Assist the woman to the bathroom to urinate at least every 2 hours during labor to prevent bladder distention.

CRITICAL THINKING EXERCISES

1. When working with a group of expectant fathers, the nurse is asked if there really is "a physical reason for all the pain that women say they feel when they're in labor." *DESCRIBE* the response this nurse should give.

2. On admission to the labor unit in the latent phase of labor, Mr. and Mrs. T. (2-0-0-1-0) tell you that they are so glad that they took Lamaze classes and did so much reading about childbirth. "We will not need any medication now that we know what to do. But, most important, our baby will be safe!" *DESCRIBE* how you would respond if you were their primary nurse for childbirth.

3. *IMAGINE* that you are the nurse manager of a labor and birth unit. Major renovations are being planned for your unit, and your input is required. You and your staff nurses believe that water therapy, including the use of showers and whirlpool baths, is a beneficial nonpharmacologic method for relieving pain and discomfort and enhancing the progress of labor. *DISCUSS* the rationale that you would use to convince planners that installation of a shower and whirlpool bath into each birthing room is a cost-effective measure.

4. Tara has been in labor for 4 hours. Her blood pressure had been stable, averaging 130/80 mm Hg when assessed between contractions, and the fetal heart rate (FHR) pattern has consistently exhibited criteria of a reassuring pattern. A lumbar epidural block is initiated. Shortly afterward, during assessment of maternal vital signs and FHR, Tara's blood pressure decreases to 102/60 mm Hg, and the FHR pattern begins to exhibit a decrease in rate and variability.

A. *STATE* what Tara is experiencing. *SUPPORT* your answer and *EXPLAIN* the physiologic basis for what is happening to Tara.

B. *WRITE* a nursing diagnosis that reflects this occurrence.

C. *LIST* the immediate nursing actions.

5. Moira, a primigravida, has chosen a continuous epidural block as her pharmacologic method of choice for pain relief during childbirth.

A. *IDENTIFY* the assessment procedures that should be used to determine Moira's readiness for initiation of the epidural block.

B. *DESCRIBE* the preparation methods that should be implemented.

C. *STATE* two position that you could help Moira to assume for the induction of the epidural block.

D. *OUTLINE* the nursing care management interventions recommended while Moira is receiving the anesthesia to ensure her well-being and that of her fetus.

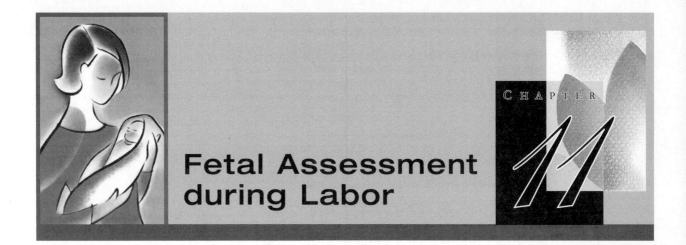

Fetal Assessment during Labor

CHAPTER 11

CHAPTER REVIEW ACTIVITIES

FILL IN THE BLANKS: Insert the term that corresponds to each of the following.

Fetal Monitoring

1. The goals of intrapartum fetal heart rate (FHR) monitoring are to identify and differentiate the _____ patterns from the _____ patterns that indicate fetal _____. Fetal _____ is a deficiency of oxygen in the arterial blood, whereas fetal _____ is an inadequate supply of oxygen at the cellular level.

2. One method to assess fetal status is intermittent _____, using a(n) _____ or _____ to listen to the FHR.

3. _____ is the method used to assess the FHR pattern continuously. Two modes can be used to accomplish this method of assessment. External monitoring uses a(n) _____ to assess the FHR pattern and (a) _____ to monitor the frequency and duration of contractions. Internal monitoring uses (a) _____ _____attached to the fetal presenting part to assess the FHR pattern and a(n) _____ to monitor the frequency, duration, and intensity of contractions.

4. Compression of the umbilical cord can result in a(n) _____ FHR pattern. _____ can be used to instill normal saline or lactated Ringer's solution into the uterine cavity via the intrauterine catheter to add fluid around the umbilical cord and thus prevent its compression during uterine contractions.

5. _____ therapy can be used when fetal compromise occurs related to increased uterine activity. _____ improves blood flow through the placenta by inhibiting uterine contractions. _____ can be administered to achieve a reduction in uterine activity.

6. It is critical that a nurse working on a labor unit be knowledgeable about factors associated with a reduction in fetal oxygen supply, characteristics of a reassuring FHR pattern, and characteristics of normal uterine activity. *LIST* the required information for each of the following:

   A. Factors associated with a reduction in fetal oxygen supply

B. Characteristics of a normal (reassuring) FHR pattern

C. Characteristics of normal uterine activity

7. *IDENTIFY* the characteristics of abnormal (nonreassuring) FHR patterns.

MATCHING: Match the definition in Column I with the appropriate term from Column II.

FHR Patterns

COLUMN I

_____ 8. Average FHR range of 110 to 160 beats/min at term as assessed during a 10-minute period that excludes periodic and episodic changes and periods of marked variability

_____ 9. Persistent (longer than 10 minutes) baseline FHR below 110 beats/min

_____ 10. Visually apparent decrease in the FHR of 15 beats/min or more below baseline that lasts longer than 2 minutes but less than 10 minutes

_____ 11. Changes from baseline patterns in FHR that occur with uterine contractions

_____ 12. Persistent (longer than 10 minutes) baseline FHR above 160 beats/min

_____ 13. Expected irregular fluctuations of the baseline FHR of two or more cycles per minute

_____ 14. FHR decrease shortly after onset of a contraction as a response to fetal head compression

_____ 15. FHR decrease after the peak of a contraction in response to uteroplacental insufficiency

_____ 16. FHR decrease at any time during a contraction in response to umbilical cord compression

_____ 17. Visually apparent abrupt increase in the FHR of 15 beats/min or more above the baseline that lasts 15 seconds or longer, with return to baseline less than 2 minutes after onset

_____ 18. Changes from baseline patterns in FHR that are not associated with uterine contractions

COLUMN II

A. Acceleration
B. Early deceleration
C. Variability
D. Late deceleration
E. Variable deceleration
F. Tachycardia
G. Prolonged deceleration
H. Bradycardia
I. Baseline FHR
J. Periodic changes
K. Episodic (nonperiodic) changes

FILL IN THE BLANKS: In general, the recommended frequency of FHR assessment depends on the risk status of the mother and the stage of labor. Insert the appropriate time for each of the following assessment recommendations.

19. Low risk patient (risk factors are absent during labor): auscultate FHR/assess tracing with _____ in the latent phase of the first stage of labor, every _____ in the active and transition phases of the first stage of labor, and every _____ in the second stage of labor.

20. High risk patient (risk factors are present during labor): auscultate FHR/assess tracing with _____ in the latent phase of the first stage of labor, every _____ in the active and transition phases of the first stage of labor, and every _____ in the second stage of labor.

21. Nurses caring for laboring women might need to use intermittent auscultation to assess fetal health and well-being during labor. *STATE* the advantages and disadvantages of intermittent auscultation as a method of fetal assessment during childbirth.

22. The nurse is preparing to auscultate fetal heart sounds as part of the admission process for a woman in labor. *OUT-LINE* the guidelines that this nurse should follow when monitoring the fetus using the intermittent auscultation method.

23. *INDICATE* the legal responsibilities related to fetal monitoring of nurses who care for women during childbirth.

TRUE OR FALSE: Circle T if true or F if false for each of the following statements. Correct the false statements.

T   F   24. An abnormal (nonreassuring) FHR pattern indicates that the fetus is compromised and is experiencing some degree of hypoxemia or hypoxia or both.

T   F   25. Auscultation should be performed during a uterine contraction and for at least 10 seconds after the end of the contraction to detect periodic changes in pattern.

T   F   26. FHR variability can temporarily decrease when the fetus is in a sleep state.

T   F   27. When external monitoring is used, the tocotransducer should be repositioned every 3 to 4 hours.

T   F   28. Maternal supine hypotensive syndrome reduces blood flow to the placenta, resulting in fetal hypoxia as reflected in fetal bradycardia, absent or minimal variability, and late decelerations.

T   F   29. Acceleration of the FHR associated with fetal movement is a reassuring sign.

T   F   30. Decelerations of the FHR can be either benign or nonreassuring in terms of fetal well-being.

T   F   31. Late deceleration patterns are characterized by a U or V shape with acceleration shoulders before and after the deceleration.

T   F   32. Early decelerations are nonreassuring patterns that typically occur when blood flow through the placenta is diminished.

T   F   33. The average intrauterine pressure during a contraction ranges from 50 to 85 mm Hg.

T   F   34. The tocotransducer should be placed on the abdomen over the fundus.

T   F   35. The intrauterine pressure catheter is able to assess uterine contraction frequency, duration, and intensity.

T   F   36. A Ritgen maneuver is used to determine the correct placement of the ultrasound transducer.

T   F   37. Late deceleration patterns are caused by uteroplacental insufficiency.

38. A nurse caring for a laboring woman in active labor notes an abnormal (nonreassuring) FHR pattern when evaluating the monitor tracing. *DESCRIBE* the action the nurse should take on the basis of this finding.

39. *OUTLINE* the nursing interventions that should be implemented when caring for a woman who is being monitored by an external monitor.

40. A woman is in labor. An external monitor is being used to assess the status of her fetus and the pattern of her uterine contractions. *SPECIFY* the data that the nurse should document on:

A. **Patient record**

B. **Monitor strip**

MULTIPLE CHOICE: Circle the one correct option and state the rationale for the option chosen.

41. A laboring woman's uterine contractions are being monitored internally. When evaluating the monitor tracing, which of the following findings would be a source of concern and require further assessment?
    A. Frequency every 2½ to 3 minutes
    B. Duration of 80 to 85 seconds
    C. Intensity during a uterine contraction of 85 to 90 mm Hg
    D. Average resting tone of 20 to 25 mm Hg

42. External electronic fetal monitoring will be used for a woman just admitted to the labor unit in active labor. A guideline that the nurse should follow when implementing this form of monitoring would be to:
    A. Use Leopold maneuvers to determine the correct placement of the tocotransducer.
    B. Apply contact gel to the ultrasound transducer before application over the point of maximum intensity.
    C. Reposition the ultrasound transducer every hour and massage the site.
    D. Apply a spiral electrode if abnormal (nonreassuring) FHR signs are noted.

43. The nurse caring for women in labor should be aware of signs characterizing normal (reassuring) FHR patterns. A reassuring sign would be:
    A. Moderate baseline variability.
    B. Average baseline FHR of 90 to 110 beats/min.
    C. Transient episodic deceleration with movement.
    D. Late deceleration patterns approximately every three or four contractions.

44. A laboring woman's temperature is elevated as a result of an upper respiratory infection. The FHR pattern that reflects maternal fever would be:
    A. Diminished variability.
    B. Variable decelerations.
    C. Tachycardia.
    D. Early decelerations.

45. A nulliparous woman is in the active phase of labor, and her cervix has progressed to 6 cm dilation. The nurse caring for this woman evaluates the external monitor tracing and notes the following: decrease in FHR shortly after onset of several uterine contractions, returning to baseline rate by the end of the contraction; shape is uniform. On the basis of these findings, the nurse should:
    A. Change the woman's position to her left side.
    B. Document the finding on the woman's chart.
    C. Notify the physician.
    D. Perform a vaginal examination to check for cord prolapse.

CRITICAL THINKING EXERCISES

1. Darlene, a primigravida in active labor, has just been admitted to the labor unit. She becomes very anxious when external electronic monitoring equipment is set up. She tells the nurse that her father had a heart attack 2 months ago. "He was so sick that they had to put him on a monitor too. Does this mean that my baby has a heart problem just like my father?" *DESCRIBE* the nurse's expected response.

2. Terry is a primigravida at 43 weeks of gestation. Her labor is being stimulated with oxytocin administered intravenously. Her contractions have been increasing in intensity, with a frequency of every 2 to 2½ minutes and a duration of 80 to 85 seconds. She is currently in a supine position with her head elevated 30 degrees. On observation of the monitor tracing, you note that during the last two contractions the FHR decreased after the contraction peaked and did not return to baseline until about 10 seconds into the rest period. A slight decrease in variability and increase in baseline rate were observed.

A. *IDENTIFY* the pattern described and the possible factors responsible for it.

B. *DESCRIBE* the actions that you would take. *STATE* the rationale for each action.

3. *ANALYZE* each of the following monitor tracings and *DOCUMENT* your findings. *DESCRIBE* each FHR pattern depicted and the criteria used to determine whether the pattern is reassuring or nonreassuring. *INDICATE* the possible causes, significance, and nursing actions required for each nonreassuring FHR pattern identified.

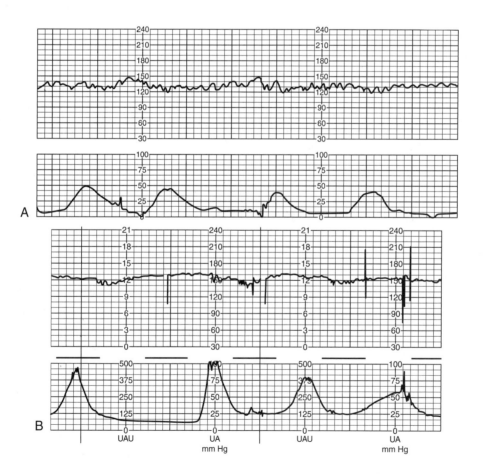

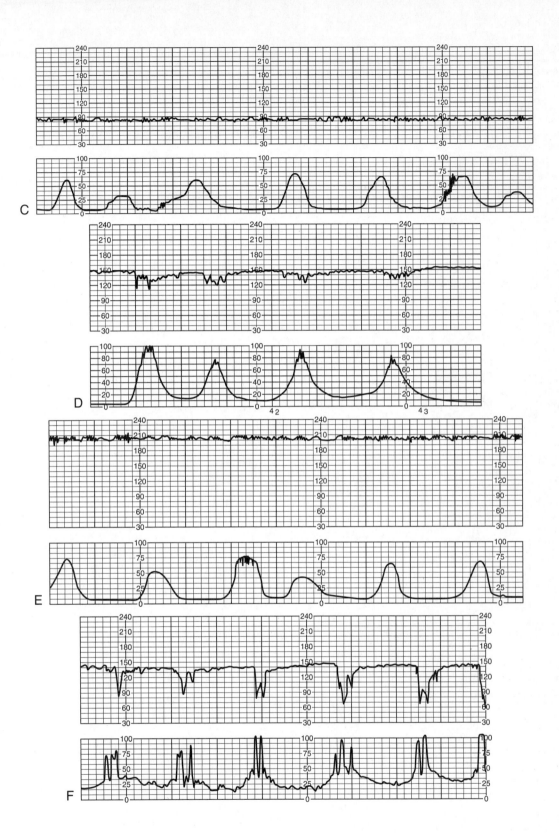

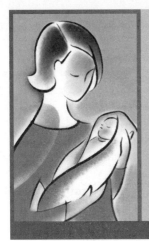

Nursing Care of the Family during Labor and Birth

CHAPTER 12

CHAPTER REVIEW ACTIVITIES

EVALUATE each of the following assessment findings used to distinguish true labor from false labor. *DESIGNATE* whether the assessment finding is associated with true labor (TL) or false labor (FL).

_____ 1. Contractions regular and progressive

_____ 2. Cervix soft and posterior

_____ 3. Contractions ceasing with ambulation

_____ 4. Cervix soft, 25%, 2 cm, midposition

_____ 5. Lightening in multiparous woman

_____ 6. Discomfort present in abdomen above umbilicus

_____ 7. Increased contraction intensity with activity and ambulation

_____ 8. Presenting part above ischial spines

_____ 9. Bloody show

_____ 10. Discomfort radiating from lower back to lower abdomen

_____ 11. Contractions continuing even after a shower or back rub

FILL IN THE BLANKS: Insert the term that corresponds to each of the following.

Stages of Labor

12. The second stage of labor is the stage when the _____. It begins with full cervical _____ and complete _____. It ends with the _____. This stage has three phases (i.e., _____, _____, and _____). A second stage that is longer than _____ hours might be considered prolonged in a woman without regional anesthesia and should be reported to the primary health care provider.

13. The third stage of labor lasts from the time the _____ until the placenta is _____. Detachment of the placenta from the wall of the uterus or _____ is indicated by a firmly contracted _____, change from a _____ shape to a _____ shape, a sudden _____ from the introitus, apparent _____ of the umbilical cord, and the finding of vaginal _____.

MATCHING: Match the description in Column I with the appropriate term from Column II.

COLUMN I

_____ 14. Prolonged breath holding while bearing down (closed-glottis pushing)

_____ 15. Artificial rupture of membranes

_____ 16. Occurrence when widest part of the head (biparietal diameter) distends the vulva just before birth

_____ 17. Incision into perineum to enlarge the vaginal outlet

_____ 18. Test to determine if membranes have ruptured by assessing pH of the fluid

_____ 19. Technique used to control birth of fetal head and protect perineal tissue

_____ 20. Expulsion of placenta with fetal side emerging first

_____ 21. Cord encircling the fetal neck

_____ 22. Occurrence when pressure of presenting part against pelvic floor stretch receptors results in a woman's perception of an urge to bear down

_____ 23. Classification of medication that stimulates the uterus to contract

_____ 24. Expulsion of placenta with maternal surface emerging first

_____ 25. Protrusion of umbilical cord in advance of the presenting part

COLUMN II

A. Ritgen maneuver
B. Episiotomy
C. Oxytocic
D. Ferguson reflex
E. Schultze mechanism
F. Valsalva maneuver
G. Crowning
H. Duncan mechanism
I. Amniotomy
J. Nuchal cord
K. Prolapse of umbilical cord
L. Nitrazine test

FILL IN THE BLANKS: Insert the term that corresponds to each of the following definitions.

Characteristics of the Powers of Labor

26. _____ Primary powers of labor that act involuntarily to expel the fetus and the placenta from the uterus

27. _____ "Building up" phase of a contraction

28. _____ Peak of a contraction

29. _____ "Letting down" phase of a contraction

30. _____ How often contractions occur, or period of time from the beginning of one contraction to the beginning of the next or from the peak of one contraction to the peak of the next

31. _____ Strength of the contraction at its peak

32. _____ Period of time that elapses between the onset and end of a contraction

33. _____ Tension of the uterine muscle during the interval between contractions

34. _____ Period of rest between contractions

35. _____ Involuntary urge to push in response to the Ferguson reflex

36. Assessment of the characteristics and patterns of uterine contractions is an important nursing responsibility.

A. *LABEL* the following illustration that depicts the characteristics of uterine contractions.

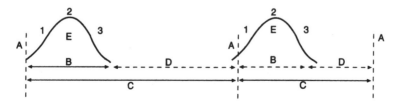

B. *DESCRIBE* how you would assess each of these characteristics using the palpation method.

37. Laura (3-1-1-0-1) has just been admitted in the latent phase of the first stage of labor. As part of the admission procedure, you review her prenatal record, interview her regarding what she has observed regarding her labor, and discuss her current health status.

A. *LIST* the data that you need to obtain from the prenatal record to plan care appropriate for Laura.

B. *IDENTIFY* the information required regarding the status of Laura's labor.

C. *STATE* the information required regarding Laura's current health status.

TRUE OR FALSE: Circle T if true or F if false for each of the following statements. Correct the false statements.

T   F   38. Amniotic fluid turns nitrazine test paper greenish-yellow.

T   F   39. A partogram is used to diagram the progress of uterine contractions.

T   F   40. A laboring woman should be encouraged to void at least every 2 hours during labor.

T   F   41. Ambulation should be encouraged only during the latent phase of the first stage of labor.

T   F   42. A hands-and-knees position is recommended during contractions to facilitate the internal rotation of an occiput posterior position to a more anterior position.

T   F   43. The nurse should perform a vaginal examination immediately, using strict sterile technique, if bright red, fresh vaginal bleeding is noted during active labor.

T   F   44. Maternal body temperature should be monitored at least every 2 hours after the amniotic membranes have ruptured.

T   F   45. Increased sensitivity to touch or hyperesthesia, which develops as labor progresses, results in a woman's rejection of her partner's or the nurse's touch with comfort measures.

T   F   46. A woman should begin pushing as soon as the second stage of labor begins.

T   F   47. For childbirth to progress safely and in a timely fashion, a woman's bearing-down efforts must be carefully regulated by the nurse and coach.

T   F   48. For pushing to be effective, the woman should maintain a push and hold her breath for at least 10 seconds.

T F 49. The only certain objective sign of the onset of the second stage of labor is the woman's perception of an urge to bear down.

T F 50. During the descent phase of the second stage of labor, pressure of the presenting part on the pelvic floor stimulates release of oxytocin from the pituitary gland, thus intensifying uterine contractions.

T F 51. During birth of the head, the woman must continue to bear down fully with uterine contractions to ensure prompt expulsion.

T F 52. If stirrups are used during birth, it is important to place the legs into the stirrups one leg at a time.

T F 53. The time of birth is recorded as the precise time when the newborn takes her or his first breath.

T F 54. The priority goal for a newborn in the immediate postbirth period is that the newborn's airway remains patent.

55. *COMPLETE* the following table by identifying the stressors that a woman and her partner or coach experience during childbirth and the nursing measures that can be supportive and reduce stress.

56. A nurse caring for a laboring woman needs to be alert for signs of potential complications. *LIST* these signs.

57. *COMPLETE* the following table by identifying two advantages for each of the labor positions.

Woman and Partner or Coach	Stressors	Support Measures
Laboring woman		
Partner or coach		

58. *OUTLINE* the critical factors that should be included in the physical assessment of the maternal-fetal unit during labor.

59. *INDICATE* the laboratory and diagnostic tests that are recommended during labor. *STATE* the purpose for each.

60. *COMPLETE* the following table by identifying two support measures that you would use during each phase of the second stage of labor. Validate your response with events and behaviors typical of that phase.

Labor Position	Advantages
Semirecumbent	
Upright	
Lateral	
Hands-and-knees	

61. *IDENTIFY* the factors that can influence the duration of the second stage of labor.

62. *DESCRIBE* the maternal positions recommended to enhance the effectiveness of a woman's bearing-down efforts during the second stage of labor. *STATE* the basis for the effectiveness of each position in facilitating the descent and birth of the fetus.

MULTIPLE CHOICE: Circle the one correct option and state the rationale for the option chosen.

63. A primigravida calls the hospital and tells a nurse on the labor unit that she knows that she is in labor. The nurse's initial response would be:
    A. "Tell me why you know that you're in labor."
    B. "How far do you live from the hospital?"
    C. "How far along are you in your pregnancy?"
    D. "Have your membranes ruptured?"

64. A woman's amniotic membranes apparently have ruptured. The nurse assesses the fluid to determine its characteristics and confirm membrane rupture. An expected assessment finding would be:
    A. pH 5.5.
    B. Absence of ferning.
    C. Pale, straw-colored fluid with white flecks.
    D. Strong odor.

65. A vaginal examination is performed on a multiparous woman who is in labor. The results of the examination have been documented as 4 cm, 75%, 2, LOT. An accurate interpretation of these data is:
    A. Woman is in the latent phase of the first stage of labor.
    B. Station is 2 cm above the ischial spines.
    C. Presentation is vertex.
    D. Lie is transverse.

66. A nulliparous woman is in active labor. She is considered to be at low risk for complications. Which of the following is a standard recommendation for assessment during this phase of labor?
    A. Maternal blood pressure, pulse, and respirations every hour
    B. Fetal heart rate (FHR) every 15 to 30 minutes
    C. Temperature twice per shift once membranes rupture
    D. Vaginal examination to determine progress of dilation and effacement every hour

67. A physical care measure for a laboring woman that has been identified as unlikely to be beneficial and that might even be harmful is:
    A. Allowing the laboring woman to drink fluids and eat light solids as tolerated.
    B. Administering a Fleet enema at admission.
    C. Having the woman ambulate periodically throughout labor as tolerated.
    D. Using a whirlpool bath once active labor has been established.

1. Alice, a primigravida, calls the labor unit. She tells the nurse that she thinks that she is in labor. "I have had some pains for about 2 hours. Should my husband bring me to the hospital now?"

    A. *DESCRIBE* how the nurse should approach this situation.

    B. *WRITE* several questions that the nurse could use to elicit the appropriate information required to determine the course of action required.

    C. Based on the data collected during the telephone interview, the nurse determines that Alice is in very early labor. Because she lives fairly close to the hospital, she is instructed to stay home until her labor progresses. *OUTLINE* the instructions and recommendations for care that Alice and her husband should be given.

2. *ANALYZE* the assessment findings documented for each of the following women.

Denise	Teresa	Danielle
5 cm	9 cm	2 cm
moderate	very strong	mild
q4min	q2-3min	q6-8min
40-55 sec	65-75 sec	30-35 sec
0	+2	−1

    A. *IDENTIFY* the phase of labor being experienced by each woman.

B. *DESCRIBE* the behavior and appearance you would expect to be exhibited by each woman.

C. *SPECIFY* the physical care and emotional support measures you would implement if you were caring for each of these women.

3. *DESCRIBE* the procedure for locating the point of maximal impulse that should be followed before auscultating the FHR or applying an ultrasound transducer to the abdomen of a laboring woman. *EXPLAIN* the rationale for using this procedure.

4. Tasha is 6 cm dilated. Her coach comes to tell you that her "water just broke with a gush!" *IDENTIFY* each action you would take in this situation, in order of priority. *STATE* the rationale for the actions that you have identified.

5. Sara, a 17-year-old primigravida, is admitted in the latent phase of labor. Her boyfriend, Dan, is with her as her only support. They appear committed to each other. During the admission interview, Sara tells you that they did not go to any classes because she was embarrassed about not being married. Both Sara and Dan appear very nervous, and assessment indicates that they know little about what is happening, what to expect, and how to work together during the process of labor. *IDENTIFY* the nursing diagnosis reflected in these data. *STATE* one expected outcome, and *LIST* nursing measures appropriate for the diagnosis you identified.

Nursing Diagnosis   **Expected Outcome**   **Nursing Measures**

6. Cori (4-3-0-0-3) is in latent labor. She and her husband are being oriented to the birthing room. Their last birth occurred in a delivery room 10 years ago. Both she and her husband are amazed by the birthing room and the birthing bed, which allows her to give birth in an upright position. They are also informed that changes in bearing-down efforts now allow a woman to follow her own body feelings and even to vocalize with pushing. Both Cori and her husband state that with every other birth they put her legs in stirrups, she held her breath for as long as she could, and she pushed quietly. "Everything turned out okay, so why should we change?" *DESCRIBE* the response that the primary nurse caring for this couple should make about their concerns.

7. Beth is in the descent phase of the second stage of labor. She is actively pushing and bearing down to facilitate birth. *INDICATE* the criteria that a nurse would use to evaluate the correctness of Beth's technique.

8. Molly is entering the second stage of labor. She states that she is experiencing some perineal pressure but refuses to start pushing because, as she states, "I'm just not ready to push yet."

   A. *DISCUSS* the factors that might be inhibiting Molly's desire to bear down and give birth to her baby.

   B. *DESCRIBE* what the nurse could do to help Molly reach the point of readiness to give birth.

9. *IMAGINE* that you are participating in a panel discussion on childbirth practices. Your topic is "Episiotomies—are they needed to ensure the safety and well-being of the laboring woman and her fetus?" *OUTLINE* the information that you would include in your presentation.

10. *IMAGINE* that you are a staff nurse on a childbirth unit. Your hospital is instituting a change in policy that would allow the participation of children in their mother's labor and birth process. You are asked to be part of the committee that will formulate the guidelines regarding sibling participation during childbirth. *DISCUSS* the suggestions that you would make to help ensure a positive outcome for parents, children, and health care providers.

11. Annie is a primipara in the fourth stage of labor following a long and difficult labor and birth process. She seems disinterested in her baby. Annie looks him over quickly and then asks if you would take him back to the nursery.

A. *IDENTIFY* the factors that might be accounting for Annie's behavior.

B. *DISCUSS* the nursing measures that you would use to encourage future maternal-newborn interactions and facilitate the attachment process.

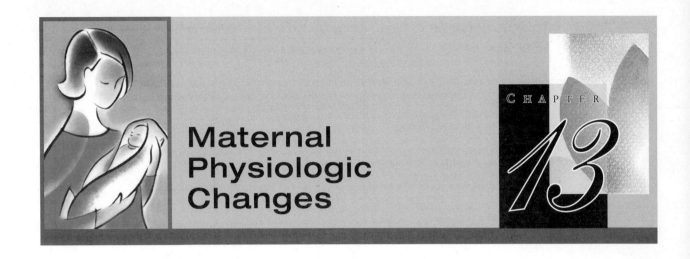

Maternal Physiologic Changes

CHAPTER 13

CHAPTER REVIEW ACTIVITIES

TRUE OR FALSE: Circle T if true or F if false for each of the following statements. Correct the false statements.

T F 1. Within 12 hours of birth the fundus of the uterus may be approximately 1 cm above the umbilicus.

T F 2. The uterus is slightly smaller after every pregnancy.

T F 3. Regeneration of the endometrium at the placental site is complete in approximately 4 weeks after birth.

T F 4. The external os of the cervix has a jagged, slitlike appearance once healing has taken place after vaginal birth.

T F 5. Until estrogen levels rise, the postpartum woman is likely to experience discomfort during intercourse (dyspareunia) associated with inadequate secretion of lubricating mucus.

T F 6. The appearance of colostrum is bluish white and thin.

T F 7. For most nonlactating women, menstruation resumes by 4 to 6 weeks after birth.

T F 8. During the first 24 hours after birth an elevated temperature of 38° C most likely indicates the onset of infection.

T F 9. By 8 weeks after childbirth the majority of women have a normal hematocrit.

T F 10. In the postpartum period a leukocytosis of 20,000/mm^3 strongly indicates uterine or bladder infection.

T F 11. During involution the process of autolysis often produces a pregnancy-associated proteinuria which resolves by 6 weeks postpartum.

T F 12. An elevated level of follicle-stimulating hormone in the postpartum period is responsible for the suppression of ovulation in lactating women.

T F 13. Lochia normally has a fleshy odor similar to that of menstrual flow.

T F 14. Women with type 1 diabetes mellitus usually require more insulin for several weeks after they give birth.

15. When caring for a woman following vaginal birth, it is critically important for the nurse to assess the woman's bladder for distention.

   A. *STATE* why bladder distention is more likely to occur during the immediate postpartum period.

B. *DISCUSS* the problems that can occur if the bladder is allowed to become distended.

16. *IDENTIFY* the factors that can interfere with bowel elimination in the postpartum period.

17. *EXPLAIN* why hypovolemic shock is less likely to occur in the postpartum woman experiencing a normal or average blood loss.

18. *INDICATE* the factors that place a postpartum woman at increased risk for the development of thromboembolism.

19. *COMPARE AND CONTRAST* the characteristics of lochial bleeding with nonlochial bleeding.

MULTIPLE CHOICE: Circle the one correct option and state the rationale for the option chosen.

20. A nurse has assessed a woman who gave birth vaginally 12 hours ago. Which of the following findings would require further assessment?
    A. Bright-to–dark red uterine discharge—three quarters of pad saturated in 2 to 3 hours
    B. Midline episiotomy—approximated, moderate edema, slight erythema, absence of ecchymosis
    C. Protrusion of abdomen with slight separation of abdominal wall muscles
    D. Fundus firm at level of umbilicus and to the right of midline

21. A woman at 24 hours after birth complains to the nurse that her sleep was interrupted the night before because of sweating and the need to have her gown and bed linen changed. The nurse's first action would be to:
    A. Assess this woman for additional clinical manifestations of infection.
    B. Explain to the woman that the sweating represents her body's attempt to eliminate the fluid that was accumulated during pregnancy.
    C. Notify her physician of the finding.
    D. Document the finding as postpartum diaphoresis.

22. Which of the following women at 24 hours following birth is least likely to experience afterpains?
    A. Primipara who is breastfeeding her twins who were born at 38 weeks of gestation
    B. Multipara who is breastfeeding her 10-pound full-term baby girl
    C. Multipara who is bottle-feeding her 8-pound baby boy
    D. Primipara who is bottle-feeding her 7-pound baby girl

CRITICAL THINKING EXERCISES

1. *DESCRIBE* how you would respond to each of the following typical questions or concerns of postpartum women.

    A. Mary is a primipara who is breastfeeding. "Why am I experiencing so many painful cramps? I thought this happens only to women who have had babies before."

    B. Susan is being discharged after giving birth 20 hours ago. "For how many days should I be able to palpate my uterus to make sure that it's firm?"

    C. June is a primipara. "My friend who had a baby last year said that she had a flow for 6 weeks. Isn't that a long time to bleed after having a baby?"

D. Jean is at 24 hours postpartum. "I cannot believe it—I look as if I'm still pregnant!! How can this be?"

E. Marion is 1 day postpartum. "I perspired so much last night, and I have so much urine when I go to the bathroom. I hope everything is okay and I can still go home!"

F. Joan is a primipara who is breastfeeding her baby. "My friend told me that I can't get pregnant as long as I continue to breastfeed. This is great because I do not like to use birth control."

G. Alice, a multiparous woman, is concerned. She states, "My doctor is not going to give me a drug to dry up my breasts like I had with my first baby. How will my breasts ever get back to normal now?"

H. Andrea, a primipara, is 1 day postpartum. While breastfeeding her baby she confides to the nurse that she does not know how long she will continue to breastfeed. "My husband and I have always had a satisfying sex life, but my friend told me that as long as I breastfeed, intercourse is painful."

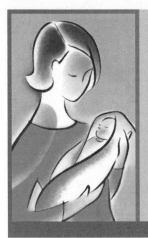

Nursing Care of the Family during the Fourth Trimester

CHAPTER REVIEW ACTIVITIES

FILL IN THE BLANKS: Insert the term that corresponds to each of the following.

Postpartum Period

1. The first 1 to 2 hours after birth are called the _____.

2. The nursing care management approach of _____ has one nurse caring for both the mother and her infant. It is also called _____ care or _____ care.

3. _____ is a classification of medications that stimulates contraction of the uterine smooth muscle.

4. _____ is the failure of the uterine muscle to contract firmly. It is the most frequent cause of _____ following childbirth.

5. A(n) _____ is a perineal treatment that involves sitting in warm water for approximately 20 minutes to soothe and cleanse the site and increase blood flow, thereby enhancing healing.

6. Painful cramps experienced by many women when the uterus contracts after childbirth are called _____.

7. _____ is the dilation of the blood vessels supplying the intestines as a result of the rapid decrease in intraabdominal pressure after birth. It causes blood to pool in the viscera and thereby contributes to the development of _____ when the woman who has recently given birth stands up.

8. A complaint of pain in calf muscles when dorsiflexion of the foot is forced is called _____. The presence of pain can be associated with the presence of a thrombophlebitis.

9. _____ exercises can assist women to regain pelvic muscle tone that is often lost when pelvic tissues are stretched and torn during pregnancy and birth.

10. _____ is the swelling of breast tissue caused by increased blood and lymph supply to the breasts preceding lactation.

11. _____ vaccine can be given to postpartum women whose antibody titer is lower than 1:8 or whose enzyme immunoassay value is lower than 0.8. It is used to prevent nonimmune women from contracting this TORCH infection during a subsequent pregnancy.

12. _____, also referred to as RhoGAM, is a medication given within 72 hours of birth to Rh-negative, antibody (Coombs')–negative women who have given birth to Rh-positive newborns to prevent the formation of maternal sensitization. The _____ test may be performed if a large fetomaternal transfusion is suspected to determine the amount of fetal blood present in the maternal circulation more accurately so the correct dosage of RhoGAM can be given.

13. *EXPLAIN* to a woman who has just given birth why breastfeeding her newborn during the fourth stage of labor is beneficial to her and her baby.

14. A postpartum woman at 6 hours after vaginal birth is having difficulty voiding. *LIST* the measures that you would try to help this woman void spontaneously.

15. *IDENTIFY* the measures that you would teach a postpartum woman in an effort to prevent the development of thrombophlebitis.

16. *IDENTIFY* the measures that you would teach a bottle-feeding mother to suppress lactation naturally and relieve discomfort during breast engorgement.

17. *STATE* the two most important interventions that can be used to prevent excessive postpartum bleeding in the early postpartum period. *INDICATE* the rationale for the effectiveness of each intervention that you identified.

122 Chapter **14** **Nursing Care of the Family during the Fourth Trimester**   Copyright © 2012, 2010, 2006 by Mosby, Inc., an affiliate of Elsevier Inc. All rights reserved.

TRUE OR FALSE: Circle T if true or F if false for each of the following statements. Correct the false statements.

T   F   18. The effectiveness of the rubella vaccine might be reduced if a postpartum woman receives both Rh immunoglobulin and a rubella vaccine.

T   F   19. Before sitting down in a sitz bath, the woman should relax her gluteal muscles to reduce discomfort when entering the bath and then tighten them after she is sitting in the bath.

T   F   20. Tucks are used to soothe sore hemorrhoids.

T   F   21. Medications such as estrogen and bromocriptine (Parlodel) are often used to suppress lactation for the bottle-feeding woman.

T   F   22. The most common cause of excessive bleeding after birth is unrepaired vaginal or cervical lacerations.

T   F   23. Ice packs are most effective in minimizing perineal edema during the first 36 hours following birth.

T   F   24. An appropriate time to administer pain medication to a breastfeeding woman would be immediately after a feeding session.

T   F   25. Rubella vaccine should not be given to a woman who is breastfeeding her infant.

T   F   26. A woman should be expected to void at least 250 ml of urine spontaneously within 2 hours following vaginal birth.

T   F   27. Chinese women often avoid the use of hormonal methods as a primary method of contraception.

T   F   28. A depressed postpartum woman who is experiencing suicidal ideation should call the warm line that she learned about at discharge.

29. Imagine that you are the nurse who cared for a woman during her labor, birth, and recovery during the fourth stage of labor. *OUTLINE* the information that you would report to the mother-baby nurse when you transfer the new mother and her baby to their room on the postpartum unit.

30. Infection control measures should guide the practice of nurses working on a postpartum unit.

A. *DISCUSS* the measures designed to prevent transmission of infection from person to person.

B. *DISCUSS* measures that a postpartum woman should be taught to reduce her risk of infection.

31. When assessing postpartum women, nurses should be alert for clinical manifestations of developing complications. *IDENTIFY* the signs of potential postpartum complications of which the nurse should be aware.

CRITICAL THINKING EXERCISES

1. Tara is a breastfeeding woman at 12 hours after birth. She requests medication for pain. *DESCRIBE* the approach that you would take when fulfilling Tara's request.

2. When caring for a woman 4 hours after birth, the nurse notes an excessive lochial flow and early signs of hypovolemic shock.

    A. *STATE* the criteria that the nurse should use to determine that the flow is lochial and excessive and that the early signs of hypovolemic shock are being exhibited.

    B. *IDENTIFY* the nurse's priority action in response to these assessment findings.

    C. *IDENTIFY* additional interventions that a nurse might need to implement to ensure this woman's safety and prevent the development of further complications.

3. Carrie is a postpartum woman awaiting discharge. Because her rubella titer indicates that she is not immune, a rubella vaccination has been ordered before discharge. *STATE* what you would tell Carrie with regard to this vaccination.

4. The physician has written the following order for a postpartum woman: "Administer Rh immunoglobulin (RhoGAM) if indicated." *DESCRIBE* the actions that the nurse should take in fulfilling this order.

5. Susan, a postpartum woman, confides to the nurse, "My partner and I have always had a very satisfying sex life, even when I was pregnant. My sister told me that this will definitely change now that I have had a baby." *DESCRIBE* what the nurse should tell Susan regarding sexual changes and sexual activity after birth.

6. *IDENTIFY* the priority nursing diagnosis and one expected outcome of care and appropriate nursing management for each of the following situations.

   A. Tina is 2 days postpartum. During a home visit the nurse notes that Tina's episiotomy is edematous and slightly reddened, with approximated wound edges and no drainage. A distinct odor is noted, and there is a buildup of secretions and the Hurricaine gel Tina uses for discomfort. During the interview, Tina reveals that she is afraid to wash the area. "I rinse with a little water in my peri bottle in the morning and again at night. I also apply plenty of my gel."

   Nursing Diagnosis   **Expected Outcome**   **Nursing Management**

B. Erin, who gave birth 3 days ago, has not had a bowel movement since 1 or 2 days before labor. She tells the visiting nurse during the interview that she has been avoiding fiber foods for fear that the baby will get diarrhea. Her activity level is low. "My family is taking good care of me. I do not have to lift a finger! Besides, I would prefer to wait until my episiotomy is less sore before trying to have a bowel movement."

Nursing Diagnosis   **Expected Outcome**   **Nursing Management**

C. Mary gave birth 24 hours ago. She complains of perineal discomfort. "My hemorrhoids and stitches are killing me, but I don't want to take any medication because it will get into my breast milk and hurt my baby."

Nursing Diagnosis   **Expected Outcome**   **Nursing Management**

7. Dawn gave birth 8 hours ago. On palpation her fundus was found to be two fingerbreadths above the umbilicus and deviated to the right of midline. It was also assessed to be less firm than previously noted.

A. *STATE* the most likely basis for these findings.

B. *DESCRIBE* the action that the nurse should take on the basis of these assessment findings.

8. Jill gave birth 3 hours ago. During labor epidural anesthesia was used for pain relief. Jill's primary health care provider has written the following order: "Out of bed and ambulating when able." *DISCUSS* the approach that the nurse should take in fulfilling this order safely.

9. Andrea gave birth 1½ hours ago. She tells the nurse that she is ravenous. You check the chart, noting that Andrea's primary health care provider has ordered: "Diet as tolerated." *STATE* the criteria that should be met before fulfilling this order.

10. Dawn, a primiparous woman at 20 hours postpartum, is preparing for discharge within the next 4 hours. She is breastfeeding her new daughter.

   A. *DESCRIBE* the nurse's legal responsibility in terms of early discharge.

   B. *LIST* the criteria that Dawn and her newborn must meet before discharge from the hospital to home.

   Maternal criteria

   Newborn criteria

   General criteria

C. *OUTLINE* the essential content that must be taught before discharge. A home visit by a nurse is planned for Dawn's third postpartum day.

11. Certain cultural beliefs and practices must be considered when planning and implementing care in the postpartum period.

   A. *DISCUSS* the importance of using a culturally sensitive approach when providing care to postpartum women and their families.

   B. Kim, a Korean-American woman, has just given birth. Assessment reveals that she and her family are guided by beliefs and practices based on a balance of heat and cold. *DESCRIBE* how the nurse would adjust typical postpartum care to respect and accommodate Kim's cultural beliefs and practices.

   C. A Muslim woman has been admitted to the postpartum unit following the birth of her second son. *DESCRIBE* the approach that you would use in managing this woman's care in a culturally sensitive manner.

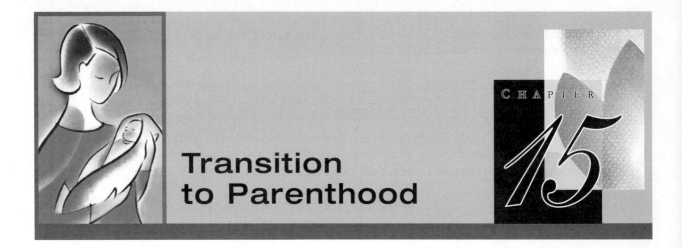

Transition to Parenthood

CHAPTER 15

CHAPTER REVIEW ACTIVITIES

1. *COMPLETE* the following table by identifying the focus, characteristics (typical behaviors and concerns), and care requirements for postpartum women in each of the following phases of maternal adjustment.

Phase	Focus	Characteristics	Requirements
Dependent (taking-in)			
Dependent-independent (taking-hold)			
Interdependent (letting-go)			
Postpartum blues			

2. Attachment of the newborn to parents and family is critical for optimum growth and development.

   A. *DEFINE* the process of attachment and bonding.

   B. *LIST* conditions that must be present for the parent-newborn attachment process to begin favorably.

   C. *DESCRIBE* the acquaintance process.

   D. *DISCUSS* how you would assess the progress of attachment between parents and their newborns.

3. *IDENTIFY* parental tasks that need to be accomplished during the process of parental adjustment to a new baby.

4. *DISCUSS* how each of the following forms of parent-infant contact can facilitate attachment and promote the family as a focus of care.

   Early contact

   Extended contact

FILL IN THE BLANKS: Insert the term that corresponds to each of the following.

Newborn-Parent Interaction

5. _____ refers to the process whereby the infant's behaviors and characteristics call forth a corresponding set of maternal behaviors and characteristics.

6. _____ is a process used by parents to get to know their infant during the immediate postpartum period. _____, _____, _____, and _____ are important actions in this process.

7. The _____ process is the identification of the new baby. The child is first identified in terms of _____ to other family members, then in terms of _____, and finally in terms of _____.

8. _____ is exhibited when newborns move in time with the structure of adult speech by _____, _____, and _____, seemingly _____ to a parent's voice.

9. One of the newborn's tasks is to establish a personal rhythm or _____. Parents can help in this process by giving consistent _____ and using their infant's _____ state to develop _____ behavior and thereby increase _____ and opportunities for _____.

10. _____ is a type of body movement or behavior that provides the observer with cues. The observer or receiver interprets these cues and responds to them. _____ refers to the "fit" between the infant's cues and the parent's response.

11. _____ refers to the face-to-face position in which the parent's and infant's faces are approximately 20 cm apart and on the same plane.

12. _____ is a term that applies to a parent's absorption, preoccupation, and interest in his or her infant; the term typically is used to describe the father's intense involvement with his newborn.

13. *COMPLETE* the following table by identifying three infant and three parent facilitating behaviors and three infant and three parent inhibiting behaviors that can affect the process of attachment.

Infant/Parent	Facilitating Behaviors	Inhibiting Behaviors
Infant		
Parent		

14. *DESCRIBE* how each of the following factors influences the manner in which parents respond to the birth of their child. *STATE* two nursing implications/actions related to each factor.

Adolescent parents

Parental age older than 35

Social support

Culture

Socioeconomic conditions

Personal aspirations

Visual impairment

Hearing impairment

MULTIPLE CHOICE: Circle the one correct option and state the rationale for the option chosen.

15. During the final phase of the claiming process of a newborn, the mother might say:
    A. "She has her grandfather's nose."
    B. "His ears lay nice and flat against his head, not like mine and his sister's that stick out."
    C. "She gave me nothing but trouble during pregnancy, and now she's so stubborn that she won't wake up to breastfeed."
    D. "He has such a sweet disposition and pleasant expression. I have never seen a baby quite like him before."

16. Which of the following nursing actions is least effective in facilitating parental attachment to their new infant?
    A. Referring the couple to a lactation consultant to ensure continuing success with breastfeeding
    B. Keeping the baby in the nursery as much as possible for the first 24 hours after birth so the mother can rest
    C. Extending visiting hours for the woman's partner or significant other as desired
    D. Providing guidance and support as the parents care for their baby's nutrition and hygiene needs

17. A behavior that illustrates engrossment is:
    A. Father is sitting in a rocking chair holding his new baby boy, touching his toes, and making eye contact.
    B. Mother tells her friends that her baby's eyes and nose are just like hers.
    C. Mother picks up and cuddles her baby girl when she begins to cry.
    D. Grandmother gazes into her new grandson's face, which she holds about 8 inches away from her own, and she and the baby make eye-to-eye contact.

18. A woman expresses a need to review her labor and birth experience with the nurse who cared for her while she was in labor. This behavior is most characteristic of which of the following phases of maternal postpartum adjustment?
    A. Taking-hold (dependent-independent phase).
    B. Taking-in (dependent phase).
    C. Letting-go (interdependent).
    D. Postpartum blues (baby blues).

19. Before discharge a postpartum woman and her partner ask the nurse about the baby blues. "Our friend said that she felt so let down after she had her baby, and we have heard that some women actually become very depressed. Is there anything we can do to prevent this from happening to us or at least to cope with the blues if they occur?" The nurse could tell this couple:
    A. "Postpartum blues usually happen in pregnancies that are high risk or unplanned, so there's no need for you to worry."
    B. "Try to become skillful in breastfeeding and caring for your baby as quickly as you can."
    C. "Get as much rest as you can and sleep when the baby sleeps because fatigue can precipitate the blues or make them worse."
    D. "I'll call your doctor before you leave to get a prescription for an antidepressant to prevent the blues from happening."

CRITICAL THINKING EXERCISES

1. Jane and Andrew are parents of a newborn girl. *DESCRIBE* what you would teach them regarding the communication process as it relates to their newborn.

    A. Techniques that they can use to communicate with their newborn effectively

    B. The manner in which the baby is able to communicate with them

2. Allison had a difficult labor, which resulted in an emergency cesarean birth under general anesthesia. She did not see her baby until 12 hours after her birth. Allison tells the nurse who brings the baby to her room, "I am so disappointed. I had planned to breastfeed my baby and hold her close, skin to skin, right after her birth just like all the books say. I know that this is so important for our relationship." *DESCRIBE* how the nurse should respond to Allison's concern.

3. Angela is the mother of a 1-day-old boy and a 3-year-old girl. As you prepare Angela for discharge, she states, "My little girl just saw her brother. She says that she loves him and cannot wait for him to come home. I'm so glad that I don't have to worry about any of that sibling rivalry business!" *INDICATE* how you would respond to Angela's comments.

4. Sara and Ben have just experienced the birth of their first baby. They are very happy with their baby boy but appear very unsure of themselves and are obviously anxious about how to tell what their baby needs. Sara is trying very hard to breastfeed and is having some success but not as much as she had hoped. Both parents express self-doubt about their ability to succeed at the "most important role in our lives."

   A. *STATE* the nursing diagnosis that is most appropriate for this couple.

   B. DESCRIBE what the nurse caring for this family can do to facilitate the attachment process.

5. Mary and Jim are the parents of three sons. They had very much wanted to have a girl this time, but after a long and difficult birth they had another son who weighed 10 pounds. His appearance reflects the difficult birth process: occipital molding, caput succedaneum, and forceps marks on each cheek. Mary and Jim express their disappointment, not only in the appearance of their son but also in the fact that they had another boy. "This was supposed to be our last child. Now we just don't know what we'll do." *DISCUSS* how you would facilitate Mary and Jim's attachment to their son and reconcile their fantasy ("dream") child with the reality of their actual child.

6. Dawn and Matthew have just given birth to their first baby. This is the first grandchild for both sets of grandparents. The grandmothers approach the nurse to ask how they can help the new family, stating, "We want to help Dawn and Matthew but at the same time not interfere with what they want to do." *DISCUSS* the role of the nurse in helping these grandparents recognize their importance to the new family and develop a mutually satisfying relationship with Dawn, Matthew, and the new baby.

7. Jane is 2 days postpartum. When the nurse makes a home visit, Jane is found crying. She states, "I have such a letdown feeling. I can't understand why I feel this way when I should be so happy about the healthy outcome for myself and my baby." Jane's husband confirms her behavior and expresses confusion as well, stating, "I wish I knew what to do to help her." *IDENTIFY* the priority nursing diagnosis and one expected outcome of care for this situation. *DESCRIBE* the recommended nursing management for the nursing diagnosis that you have identified.

Nursing Diagnosis   **Expected Outcome**   **Nursing Management**

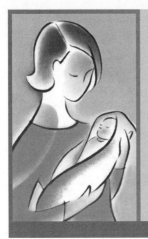

Physiologic and Behavioral Adaptations of the Newborn

CHAPTER 16

CHAPTER REVIEW ACTIVITIES

Neonatal nurses are responsible for the assessment of the physiologic integrity of newborns. As part of this responsibility the nurse must be aware of the significance of data collected. *LABEL* each of the following assessment findings, if present in a group of three full-term newborns who were born 12 hours ago, as N (reflective of normal adaptation or acceptable variation to extrauterine life) or P (reflective of potential problems with adaptation to extrauterine life). (Use Chapters 16 and 17 to assist you in completing this activity.)

Assessment Finding	Evaluation
1. Crackles on auscultation of the lungs	_____
2. Respirations: 36, irregular, shallow	_____
3. Episodic apnea lasting 5 to 10 seconds	_____
4. Nasal flaring and sternal retractions	_____
5. Slight bluish discoloration of feet and hands	_____
6. Blood pressure: 76/43 mm Hg	_____
7. Apical rate: 126, with murmurs	_____
8. Temperature 37.1° C axillary	_____
9. Head, 34 cm; chest, 36 cm	_____
10. Boggy edematous swelling over occiput	_____
11. Overlapping of parietal bones	_____
12. White, pimplelike spots on nose and chin	_____
13. Yellowish coloration on face and chest	_____
14. Regurgitation of small amount of milk after feedings	_____
15. Liver palpated 3 cm below right costal margin	_____
16. Absence of bowel elimination since birth	_____
17. Spine straight with dimple at base	_____
18. Tight prepuce, unable to fully retract	_____
19. Edema of scrotum and labia	_____
20. Toes hyperextended and flared when sole is stroked upward	_____
21. Hematocrit, 36%; hemoglobin, 12 g/dl	_____
22. White blood cell count: 23,000/mm^3	_____
23. Blood glucose: 40 mg/dl	_____

24. The most critical adjustment a newborn must make at birth is establishing respirations.

A. *LIST* the factors responsible for the initiation of breathing after birth.

B. *LIST* the four conditions essential for maintaining an adequate oxygen supply in the newborn.

C. *DESCRIBE* the expected respiratory pattern in a newborn.

D. *STATE* four signs indicating respiratory distress in the newborn.

25. *COMPLETE* the following table by identifying the purpose and location of each of the following fetal circulatory shunts and describing the mechanisms responsible for their closure.

Shunt	Purpose/Location	Closure Mechanism
Foramen ovale		
Ductus arteriosus		
Ductus venosus		

26. Cold stress presents a danger if experienced by the newborn during the postbirth period.

A. *LIST* the dangers that the newborn faces if he or she experiences cold stress.

B. *IDENTIFY* the characteristic newborn behaviors associated with cold stress.

C. *IDENTIFY* several measures that the nurse can use to stabilize a newborn's temperature.

27. *COMPLETE* the following table by defining each of the heat loss mechanisms and identifying one nursing measure that can be used to prevent heat loss as a result of each mechanism.

Heat Loss Mechanism	Definition of Heat Loss Mechanism	Nursing Measure to Prevent Heat Loss
Convection		
Radiation		
Evaporation		
Conduction		

28. *IDENTIFY* the specific criteria or assessment findings that characterize physiologic jaundice.

FILL IN THE BLANKS: Insert the term that corresponds to each of the following.

Behavioral Adaptations of the Newborn

29. Variations in the state of consciousness of newborn infants are called the _____ states. The sleep states are _____ sleep and _____ sleep. The wake states are _____, _____, _____, and _____. The optimum state of arousal is the _____ state in which infants _____, _____, _____, _____, and _____.

30. _____ is the ability of the infant to respond to and then inhibit responding to discrete stimuli (e.g., light, rattle, bell, pinprick) while asleep. It is a protective mechanism that allows the infant to be accustomed to _____. It is a psychologic/physiologic phenomenon whereby the response to a(n) _____ or _____ stimulus is _____.

31. _____, the individual variations in the primary reaction patterns of newborns, guides an infant's style of behavior to stimuli.

32. _____ refers to the ability of newborns to comfort themselves or be comforted by others. In the crying state most newborns initiate one of several ways to reduce their distress, including using _____ movements and alerting to _____, _____, or _____ stimuli.

33. _____ refers to the ability of newborns to mold into the contours of the persons holding them.

34. During the first 6 to 8 hours after birth, newborns experience a transition period characterized by three phases of instability. *COMPLETE* the following table by identifying the timing or duration and typical behaviors for each phase of this transitional period.

Phase	Time/Duration	Typical Behaviors
First period of reactivity		
Period of diminished response		
Second period of reactivity		

TRUE OR FALSE: Circle T if true or F if false for each of the following statements. Correct the false statements.

T　F　35. During the first 1 to 2 days of life, the newborn should void two to six times.

T　F　36. Crackles, grunting, nasal flaring, and chest retractions are often noted during the second period of reactivity.

T　F　37. Vitamin B_{12} is often given by injection to newborns immediately after birth to enhance clotting and prevent hemorrhage.

T　F　38. Blood-tinged mucus on the diaper of the female newborn should be documented by the nurse as pseudomenstruation and recognized as an expected assessment finding related to the withdrawal of maternal hormones.

T　F　39. Physiologic jaundice in the full-term newborn disappears by 7 to 10 days of life.

T　F　40. A decrease of 20 mm Hg in the systolic blood pressure is an expected finding during the first hour after birth.

T　F　41. Meconium stool often has a strong odor as a result of bacteria present in the fetal intestine during intrauterine life.

T　F　42. Breast tissue in full-term male and female newborns can be swollen and secrete a thin milky-type discharge.

T　F　43. A newborn can be expected to lose up to 15% of his or her birth weight in the first 3 to 5 days after birth.

T　F　44. A newborn achieves active immunity from the mother by transplacental transfer of antibodies.

MATCHING: Match the description in Column I with the appropriate newborn reflex from Column II.

COLUMN I

_____ 45. Applying pressure to feet with fingers when infant's lower limbs are semiflexed and legs are extended

_____ 46. Placing infant on flat surface and striking surface—infant shows symmetric abduction and extension of arms, fingers fan out, thumb and forefinger form a "C," slight tremor can occur

_____ 47. Placing finger in palm of hand or at base of toes—infant's fingers curl around examiner's finger, and toes curl

_____ 48. Placing infant prone on flat surface and running finger down side of back 4 to 5 cm lateral to spine—infant's body flexes and pelvis swings toward stimulated side

_____ 49. Tapping over forehead, bridge of nose, or maxilla when eyes are open—infant blinks for first four to five taps

_____ 50. Using finger to stroke sole of foot beginning at heel, moving upward along lateral aspect of sole, then crossing ball of foot—all of infant's toes hyperextend, with dorsiflexion of big toe

_____ 51. Clapping hands sharply—infant's arms abduct, with flexion of elbows, and hands remain clenched

_____ 52. Testes retract when infant is chilled

_____ 53. Touching infant's lip, cheek, or corner of mouth with nipple—infant turns head toward stimulus, opens mouth, takes hold, and sucks

_____ 54. Placing infant in a supine position and turning head quickly to one side as infant is falling asleep or is asleep—infant's arm and leg extend on side to which head is turned while opposite arm and leg flex

_____ 55. Holding infant vertically and allowing one foot to touch surface—infant alternates flexion and extension of feet on table

_____ 56. Touching or depressing tip of tongue—infant's tongue is forced outward

COLUMN II

A. Rooting

B. Grasp

C. Extrusion

D. Glabellar

E. Tonic neck

F. Moro

G. Stepping (walking)

H. Startle downward

I. Babinski

J. Trunk incurvation

K. Magnet

L. Cremasteric

57. *DESCRIBE* how each of the following factors can influence a newborn's behavior.

Gestational age

Time

Stimuli

Medication

MULTIPLE CHOICE: Circle the one correct option and state the rationale for the option chosen.

58. A newborn at 5 hours old wakes from a sound sleep and becomes very active. He exhibits the following signs when assessed. Which one would require further assessment?

A. Increased mucus production

B. Passage of meconium

C. Heart rate of 160 beats/min

D. Two apneic episodes of 16 and 20 seconds in duration

59. When assessing a newborn boy at 12 hours of age, the nurse notes a rash on his abdomen and thighs. The rash appears as irregular reddish blotches with pale centers. The nurse would:

A. Document the finding as erythema toxicum.

B. Isolate the newborn and his mother until infection is ruled out.

C. Apply an antiseptic ointment to each lesion.

D. Request nonallergenic linen from the laundry.

60. As part of a thorough assessment of a newborn, the nurse practitioner should check for hip dislocation and dysplasia. The technique the nurse would most likely use would be:

A. Measurement of each leg from hip to heel.

B. Stepping or walking reflex.

C. Magnet reflex.

D. Ortolani maneuver.

61. When assessing a newborn after birth, the nurse notes flat, irregular pinkish marks on the bridge of the nose, the nape of the neck, and over the eyelids. The areas blanch when pressed with a finger. The nurse would document this finding as:

A. Milia.

B. Nevus vasculosus.

C. Telangiectatic nevi.

D. Nevus flammeus.

CRITICAL THINKING EXERCISES

1. Significant variations occur in physiologic functioning of the newborn and adult. *COMPLETE* the following table by identifying these variations and the implications for newborn care.

Physiologic Function	Variations	Implications for Care
Respiratory patterns		
Cardiovascular patterns		
Thermoregulation		
Hematopoietic characteristics		
Renal function		

2. After a long and difficult labor, baby boy James was born with a caput succedaneum, a single small cephalohematoma on the left parietal bone, and significant molding over the occipital area. Low forceps were used for the birth, resulting in ecchymotic areas on both cheeks. *DESCRIBE* what you would tell James' parents about these assessment findings.

3. Tonya and Sam, an African-American couple, express concern that their new baby girl has several bruises on her back and buttocks. They ask if their baby was injured during birth or in the nursery. *DESCRIBE* the nurse's appropriate response to Tonya and Sam's concern.

4. Susan and Allen are first-time parents of a baby girl. They ask the nurse about their baby's ability to see and hear things around her and interact with them.

   A. *SPECIFY* what the nurse should tell these parents about the sensory capabilities of their healthy full-term newborn.

   B. *NAME* four stimuli that Susan and Allen could provide for their baby to help foster her development.

5. Mary and Jim are concerned that their baby boy, who weighed 8 lb 6 oz at birth, now at 2 days of age weighs only 7 lb 14 oz. *DESCRIBE* how you would respond to their concern.

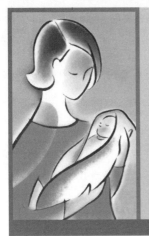

Assessment and Care of the Newborn and Family

CHAPTER 17

CHAPTER REVIEW ACTIVITIES

TRUE OR FALSE: Circle T if true or F if false for each of the following statements. Correct the false statements.

T F 1. Cardiopulmonary resuscitation for infants recommends performing ten cycles of five compressions and one ventilation (a 5:1 ratio) and then checking the brachial artery for a pulse.

T F 2. A delay of up to 2 hours for instilling a prophylactic antibiotic ointment into a newborn's eyes is acceptable to facilitate parent-infant attachment and bonding.

T F 3. If an infant's airway is obstructed by a foreign body, the infant should receive three chest thrusts followed by two back blows.

T F 4. Placing a dressed newborn under a radiant heat panel facilitates a more rapid stabilization of body temperature after birth.

T F 5. The thermistor probe of a radiant heat panel should be taped to the right upper quadrant just below the costal margin (ribs).

T F 6. For the first 12 hours after birth a newborn's temperature should be taken rectally until it has stabilized.

T F 7. Penicillin ointment is instilled into the newborn's lower conjunctiva to prevent ophthalmia neonatorum.

T F 8. Tympanic thermometers should not be used until after the first month of life.

T F 9. Both breastfed and bottle-fed babies should be fed every 3 to 4 hours during the day and throughout the night.

T F 10. The recommended site for intramuscular injections in the newborn is the vastus lateralis muscle.

T F 11. If bleeding is noted after a circumcision, the nurse should apply firm, constant pressure to the site until the physician arrives.

T F 12. To facilitate obtaining a heel stick blood sample, the loose application of a warm, wet washcloth around the foot for 5 to 10 minutes is sufficient to dilate the blood vessels in the heel.

T F 13. An alcohol swab should be used to apply pressure to the heel after a blood sample is obtained.

T F 14. Pressure should be applied over an arterial or femoral vein puncture for at least 3 to 5 minutes to prevent bleeding from the site.

T F 15. Before application of a U bag, the genitalia, perineum, and surrounding skin should be washed, dried, and sprinkled with talcum powder to prevent excoriation.

T F 16. Nonnutritive sucking with a pacifier or finger should be discouraged in the newborn because it leads to malformation of the jaw and dependency.

T F 17. A newborn's serum glucose level should be 40 mg/dl or higher.

T F 18. Hepatitis B vaccine should only be administered to newborns exposed to the hepatitis B virus.

T   F   19. The prone position should not be used for the first few months of life because it has been associated with an increase in the risk for sudden infant death syndrome.

T   F   20. Late preterm infants are those born at 39 0/7 weeks of gestation or more.

T   F   21. An Apgar score of 9 indicates that the newborn is having minimal or no difficulty adjusting to extrauterine life.

T   F   22. The wink reflex can be used to assess anal sphincter response.

T   F   23. Screening for hypothyroidism involves assessing the newborn's level of T_4.

T   F   24. When caring for the newborn, wearing gloves is the single most important measure in preventing neonatal infection.

T   F   25. When using a bulb syringe after birth, the newborn's nose should be suctioned before her or his mouth.

T   F   26. The ointment used for prevention of newborn ophthalmic infection should be flushed out of the eyes with normal saline 5 minutes after instillation.

T   F   27. Infants should be placed in a rear-facing car seat that is secured in the back seat of the car.

FILL IN THE BLANKS: Insert the term that corresponds to each of the following.

Newborns and Their Care

28. During a circumcision the _____ of the glans penis is removed. Currently the decision to perform this elective procedure is left up to the _____.

29. _____ or _____ ointment is used to prevent ophthalmia neonatorum. It should be instilled into the _____ of each eye.

30. _____ is administered intramuscularly to newborns to prevent hemorrhage. It is administered in a dose of _____ using a(n) _____-gauge, _____-inch needle.

31. The umbilical cord site should be assessed for _____, _____, and _____ at each diaper change.

32. An infant born before completion of 37 weeks of gestation, regardless of birth weight, is referred to as _____ or _____.

33. An infant born between the beginning of week 38 and the end of week 42 of gestation is referred to as _____.

34. An infant who is born after the completion of week 42 of gestation is referred to as _____ or _____.

35. An infant born after 42 weeks of gestation and showing the effects of progressive placental insufficiency is referred to as _____.

36. An infant whose weight is above the 90th percentile (or 2 or more standard deviations above the norm) at any week is referred to as _____.

37. An infant whose weight falls between the 10th and the 90th percentiles for his or her gestational age is referred to as _____.

38. An infant whose weight is below the 10th percentile (or 2 or more standard deviations below the norm) at any week is referred to as _____.

39. The New Ballard Scale is used to assess clinical gestational age of the newborn.

   A. *LIST* the signs assessed to determine neuromuscular maturity. *INDICATE* the expected finding for a full-term newborn for each sign listed.

   B. *LIST* the signs assessed to determine physical maturity. *INDICATE* the expected finding for a full-term newborn for each sign listed.

   C. *EXPLAIN* how the designations appropriate for gestational age, large for gestational age, and small for gestational age are made.

40. Preparing parents for the discharge of their newborn requires informing them about the essential aspects of newborn care. *IDENTIFY* the information that you would teach parents regarding each of the following areas.

   Infant positioning and holding

   Umbilical cord

   Car seat safety

Temperature

Elimination

Bathing

41. *LIST* the safety and medical aseptic principles that should be followed when sponge bathing a newborn.

42. *DESCRIBE* how the nurse would meet the prescribed standards for a newborn protective environment in terms of each of the following areas.

Environment

Infection control

Safety

MULTIPLE CHOICE: Circle the one correct option and state the rationale for the option chosen.

43. A newborn male is estimated to be 40 weeks of gestation following an assessment using the New Ballard Scale. A Ballard Scale finding consistent with this newborn's full-term status would be:
    A. Apical pulse rate of 120 beats/min, regular, and strong.
    B. Popliteal angle of 160 degrees.
    C. Weight of 3200 g, placing him at the 50th percentile.
    D. Thinning of lanugo with some bald areas.

44. The nurse evaluates the laboratory test results of a newborn who is 4 hours old. Which of the following results would require notification of the pediatrician?
    A. Hemoglobin, 20 g/dl.
    B. Hematocrit, 54%.
    C. Glucose, 34 mg/dl.
    D. Direct bilirubin, 0.6 mg/dl.

45. A newborn male has been designated as large for gestational age. His mother was diagnosed with gestational diabetes late in her pregnancy. The nurse should be alert for signs of hypoglycemia. Which of the following assessment findings are consistent with a diagnosis of hypoglycemia?
    A. Unstable body temperature
    B. Cyanosis
    C. Edema of the extremities
    D. Abdominal distention

46. A radiant warmer will be used to help a newborn girl stabilize her temperature. The nurse implementing this care measure should:
    A. Undress and dry the infant before placing her under the warmer.
    B. Set the control panel between 35° and 38° C.
    C. Place the thermistor probe on the left side of her chest just below her nipple.
    D. Assess her rectal temperature every hour until her temperature stabilizes.

47. A newborn male has been scheduled for a circumcision using the Gomco clamp technique. Essential nursing measures as part of this surgical procedure include which one of the following?
    A. Feed the infant just before the procedure to help him remain relaxed and quiet.
    B. Apply petroleum jelly to the site with each diaper change.
    C. Check the penis for bleeding every 15 minutes for the first 4 hours.
    D. Teach the parents to remove the yellowish exudate that forms over the glans using a diaper wipe.

1. Apgar scoring is a method of newborn assessment used in the immediate postbirth period at 1 and 5 minutes. *INDICATE* the Apgar score for each of the following newborns.

A. Baby boy Smith at 1 minute after birth:
    Heart rate—160 beats/min
    Respiratory effort—good; vigorous crying
    Muscle tone—active movement, well flexed
    Reflex irritability—crying with stimulus to soles of feet
    Color—body pink, feet and hands cyanotic

    Score: _____
    Interpretation:

B. Baby girl Doe at 5 minutes after birth:
    Heart rate—102 beat/min
    Respiratory effort—slow, irregular, weak crying
    Muscle tone—some flexion of extremities
    Reflex irritability—grimace with stimulus to soles of feet
    Color—pale

    Score: _____
    Interpretation:

2. Baby girl June was just born.

A. *OUTLINE* the protocol that the nurse should follow when assessing June's physical status during the 2 hours after her birth.

B. *STATE* the nurse's legal responsibility regarding identification of June and her mother after birth.

C. *CITE* two priority nursing diagnoses appropriate for June during the first 2 hours after birth.

D. *IDENTIFY* the priority nursing care measures the nurse must implement to ensure June's well-being and safety during the first 2 hours after birth.

3. Susan and James are taking their newly circumcised (6 hours postprocedure) baby home. This is their first baby, and they express anxiety concerning care of both the circumcision and the umbilical cord.

   A. *STATE* one nursing diagnosis related to this situation.

   B. *STATE* one expected outcome related to the nursing diagnosis identified.

   C. *SPECIFY* the instructions that the nurse should give to Susan and James regarding assessment of both sites and the care measures required to facilitate healing.

4. Andrew and Marion are parents of a newborn, 30 hours old, who has developed hyperbilirubinemia. They are very concerned about the color of their baby and the need to put the baby under special lights. "Andrew's uncle was yellow just like our baby and later died of liver cancer!"

   A. *DESCRIBE* how the nurse should respond to Andrew and Marion's concern.

B. *IDENTIFY* the expected assessment findings and physiologic effects related to hyperbilirubinemia.

C. *LIST* the precautions and care measures required by the newborn undergoing phototherapy to prevent injury to the newborn and yet maintain the effectiveness of the treatment. *STATE* the rationale for each action identified.

5. Baby girl Susan has an accumulation of mucus in her nasal passages and mouth, making breathing difficult.

A. *INDICATE* signs of abnormal breathing that baby girl Susan might exhibit as a result of difficulty breathing.

B. *STATE* the nursing diagnosis represented by the assessment findings.

C. *LIST* the steps that the nurse should follow when clearing the baby's airway with a bulb syringe.

D. If mucus accumulation continues and breathing is compromised, a nasopharyngeal catheter with mechanical suction might be required. *LIST* the guidelines that the nurse should follow when using this method to clear the newborn's airway.

6. Angela, the mother of a newborn, tells the nurse, "I know that I should get my baby immunized, but I have heard that each shot is so expensive, and there are so many. Because I am breastfeeding, my baby is protected from infection anyway. Do you think it would be all right to wait until the baby's first birthday? Then he'll need fewer shots." *DESCRIBE* how the nurse should reply to Angela.

7. A newborn is scheduled for a circumcision. The nurse caring for this newborn is aware that he will experience pain as a result of this procedure.

   A. *DESCRIBE* the most common behavioral responses to pain.

   B. *INDICATE* how a newborn's vital signs and integument change when he experiences pain.

   C. *STATE* the nursing diagnosis reflective of this pain experience.

   D. *OUTLINE* the nonpharmacologic and pharmacologic measures that the nurse could use or suggest to be used to minimize the pain experience and its effects and maximize the newborn's ability to cope with the pain and recover more quickly.

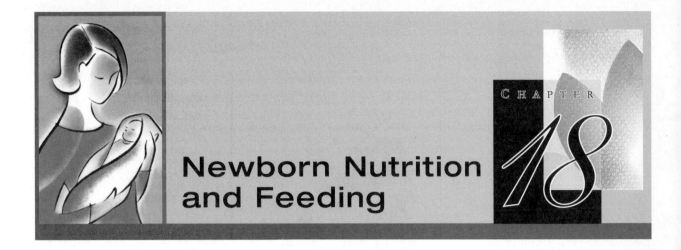

Newborn Nutrition and Feeding

CHAPTER 18

CHAPTER REVIEW ACTIVITIES

It is critical that infants ingest an appropriate amount of calories and fluid each day to support their rapid growth and development.

FILL IN THE BLANKS: Insert the term that corresponds to each of the following.

1. A. The daily energy requirement for the first 3 months of life is _____ kcal/kg; for 3 to 6 months the daily requirement is _____ kcal/kg; for 6 to 9 months it is _____ kcal/kg/day, and it is _____ kcal/kg/day from 9 months to 1 year.

   Human milk provides _____ kcal/100 ml or _____ kcal/oz. Standard formula also contains _____ kcal/oz.

   B. *CALCULATE* the daily energy requirement(in kcal) for each of the following infants.

   Infant   **Calories**

   Jim:
   1 month
   4 kg

   Sue:
   4 months
   6 kg

   Sam:
   7 months
   7.5 kg

   Jean:
   10 months
   10.5 kg

2. Development and function of lactation structures within the breast are critical to the success of lactogenesis.

   A. *LABEL* the following illustration as indicated.

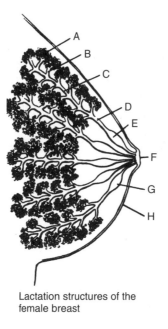

Lactation structures of the
female breast

B. Insert the term that corresponds to each of the following.
   1. _____ Structures in the breast composed of alveoli, milk ductules, and myoepithelial cells
   2. _____ Cluster of milk-producing cells
   3. Each lobe contains _____, consisting of alveoli surrounded by myoepithelial cells.
   4. Each nipple has multiple _____ that transfer milk to the suckling infant.
   5. Within each breast is a complex intertwining network of _____ that transport milk from the alveoli to the nipple.
   6. _____ Cells surrounding alveoli that contract in response to oxytocin, resulting in the milk ejection reflex or let-down
   7. _____ Rounded pigmented section of tissue surrounding the nipple

3. A nurse has been asked to participate in a women's health seminar for women of childbearing age in the community. Her topic will be "Breastfeeding—the Goals for Healthy People 2010 and Beyond." *OUTLINE* the points that this nurse should emphasize to help women appreciate the benefits of breastfeeding and seriously consider breastfeeding when they have a baby.

4. It is important that a breastfeeding woman alter the position she uses for breastfeeding as one means of preserving nipple and areolar integrity. *DESCRIBE* four breastfeeding positions that the nurse should demonstrate to a woman who is breastfeeding her newborn.

5. Infants exhibit feeding readiness cues as they recognize and express their hunger.

   A. *IDENTIFY* feeding readiness cues of the infant.

   B. *STATE* why the new mother should be guided by these cues when determining the timing of feeding sessions.

6. *INDICATE* the differences between foremilk and hindmilk.

7. *LABEL* each of the following illustrations depicting the maternal breastfeeding reflexes.

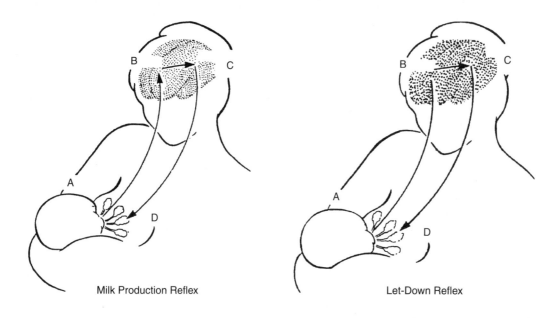

Milk Production Reflex   Let-Down Reflex

8. There are three stages of lactogenesis. *STATE* the expected time of occurrence for each stage and *DESCRIBE* the events typical of each stage.

Stage I

Stage II

Stage III

9. Proper latch-on is essential for effective breastfeeding and preservation of nipple and areolar tissue integrity.

A. *INDICATE* the steps that the nurse should teach a breastfeeding woman to follow to ensure a proper latch-on.

B. When observing a woman breastfeeding, it is essential that the nurse determine the effectiveness of the latch-on. *STATE* the signs that a nurse should look for that indicate a proper latch-on.

C. *DESCRIBE* how a woman should remove her baby from her breast after feeding is completed.

TRUE OR FALSE: Circle T if true or F if false for each of the following statements. Correct the false statements.

T   F   10. Approximately 77% of infants in the United States are breastfed.

T   F   11. A newborn should lose no more than 15% to 20% of his or her birth weight.

T   F   12. The birth weight of a full-term newborn is usually regained within 14 days of life.

T   F   13. To prevent fat-related cardiovascular problems later in life, bottle-fed infants should be given low-fat or skim milk beginning at 6 months of life.

T   F   14. Infants who are entirely breastfed should receive iron supplementation in the form of iron-containing foods such as cereals after the first 6 months of life.

T   F   15. Women who have large breasts produce more milk than women who have small breasts.

T   F   16. Milk production primarily depends on increased secretion of estrogen and progesterone.

T   F   17. Human milk contains a higher level of protein than unmodified cow's milk.

T   F   18. Women from some cultures avoid breastfeeding until their milk comes in.

T   F   19. Early and frequent feedings facilitate the elimination of bilirubin in feces, thereby reducing the incidence or severity of hyperbilirubinemia.

T   F   20. Women with diabetes should avoid breastfeeding because insulin requirements are increased.

T   F   21. Colostrum acts as a laxative to remove meconium from the newborn's intestine.

T   F   22. Breastfed babies require vitamin C supplementation.

T   F   23. Smoking can inhibit milk production.

T   F   24. When a newborn is breastfeeding, pacifiers should be avoided until the newborn becomes proficient with breastfeeding.

T   F   25. Uterine cramping during breastfeeding indicates that oxytocin is being secreted.

T   F   26. Fluoride supplementation should begin at 2 months for breastfed and bottle-fed babies not receiving fluoridated water.

T   F   27. A woman with mastitis should stop breastfeeding temporarily as soon as the diagnosis of infection is made.

T   F   28. Lettuce leaves are very helpful in reducing the pain and swelling that accompany engorgement.

29. A breastfeeding woman has been having difficulty calming her fussy baby daughter to feed her. *IDENTIFY* several techniques that the nurse could teach this woman to calm her baby in preparation for feeding.

30. *COMPLETE* the following table by identifying the factors that should be assessed before and during breastfeeding and the factors for ongoing assessment as related to the infant and breastfeeding mother.

Infant/Mother	Assessment Before and During Breastfeeding	Ongoing Assessment
Infant		
Mother		

MULTIPLE CHOICE: Circle the one correct option and state the rationale for the option chosen.

31. During a home visit the mother of a 1-week-old infant son tells the nurse that she is very concerned about whether her baby is getting enough breast milk. The nurse tells this mother that at 1 week of age a well-nourished newborn should exhibit:
   A. Weight gain sufficient to reach his birth weight.
   B. A minimum of three bowel movements each day.
   C. Approximately 10 to 12 wet diapers each day.
   D. Sufficient nutrition from breastfeeding at a frequency of every 4 hours or about six times each day.

32. A woman is trying to calm her fussy baby daughter in preparation for feeding. She exhibits a need for further instruction if she:
   A. Removes all clothing from her infant except the diaper.
   B. Dims lights in the room and turns off the television.
   C. Gently rocks the baby and talks to her in a low voice.
   D. Allows the baby to suck on her finger.

33. The nurse should teach breastfeeding mothers about breast care measures to preserve the integrity of the nipples and areola. Which of the following should the nurse include in these instructions?
    A. Cleanse nipples and areola twice a day with mild soap and water.
    B. Apply vitamin E cream to nipples and areola at least four times each day before a feeding.
    C. Insert plastic-lined pads into the bra to absorb leakage and protect clothing.
    D. Rub expressed colostrum or breast milk on sore nipples after feeding.

34. A breastfeeding woman asks the nurse about birth control that she should use during the postpartum period. Which is the best recommendation for a safe yet effective method during the first 6 weeks after birth?
    A. Combination oral contraceptive that she used before she was pregnant
    B. Barrier method using a combination of a condom and spermicide foam
    C. Progestin-only contraceptive such as Norplant or Depo-Provera
    D. Complete breastfeeding (baby only receives breast milk for nourishment)

35. A woman has determined that bottle-feeding is the best feeding method for her. Instructions that the woman should receive regarding this feeding method include which of the the following?
    A. Place baby in a prone position after a feeding to facilitate passage of air bubbles.
    B. Sterilize water by boiling and then cool and mix with formula powder or concentrate.
    C. Expect a 1-week-old newborn to drink approximately 30 to 60 ml of formula at each feeding.
    D. Microwave refrigerated formula before feeding the newborn.

CRITICAL THINKING EXERCISES

1. *EVALUATE* each of the following actions of Janet, a breastfeeding mother. *DETERMINE* whether the action indicates competency (+) or a need for further instruction (−). *INDICATE* the information that you would give Janet to correct actions that require further instruction.

    A. _____ Washes her breasts and nipples thoroughly with soap and water twice a day.

    B. _____ Massages a small amount of breast milk into her nipple and areola before and after each feeding.

    C. _____ Lines her bra with a thick, plastic-lined pad to absorb leakage.

    D. _____ Positions baby by supporting his or her back and shoulders securely and brings her breast toward the baby, putting the nipple in the baby's mouth.

    E. _____ Alternates breastfeeding positions among football, cradle, modified cradle, and lying-down holds.

    F. _____ Limits breastfeeding at the first breast to a maximum of 10 minutes and then switches to the second breast.

    G. _____ Supports her breast with four fingers underneath the breast and thumb on the top at the back edge of the areola.

    H. _____ Inserts her finger into the corner of her baby's mouth between the gums before removing from the breast.

    I. _____ Awakens the baby every 2 to 3 hours day and night for a feeding.

    J. _____ Increases her fluid intake to 3 L/day by drinking water, coffee, herbal teas, juice, milk, cola, and wine.

    K. _____ Increases her caloric intake by approximately 500 cal/day, with a gradual weight loss noted.

    L. _____ Plans to use the pill for birth control beginning at 3 weeks postpartum.

    M. _____ States that she will resume her monthly performance of breast self-examination as soon as she weans her baby in 6 months.

2. Elise and her husband, Mark, are experiencing their first pregnancy. During one of their prenatal visits they tell the nurse that they are not sure about the method they want to use for feeding their baby. "Everyone has an opinion. Some say that breastfeeding is best, and others tell us that bottle-feeding is more convenient, especially because the father can help. What should we do?"

A. *IDENTIFY* one nursing diagnosis and one expected outcome appropriate for this situation.

B. *DISCUSS* why it is important for the pregnant couple to make this decision together.

C. *INDICATE* why it is preferable to make this decision during the prenatal period rather than waiting until the baby is born.

D. *DESCRIBE* how the nurse could use the decision-making process to help Elise and Mark to choose the method that is best for them.

3. As a first-time breastfeeding mother, Mary has many questions. *DESCRIBE* how you would respond to the following questions and comments.

A. "I'm so afraid that I won't make enough milk for my baby. My breasts are not as large as some of my friends who breastfeed."

B. "Everyone keeps talking about the let-down that is supposed to happen. What is it, and how will I know that I have it?"

C. "How can I possibly know if breastfeeding is going well and my baby is getting enough if I can't tell how many ounces he gets with each feeding?"

D. "It's only the first day that I'm breastfeeding and my nipples already feel sore. What can I do to relieve this soreness and prevent it from getting worse?"

E. "My friends all told me to watch out for the fourth day and engorgement. What can I do to keep it from happening or at least take care of myself when it does?"

F. "Every time I breastfeed, I get cramps, and my flow seems to get heavier. Is there something wrong with me?"

G. "I'm so glad that I don't have to worry about getting pregnant again as long as I'm breastfeeding. I hate using birth control, and my friend told me I don't have to use it as long as I'm breastfeeding."

H. "What should I do when I'm ready to stop breastfeeding my baby?"

4. Before discharge with her healthy full-term baby boy, Jane, a primiparous woman, asks the nurse about when she should start solid foods such as cereals so her baby will sleep through the night. DESCRIBE how the nurse should respond to Jane's request for information.

5. Susan is 2 days old. She last fed 5 hours ago. Her mother tells the nurse that Susan is so sleepy that she just doesn't have the heart to wake her.

A. *IDENTIFY* one nursing diagnosis and one expected outcome appropriate for this newborn.

B. *DISCUSS* the approach the nurse should take with regard to this situation.

6. Alice has decided that, for personal and professional reasons, bottle-feeding with a commercially prepared formula is the feeding method that is best for her. She tells the nurse that she hopes that she made a good decision for her baby. "I hope she'll be well nourished and feel that I love her even though I am bottle-feeding."

A. *DESCRIBE* how the nurse should respond to Alice's concern.

B. *STATE* three guidelines for bottle-feeding technique that the nurse should teach Alice to ensure the safety and health of her baby.

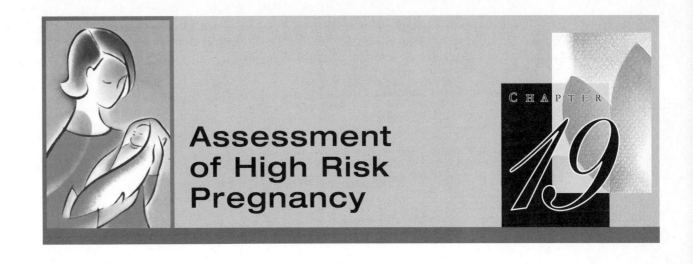

Assessment of High Risk Pregnancy

CHAPTER 19

CHAPTER REVIEW ACTIVITIES

TRUE OR FALSE: Circle T if true or F if false for each of the following statements. Correct the false statements.

T   F   1. The major outcome of antepartum testing is the detection of potential fetal compromise.

T   F   2. Oligohydramnios or a decrease in amniotic fluid amount has been associated with neural tube defects.

T   F   3. After amniocentesis or chorionic villi sampling (CVS), an Rh-negative woman should receive $Rh_o(D)$ immunoglobulin (RhoGAM).

T   F   4. The major disadvantage of a nonstress test (NST) relates to its high rate of false-negative results.

T   F   5. Research indicates that giving a woman orange juice or glucose during NST stimulates her baby to move.

T   F   6. A lower than normal alpha-fetoprotein level in the maternal serum and amniotic fluid has been associated with Down syndrome.

T   F   7. To conduct a contraction stress test (CST), four uterine contractions in a 15-minute period are required.

T   F   8. A negative result on a CST means that at least three uterine contractions occurred in a 10-minute period, with no associated late or significant variable decelerations.

T   F   9. When performing a daily fetal movement count, a pregnant woman should call her health care provider if she notes eight or fewer fetal movements in 1 hour.

T   F   10. Fetal movements decrease temporarily if the mother smokes.

11. ***DISCUSS*** the role of the nurse when caring for high risk pregnant women and their families who are required to undergo antepartal testing to determine fetal well-being.

12. Annie is a primigravida who is at 10 weeks of gestation. Her prenatal history reveals that she was treated for pelvic inflammatory disease 2 years ago. She describes irregular menstrual cycles and therefore is unsure about the first day of her last menstrual period. Annie is scheduled for a vaginal ultrasound.

   A. *CITE* the probable reason for the performance of this test.

   B. *DESCRIBE* how the nurse should prepare Annie for this test.

13. Ally, a pregnant woman at 20 weeks of gestation, is scheduled for a series of abdominal ultrasound tests to monitor the growth of her fetus. *DESCRIBE* the nursing role as it applies to Ally and to ultrasound examinations.

14. *STATE* two risk factors for each of the following pregnancy problems.

   Polyhydramnios

   Oligohydramnios

   Intrauterine growth restriction

   Chromosome abnormalities

FILL IN THE BLANKS: Insert the term that corresponds to each of the following.

Risk Assessment during Pregnancy

15. A(n) _____ is a pregnancy in which the life or health of the mother or her fetus is jeopardized by a disorder coincidental with or unique to pregnancy.

16. The major expected outcome of antepartum testing is the _____, ideally before intrauterine _____ of the fetus occurs, so the health care provider can take measures to _____ or _____ adverse perinatal outcomes.

17. _____ or _____ is the assessment of fetal activity by the mother. It is a simple yet valuable method for monitoring the condition of the fetus. The fetal alarm signal refers to the cessation of fetal movements entirely for _____. A count of less than _____ warrants further evaluation by _____, _____, _____, or a combination of these. Fetal movements are usually not present during the _____; they might be temporarily reduced if the woman is taking _____, drinking _____, or _____; they do not _____ as the woman nears term.

18. _____ is the use of sound having a frequency higher than that detectable by humans to examine structures inside the body. It can be done _____ or _____ during pregnancy. _____ is more useful after the first trimester when the pregnant uterus rises out of the pelvis. _____, in which the probe is inserted into the _____, allows _____ anatomy to be evaluated in greater detail and _____ to be diagnosed earlier. It is optimally used in the first trimester to detect _____ pregnancies, monitor the developing _____, help identify _____, and help establish _____.

19. _____ is the noninvasive study of blood flow in the fetus and placenta. It is a helpful adjunct in the management of pregnancies at risk because of _____, _____, _____, _____, or _____.

20. _____ is a noninvasive dynamic assessment of the fetus and his or her environment by _____ and external _____. This test includes assessment of five variables (i.e., _____, _____, _____, _____, and _____).

21. _____ is a noninvasive radiologic technique used for obstetric and gynecologic diagnosis. It provides excellent pictures of soft tissue without _____.

22. _____ is performed to obtain amniotic fluid, which contains fetal cells. A needle is inserted _____ into the uterus, _____ is withdrawn, and various assessments are performed. Indications for this procedure are prenatal diagnosis of _____, assessment of _____, and diagnosis of _____.

23. Direct access to the fetal circulation during the second and third trimesters is possible through _____ or _____, which is the most widely used method for fetal _____ and _____. It involves the insertion of a needle directly into a fetal _____ under ultrasound guidance.

24. _____ is a procedure that involves the removal of a small tissue specimen from the fetal portion of the placenta. Because this tissue originates from the zygote, it reflects the _____ of the fetus. It is performed between _____ and _____ weeks of gestation.

25. Determination of the _____ level is used as a screening tool for neural tube defects in pregnancy. The test is ideally performed between _____ and _____ weeks of gestation.

26. The _____ is a screening test for Down syndrome. It is performed between _____ and _____ weeks of gestation. The levels of three markers (i.e., _____, _____, and _____) in combination with maternal _____ are used to determine degree of risk.

27. A(n) _____ test is based on the fact that the heart rate of a healthy fetus with an intact central nervous system will _____ in response to fetal movement.

28. The purpose of a(n) _____ test is to identify the jeopardized fetus who is stable at rest but shows evidence of compromise when exposed to the stress of uterine contractions. If the resultant hypoxia of the fetus is sufficient, a(n) _____ of the FHR results. Two methods used for this test are the _____ test and the _____ test.

MULTIPLE CHOICE: Circle the one correct option and state the rationale for the option chosen.

29. A 34-year-old woman at 36 weeks of gestation has been scheduled for a biophysical profile. She asks the nurse why the test needs to be performed. The nurse tells her that the test:
    A. Determines how well her baby breathes after he or she is born.
    B. Evaluates the response of her baby's heart to uterine contractions.
    C. Measures her baby's head and length.
    D. Observes her baby's activities to ensure that he or she is getting enough oxygen.

30. As part of preparing a 24-year-old woman at 42 weeks of gestation for an NST, the nurse:
    A. Tells the woman to fast for 8 hours before the test.
    B. Explains that the test evaluates how well her baby is moving inside her uterus.
    C. Shows her how to indicate when her baby moves.
    D. Attaches a spiral electrode to the presenting part to determine FHR patterns.

31. A 40-year-old woman at 18 weeks of gestation is having a triple marker test performed. She is obese, and her health history reveals that she is Rh negative. The primary purpose of this test is to screen for:
    A. Spina bifida.
    B. Down syndrome.
    C. Gestational diabetes.
    D. Rh antibodies.

32. During a CST four contractions lasting 45 to 55 seconds were recorded in a 10-minute period. A late deceleration was noted during the third contraction. The nurse conducting the test documents which of the following results?
    A. Negative
    B. Positive
    C. Suspicious
    D. Unsatisfactory

33. A pregnant woman is scheduled for a transvaginal ultrasound test to establish gestational age. In preparing this woman for the test, the nurse:
    A. Places the woman in a supine position with her hips elevated on a folded pillow.
    B. Instructs her to come for the test with a full bladder.
    C. Administers an analgesic 30 minutes before the test.
    D. Lubricates the vaginal probe with transmission gel.

CRITICAL THINKING EXERCISES

1. Mary is at 42 weeks of gestation. Her physician has ordered a biophysical profile (BPP). She is very upset and tells the nurse, "All my doctor told me is that this test will see if my baby is okay. I don't know what's going to happen and if it will be painful to me or harmful for my baby."

    A. *STATE* a nursing diagnosis that reflects this situation.

B. *DESCRIBE* how the nurse should respond to Mary's concerns.

C. Mary receives a score of 8 for the BPP. *LIST* the factors that were evaluated to obtain this score and *SPECIFY* the meaning of Mary's test result of 8.

2. Jan, age 42, is 18 weeks pregnant. Because of her age, her fetus is at risk for genetic anomalies. Jan's blood type is A negative, and her partner's, the father of her baby, is B positive. Her primary health care provider has suggested an amniocentesis. *DESCRIBE* the nurse's role in terms of each of the following.

Preparing Jan for the amniocentesis

Supporting Jan during the procedure

Providing Jan with postprocedure care and instructions

3. Susan, who has diabetes and is in week 36 of pregnancy, has been scheduled for an NST.

A. *DISCUSS* what you would tell Susan about the purpose of this test and what will be learned about her baby's well-being.

B. *DESCRIBE* how you would prepare Susan for this test.

C. *INDICATE* how you would conduct the test.

D. *ANALYZE* the following tracings. *DESIGNATE* the result that each represents and *INDICATE* the criteria that you used to determine the result.

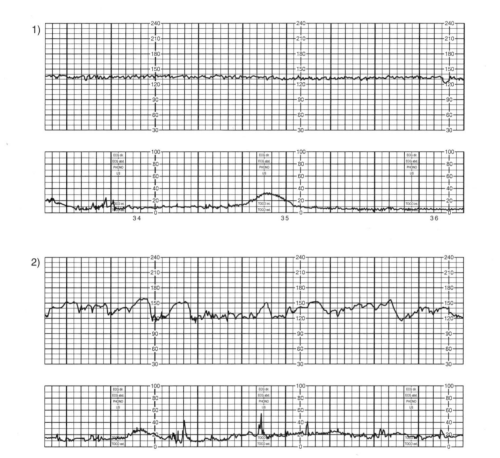

4. Beth is scheduled for a CST following a nonreactive result on an NST. Nipple stimulation is used to produce the required contraction pattern.

A. *DISCUSS* what you would tell Beth about the purpose of this test and what will be learned about the well-being of her fetus.

B. *DESCRIBE* how you would prepare Beth for the test.

C. *INDICATE* how you would conduct the test.

D. *STATE* how you would conduct the test differently if exogenous oxytocin (Pitocin) is used instead of nipple stimulation.

E. *ANALYZE* the following tracings. *DESIGNATE* the result that each represents and *INDICATE* the criteria that you used to determine the results.

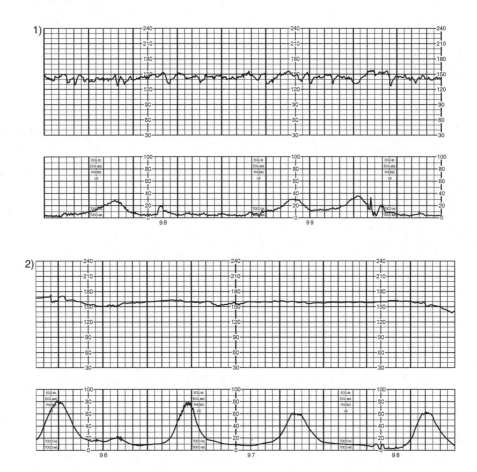

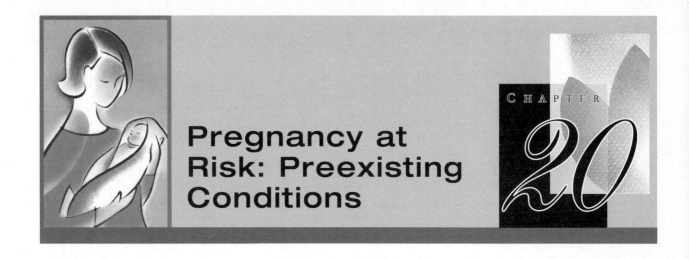

Pregnancy at Risk: Preexisting Conditions

CHAPTER 20

CHAPTER REVIEW ACTIVITIES

1. *DESCRIBE* the physiologic basis for the major clinical manifestations associated with diabetes mellitus.

    Hyperglycemia

    Polyuria

    Glycosuria

    Polydipsia

    Weight loss

Ketoacidosis and acetonuria

Polyphagia

FILL IN THE BLANKS: Insert the term that corresponds to each of the following.

Diabetes Mellitus during Pregnancy

2. Diabetes mellitus is a group of metabolic diseases characterized by _____ resulting from defects in _____, _____, or both.

3. _____ refers to excretion of large volumes of urine. _____ refers to excessive thirst, and _____ refers to excessive eating. Excretion of unusable glucose results in _____.

4. _____ is the label given to type 1 or type 2 diabetes that existed before pregnancy. _____ is any degree of glucose intolerance with onset or first recognition occurring during pregnancy.

5. The key to optimal outcome of a diabetic pregnancy is strict maternal _____ or _____ before and during pregnancy.

6. During the first trimester insulin dosage for well-controlled diabetes might need to be reduced to avoid _____. There is an increased incidence of _____ episodes in women with type 1 diabetes during early pregnancy because _____, _____, and _____ result in dietary fluctuations, which influence maternal _____ levels and necessitate a reduction in insulin dosage.

7. During the second and third trimesters the dosage of insulin must be increased to avoid _____ and _____. _____ resistance begins as early as _____ and continues to increase until it stabilizes during the last few weeks of pregnancy.

8. For the pregnancy complicated by diabetes, fetal lung maturation is best predicted by the presence of _____ in the amniotic fluid.

9. Glycemic control over the previous 4 to 6 weeks can be evaluated based on the determination of the level of _____ in the blood.

10. Dietary management during a diabetic pregnancy must be based on _____ levels. Energy needs are usually estimated based on _____ cal/kg of ideal body weight. _____% of total calories should be from carbohydrates. _____-type carbohydrates should be limited, whereas _____-type carbohydrates should be emphasized when food choices are made.

11. Blood glucose levels are measured throughout each day: before _____, _____, and _____; at _____; and sometimes in the middle of the _____. _____ measurements 2 hours after meals can also be done. More frequent testing is required when there are readjustments in _____ or if the woman is experiencing _____, _____, _____, or _____.

12. Urine should be tested for _____. The test should be performed _____ using the _____ urine. It should also be done if a(n) _____ is missed, when _____ occurs, or when the blood glucose level is higher than _____.

13. Typically _____ of the daily insulin dose is given in the morning _____ using a combination of _____ and _____ insulin. The remaining _____ is administered in the evening _____. To reduce the risk of _____ during the night, often separate injections are given with _____ insulin _____ followed by _____ insulin at _____. Another regimen is to administer _____ insulin before each meal and _____ insulin at bedtime.

14. *COMPLETE* the following table by identifying the major maternal and fetal or neonatal risks and complications associated with diabetic pregnancies.

Maternal Risks/Complications	Fetal/Neonatal Risks/Complications

15. *COMPLETE* the following table by identifying the metabolic changes that occur during pregnancy and indicating how these changes affect the woman with pregestational diabetes during the first trimester, the second and third trimesters, and the postpartum period.

Stage of Pregnancy	Metabolic Changes of Pregnancy	Impact on Diabetes
First Trimester		
Second and third trimesters		
Postpartum period		

TRUE OR FALSE: Circle T if true or F if false for each of the following statements. Correct the false statements.

Diabetes Mellitus during Pregnancy

T   F   16. Insulin requirements might decrease during the first trimester but need to increase during the second and third trimesters.

T   F   17. Fasting blood glucose levels should be between 40 and 75 mg/dl.

T   F   18. Injections of both longer acting (NPH) and shorter acting (regular insulin) are usually required to maintain glucose control for the woman with pregestational diabetes.

T   F   19. Ketoacidosis occurring at any time during pregnancy can lead to intrauterine fetal death.

T   F   20. Congenital anomalies commonly associated with pregestational diabetes include malformations of the respiratory tract and sensory deficits.

T   F   21. A glycosylated hemoglobin level of 13% to 20% indicates good glycemic control.

T   F   22. Women with diabetes should avoid a bedtime snack when they are pregnant.

T F 23. It is recommended that the 2-hour postprandial blood glucose level be lower than 130 mg/dl.

T F 24. Many women diagnosed with gestational diabetes require the use of oral hypoglycemic medications.

T F 25. Gestational diabetes is primarily a condition that complicates the pregnancies of Caucasian women.

T F 26. The incidence of congenital anomalies among infants of mothers with gestational diabetes is nearly the same as for infants of mothers in the general population.

T F 27. A 1-hour, 50-g glucose tolerance test result higher than 140 mg/dl is diagnostic for gestational diabetes.

T F 28. Pregnant women with diabetes should test their urine for glucose to determine whether the dosage of insulin needs to be adjusted.

T F 29. To avoid the risk of fetal intrauterine death, labor should be induced as soon as the fetal lungs are mature, usually at approximately 36 weeks of gestation.

T F 30. Euglycemia reflects blood glucose levels ranging between 65 and 140 mg/dl.

31. *STATE* how hyperthyroidism and hypothyroidism can affect reproductive well-being and pregnancy.

32. *IDENTIFY* the maternal and fetal complications most commonly seen in pregnant women who have cardiac problems.

TRUE OR FALSE: Circle T if true or F if false for each of the following statements. Correct the false statements.

Medical Problems Complicating Pregnancy

T F 33. Anemia is the most common medical disorder of pregnancy.

T F 34. Folic acid anemia is the most common type of anemia in pregnancy.

T F 35. Anemia increases the postpartum woman's risk for infection.

T F 36. A well-balanced diet alone is unable to prevent iron deficiency anemia in pregnancy.

T F 37. Oral iron supplementation should be taken in a dose of 60 mg three times a day, beginning in the first trimester.

T F 38. Exacerbations of sickle cell crises are diminished in pregnant women with sickle cell disease.

T F 39. Preeclampsia is more common in pregnancies complicated by thalassemia major.

T F 40. Asthma increases the incidence of miscarriage and preterm labor.

T F 41. Morphine should not be used to provide analgesia for laboring women with bronchial asthma because it releases histamine.

T F 42. In the management of care for a laboring woman with cystic fibrosis, close monitoring of the serum sodium level and fluid balance is critical.

T F 43. Infection is the leading complication among pregnant women with systemic lupus erythematosus.

T   F   44. A pregnant woman with a cardiac problem might be experiencing cardiovascular decompensation if she notices a sudden inability to perform her usual activities as a result of fatigue and dyspnea.

T   F   45. Epidural anesthesia is more effective than narcotics for providing pain relief for a woman with cardiac problems who is in labor.

TRUE OR FALSE: Circle T if true or F if false for each of the following statements. Correct the false statements.

Substance Abuse during Pregnancy

T   F   46. Health care providers are required by federal law to test the urine of all newborns for the presence of alcohol and drugs.

T   F   47. Every pregnant woman should be screened at least verbally for substance abuse at the first prenatal visit.

T   F   48. Meconium from the newborn can be analyzed to determine past drug use over a longer period of time.

T   F   49. Disulfiram (Antabuse) is an effective substance to use during pregnancy for alcohol detoxification.

T   F   50. A woman dependent on a drug tends to exhibit a high degree of depression with the abuse because drugs are a way for women to blunt feelings and relieve psychologic distress.

T   F   51. Breastfeeding is safe for women who smoke marijuana.

T   F   52. Substance abusers often exhibit poor control over their behavior and a low threshold of pain during labor.

MULTIPLE CHOICE: Circle the one correct option and state the rationale for the option chosen.

53. A woman with pregestational diabetes at 20 weeks of gestation exhibits the following: thirst, nausea and vomiting, abdominal pain, drowsiness, and increased urination. Her skin is flushed and dry, and her breathing is rapid with a fruity odor. A priority nursing action when caring for this woman is to:
    A. Provide her with a simple carbohydrate immediately.
    B. Request an order for an antiemetic.
    C. Assist her into a lateral position to rest.
    D. Administer insulin according to her blood glucose level.

54. During her pregnancy a woman with pregestational diabetes has been monitoring her blood glucose level several times a day. Which of the following levels would require further assessment?
    A. 85 mg/dl before breakfast
    B. 90 mg/dl before lunch
    C. 135 mg/dl 2 hours after supper
    D. 100 mg/dl at bedtime

55. Specific guidelines should be followed when planning a diet with a woman with pregestational diabetes to ensure a euglycemic state. An appropriate diet reflects:
    A. About 40 cal/kg of prepregnancy weight daily.
    B. A caloric distribution among three meals and at least two snacks.
    C. A minimum of 350 mg of carbohydrate daily.
    D. A protein intake of at least 30% of the total kilocalories in a day.

56. An obese pregnant woman with gestational diabetes is learning self-injection of insulin. While evaluating the woman's technique for self-injection, the nurse recognizes that the woman understands the instructions when she:
    A. Washes her hands and puts on a pair of clean gloves.
    B. Shakes the NPH insulin vial vigorously to mix the insulin fully.
    C. Draws the NPH insulin into her syringe first.
    D. Spreads her skin taut and punctures the skin at a 90-degree angle.

57. When assessing a pregnant woman at 28 weeks of gestation who is diagnosed with rheumatic heart disease, it is important that the nurse be alert for signs indicating cardiac decompensation. A sign of cardiac decompensation is:

A. Dry, hacking cough.

B. Supine hypotension.

C. Wheezing with inspiration and expiration.

D. Rapid, irregular, weak pulse.

58. A woman at 30 weeks of gestation with a class II cardiac disorder calls her primary health care provider's office and speaks to the nurse practitioner. She tells the nurse that she has been experiencing a frequent moist cough for the past few days. In addition, she has been feeling more tired and is having difficulty completing her routine activities as a result of some difficulty with breathing. The nurse's best response is:

A. "Have someone bring you to the office so we can assess your cardiac status."

B. "Try to get more rest during the day because this is a difficult time for your heart."

C. "Take an extra diuretic tonight before you go to bed because you might be developing some fluid in your lungs."

D. "Ask your family to come over and do your housework for the next few days so you can rest."

59. At a previous antepartal visit, the nurse taught a pregnant woman diagnosed with a class II cardiac disorder about measures to use to lower her risk for cardiac decompensation. This woman demonstrates a need for further instruction if she:

A. Increases roughage in her diet.

B. Remains on bed rest, only getting out of bed to go to the bathroom.

C. Sleeps 10 hours every night and rests after meals.

D. States that she will call the nurse immediately if she experiences any pain or swelling in her legs.

CRITICAL THINKING EXERCISES

1. Mary is a 24-year-old woman with diabetes. When Mary informed her gynecologist that she and her husband were trying to get pregnant, she was referred to an endocrinologist for preconception counseling. Mary tells the nurse that she just cannot understand why this is necessary. "I have had diabetes since I was 12 years old, and I have not had many problems. All I want to do is get pregnant!" *DISCUSS* how the nurse should respond to Mary's comments.

2. Luann is a 25-year-old nulliparous woman in her first trimester of pregnancy (fourth week of gestation). She has had type 1 diabetes since she was 15 years old. Recently she has been experiencing some nausea and is eating less as a result. She took her usual dose of regular and NPH insulin before eating a very light breakfast of tea and a piece of toast. Just before her midmorning snack at work, she began to experience nervousness and tremors. She felt faint and became diaphoretic and pale.

A. *IDENTIFY* the problem that Luann is experiencing. *INDICATE* the basis for her symptoms.

B. *STATE* the action that Luann should take.

3. Judy's pregnancy has just been confirmed. She also has type 1 diabetes.

A. As a result of her high risk status, a variety of additional assessment measures are emphasized during her prenatal period to evaluate the status of her fetus. *IDENTIFY* these additional assessment measures and their relevance for a diabetic pregnancy.

B. *DISCUSS* the stressors that might confront Judy and her family as a result of her status as a woman with diabetes who is pregnant.

C. *COMPLETE* the following table by inserting the diet, glucose, and insulin guidelines for each stage of Judy's pregnancy.

Care Component	Antepartum	Intrapartum	Postpartum
Diet			
Glucose monitoring			
Insulin requirements			

D. *INDICATE* the activity and exercise recommendations that Judy should be given.

4. Elena (2-1-0-0-1) is a 32-year-old Hispanic-American woman in week 28 of her pregnancy. She is obese. Her mother, who is 59, was recently diagnosed with type 2 diabetes. Elena's first pregnancy resulted in the birth of a 10-pound, 6-ounce daughter who is now 2 years old. A 1-hour, 50-g glucose screen last week revealed a glucose level of 152 mg/dl. A 3-hour glucose tolerance test was done yesterday, with the following results: fasting, 108 mg/dl; 1 hour, 189 mg/dl; 2 hours, 170 mg/dl; 3 hours, 150 mg/dl.

A. *IDENTIFY* the complication of pregnancy that Elena is exhibiting. *STATE* the rationale for your answer.

B. *LIST* the risk factors for this health problem that are present in Elena's assessment data.

C. *DESCRIBE* the pathophysiology involved in creating Elena's problem.

D. *IDENTIFY* the maternal and fetal or neonatal risks and complications that are possible in this situation.

E. *OUTLINE* the ongoing assessment measures necessitated by Elena's health problem.

F. *STATE* the dietary changes that Elena has to make to maintain glycemic control during the rest of her pregnancy.

G. Before discharge after the birth of her second daughter, Elena asks the nurse if the health problem she experienced during this pregnancy will continue now that she has had her baby. She also wonders if it will happen with her next pregnancy because she wants to get pregnant again soon so she can "try for a son." *DISCUSS* the response that the nurse should give to Elena's concerns.

5. Jennifer's pregnancy has just been confirmed. She has type 2 diabetes and is told that she now must learn how to give herself insulin. Jennifer becomes very upset and states, "I can't possibly give myself a shot. Why not let me continue to take my pills since they've been working fine so far?" *DESCRIBE* how you would respond to Jennifer.

6. Linda, a 26-year-old pregnant woman, had rheumatic fever as a child and subsequently developed mitral valve stenosis. She is presently 6 weeks pregnant. This is the first pregnancy for Linda and her husband, Sam. As part of her medical regimen, her primary health care provider substituted subcutaneous heparin for the oral warfarin sodium (Coumadin) she had been taking before pregnancy.

A. Linda states, "I can't give myself a shot! Why can't I just take the medication orally?" *DISCUSS* how you would respond about the purpose of heparin and why it must be used instead of warfarin.

B. *INDICATE* the information that the nurse should give Linda to ensure safe use of the heparin.

C. At 3 months Linda's cardiac condition is classified as class II according to the New York Heart Association's functional classification of organic heart disease. The classification, class II, means _____. *DISCUSS* the therapeutic plan for this classification in terms of the following.

Rest, sleep, and activity patterns

Prevention of infection

Nutrition

Bowel elimination

D. *IDENTIFY* physiologic and psychosocial factors that might increase the stress placed on Linda's heart during her pregnancy.

Physiologic Factors   **Psychosocial Factors**

E. *LIST* the symptoms that the nurse should teach Linda and her family to look for as indicators of possible cardiac decompensation.

F. *LIST* the objective signs indicating that Linda might be experiencing cardiac decompensation and heart failure.

G. Physiologic cardiac stress is greatest between _____ and _____ weeks of gestation because _____.

H. *IDENTIFY* three nursing interventions related to the prevention of cardiac decompensation in Linda.

I. Linda is admitted to the labor unit. Her cardiac condition is still classified as class II. *OUTLINE* the nursing measures designed to assess Linda and promote optimum cardiac function during her labor and birth process.

J. Linda should be observed carefully during the postpartum period because cardiac risk continues. The first _____ to _____ hours after birth are the most hemodynamically difficult for Linda. *INDICATE* the physiologic events after birth that place Linda at risk for cardiac decompensation.

K. *DISCUSS* the measures that the nurse can use to reduce the stress placed on Linda's heart during the postpartum period.

L. Linda indicates that she wishes to breastfeed her infant. *DESCRIBE* the nurse's response.

M. *IDENTIFY* the important factors to be considered when preparing Linda's discharge plan.

7. Jean is a primigravida at 4 weeks of gestation. She has had epilepsy for several years, and her seizures have been controlled with phenytoin (Dilantin). Jean expresses concern regarding how her medication use will affect her pregnancy and her baby. She wants to stop taking the phenytoin. *DESCRIBE* the approach that you would take in addressing Jean's concern and the course of action that she is contemplating.

8. Abuse of and dependence on psychoactive substances and alcohol have become pandemic.

   A. *DISCUSS* the approach that the nurse should take during the first prenatal health history interview to screen a pregnant woman for alcohol and drug abuse.

   B. *IDENTIFY* the factors that the nurse should consider when planning care and setting expected outcomes for the pregnant woman who is dependent on psychoactive substances.

   C. *INDICATE* the nursing measures appropriate for the woman who is dependent on drugs and alcohol during pregnancy, childbirth, and the postpartum period.

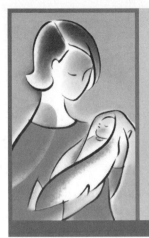

Pregnancy at Risk: Gestational Conditions

CHAPTER REVIEW ACTIVITIES

FILL IN THE BLANKS: Insert the term that corresponds to each of the following.

Hypertensive Disorders during Pregnancy

1. _____, a pregnancy-specific condition in which hypertension and proteinuria develop after _____ in a previously normotensive woman, is a multisystem vasospastic disease process. It is usually categorized as _____ or _____ in terms of management.

2. _____ is defined as a blood pressure (BP) greater than or equal to _____. The elevated values must be present on _____ occasions at least _____ hours apart.

3. _____ is defined as a protein concentration of _____ g/L (_____ on a dipstick measurement) or more in at least _____ random urine samples collected at least _____ hours apart.

4. Although edema is no longer included in the definition of preeclampsia, if present it is assessed for _____, _____, and _____, _____ is edema of the _____, or most dependent, parts of the body.

5. _____ is the presence of at least one of the following in women diagnosed with preeclampsia: systolic BP of at least _____ or a diastolic pressure of at least _____; proteinuria of _____ or more in a 24-hour collection; _____, less than 400 to 500 ml of urine output over 24 hours; _____ or _____ disturbances; and _____ with a platelet count less than _____, _____ or _____ may also be present.

6. _____ is the onset of seizure activity or coma in the woman diagnosed with preeclampsia that cannot be attributed to other causes.

7. _____ syndrome is a laboratory diagnosis for a variant of severe preeclampsia characterized by _____, _____, and _____.

8. The pathologic changes that occur in preeclampsia are caused by _____ and _____.

9. *STATE* the principles that you would follow to ensure the accuracy of BP measurement during pregnancy.

TRUE OR FALSE: Circle T if true or F if false for each of the following statements. Correct the false statements.

Hypertension in Pregnancy

T F 10. Preeclampsia complicates more than 15% of all pregnancies that progress beyond the first trimester.

T F 11. The major maternal hazard of preeclampsia is liver failure.

T F 12. A genetic predisposition might be partly responsible for the development of preeclampsia in some women.

T F 13. HELLP syndrome occurs in approximately 2% to 12% of women with severe preeclampsia.

T F 14. Calcium gluconate is the antidote for magnesium sulfate toxicity.

T F 15. The therapeutic serum magnesium level for the treatment of severe preeclampsia is 10 to 12 mg/dl.

T F 16. Pregnant women with chronic renal disease are at increased risk for developing pregnancy-induced hypertension.

T F 17. When on bed rest, the woman with preeclampsia should maintain a dorsal recumbent position.

T F 18. Sodium should be restricted to a minimal level when a woman has preeclampsia.

T F 19. Women experiencing the HELLP syndrome often exhibit a platelet count of 400,000/mm^3 or higher.

T F 20. Administration of magnesium sulfate to a woman with severe preeclampsia might precipitate labor by stimulating the uterus to contract.

T F 21. An expected outcome for the use of magnesium sulfate is the prevention of progression from preeclampsia to eclampsia.

T F 22. Hydralazine (Apresoline) can be used to lower the BP of a woman with preeclampsia.

T F 23. Epigastric or right upper quadrant pain is one symptom of impending eclampsia.

T F 24. Protein restriction is recommended for women with preeclampsia.

T F 25. Prompt treatment of a woman using appropriate medications, bed rest, and proper diet can cure preeclampsia.

T F 26. Methergine is the oxytocic of choice to prevent or treat postpartum hemorrhage for women with preeclampsia.

27. Preeclampsia is a serious complication of pregnancy. *STATE* the risk factors associated with preeclampsia for which the nurse should be alert when doing the health history interview at the first prenatal visit.

28. *DESCRIBE* the assessment technique used to determine whether the following findings are present in women with preeclampsia. (NOTE: You might wish to review this information in a physical assessment textbook for a complete explanation of each technique.)

Hyperreflexia

Ankle clonus

Proteinuria

Pitting edema

29. Preeclampsia and eclampsia affect both maternal and fetal well-being.

A. *DESCRIBE* how preeclampsia and eclampsia can adversely affect the health and well-being of the fetus.

B. *INDICATE* the fetal surveillance measures recommended for women experiencing preeclampsia.

MATCHING: Match the patient description in Column I with the appropriate diagnosis from Column II.

COLUMN I

_____ 30. At 30 weeks of gestation Angela's blood pressure was 152/96 mm Hg and her 24-hour urine collection contained 2 grams of protein.

_____ 31. At 38 weeks of gestation Mary's BP rose to 150/92 mm Hg. A urine dipstick was negative for protein.

_____ 32. Susan, a 34-year-old pregnant woman, has had a consistently high BP, ranging from 148/92 to 160/98 mm Hg since she was 28 years old. She does not have proteinuria.

_____ 33. At 32 weeks of gestation, Maria, with hypertension since 28 weeks, generalized edema, and proteinuria of 4, has a convulsion.

_____ 34. Dawn has been hypertensive since her 24th week of pregnancy. Urinalysis indicates a protein content of 3 grams. Further testing reveals a platelet count of 95,000/mm^3 and elevated aspartate aminotansferase and alanine aminotransferase levels, hematocrit is decreased, and burr cells appear on a peripheral smear.

COLUMN II

A. Eclampsia
B. Chronic hypertension
C. Gestational hypertension
D. HELLP syndrome
E. Preeclampsia

TRUE OR FALSE: Circle T if true or F if false for each of the following statements. Correct the false statements.

Hemorrhagic Complications during Pregnancy

T F 35. Miscarriages are often related to maternal behavior.

T F 36. A missed miscarriage refers to a pregnancy in which the fetus has died but miscarriage does not occur.

T F 37. An etiologic factor for incompetent cervix is use of diethylstilbestrol by the woman's mother during pregnancy.

T F 38. The most common site for an ectopic pregnancy is the ampulla of the uterine tube.

T F 39. Ectopic pregnancy is the leading pregnancy-related cause of second-trimester maternal death.

T F 40. Ectopic pregnancy is a leading cause of infertility.

T F 41. Infertile women who use clomiphene (Clomid) to stimulate ovulation are at higher risk for development of hydatidiform mole.

T F 42. Previous cesarean birth is an important risk factor for placenta previa.

T F 43. A vaginal examination performed when a woman is exhibiting signs of placenta previa can result in profound hemorrhage.

T F 44. Premature separation of the placenta (abruptio placentae) is associated with a perinatal mortality rate of 20% to 30%.

T F 45. Abdominal trauma is the most consistently identified risk factor for premature separation of the placenta.

T F 46. The urinary output of women diagnosed with disseminated intravascular coagulation should be monitored carefully because renal failure is a potential complication.

FILL IN THE BLANKS: Insert the term that corresponds to each of the following.

Bleeding during Pregnancy

47. Common early pregnancy bleeding disorders are _____, _____, _____, and _____.

48. Common late pregnancy bleeding disorders are _____, _____, or _____, _____ and _____ variations.

49. _____ is a pregnancy that ends before _____ weeks of gestation, before the fetus is _____. A fetal weight of less than _____ may also be used to define this type of pregnancy loss. There are five types of this form of pregnancy loss: _____, _____, _____, _____, and _____.

50. Evaluation of the serum level of the placental hormone _____ is performed at _____ hours apart. If normal pregnancy is present, the B-hCG level _____; a _____ or _____ rising B-hCG level indicates _____ _____.

51. Placenta previa is described as total or complete if the _____ is _____ covered by the placenta when the cervix is fully dilated and as marginal if only a(n) _____ of the placenta extends to within 2.5 cm of the _____ or the exact relationship of the placenta to the internal os has not been determined. Risk for postpartum hemorrhage is increased because the _____ is unable to _____ around the open blood vessels of the placental site.

52. _____ or abruptio placentae is the _____ of _____ or _____ of the placenta from the _____ .

53. Disseminated intravascular coagulation (DIC) can result from a number of obstetric problems.

   A. *IDENTIFY* three predisposing conditions for DIC.

   B. *INDICATE* the clinical manifestations of DIC that were noted during physical examination and with laboratory testing.

   C. *DESCRIBE* four priority nursing measures that should be used when caring for a woman experiencing DIC.

MATCHING: Match the description in Column I with the appropriate diagnosis in Column II.

COLUMN I

_____ 54. Placental anomaly in which the cord vessels begin to branch at the membranes and then course out at the placenta

_____ 55. Fertilized ovum implanted outside the uterine cavity

_____ 56. Termination of pregnancy before fetal viability as a result of natural causes

_____ 57. Complication of abruptio placentae that occurs when blood accumulates between the placenta and the uterine wall, thereby reducing uterine contractility

_____ 58. Placental implantation in the lower uterine segment

_____ 59. Painless dilation of the cervical os without uterine contractions, often resulting in inability to carry the pregnancy to term

_____ 60. Fertilization of an ovum, the nucleus of which has been lost or inactivated, resulting in the formation of a mass of fluid-filled vesicles that resembles a bunch of white grapes

_____ 61. Premature separation of part or all of the placenta from its implantation site

_____ 62. Cord insertion at the margin of the placenta

_____ 63. Placenta divided into two or more separate lobes

COLUMN II

A. Incompetent cervix
B. Abruptio placentae
C. Hydatidiform mole (complete)
D. Battledore placenta
E. Ectopic pregnancy
F. Succenturiate placenta
G. Placenta previa
H. Miscarriage
I. Couvelaire
J. Velamentous cord insertion

64. Trauma continues to be a common complication during pregnancy that might require obstetric critical care.

A. *DISCUSS* the significance of this complication using statistical data to describe the scope of the problem in terms of incidence, timing during pregnancy, and forms of trauma.

B. *INDICATE* the effects that trauma can have on pregnancy.

C. *DESCRIBE* the potential effect of trauma on the fetus.

D. *EXPLAIN* why the nurse must be alert for signs and symptoms of abruptio placentae for at least 48 hours after the trauma has occurred.

FILL IN THE BLANKS: Insert the term that corresponds to each of the following.

65. Priorities of care for the pregnant woman following trauma must be to _____ and _____. This method of approach in care management is important because _____ survival is dependent on _____ survival. In cases of minor trauma the woman is evaluated for vaginal _____; uterine _____; abdominal _____, _____, or _____; and evidence of _____. A change in or absence of _____ or _____, leakage of _____, and presence of _____ in maternal circulation are also included in the assessment. In cases of major trauma the systematic evaluation begins with a(n) _____ and the initial ABCDs of resuscitation: _____, _____, _____, and _____.

66. COMPLETE the following table by identifying recommended treatment measures and nursing considerations for each infection.

Infection	Treatment Measures	Nursing Considerations
Bacterial vaginosis		
Candidiasis		
Chlamydia		
Gonorrhea		
Group B streptococcus		
Hepatitis B		
Herpes		
Human papillomavirus		
Syphilis		
Trichomoniasis		

FILL IN THE BLANKS: Insert the term that corresponds to each of the following.

TORCH Infections

67. A viral infection of the liver that is transmitted by droplets or hands improperly washed after defecation is _____.

68. _____ is a viral infection, also known as the three-day or German measles, that can produce major congenital anomalies during the first trimester and intrauterine growth restriction and systemic infection after the fourth month.

69. A protozoan infection transmitted by consumption of infected raw or undercooked meat or with poor handwashing after handling infected cat litter is called _____. Adverse fetal effects are more common with maternal acute infection.

70. _____ is a viral infection transmitted via contact with body secretions and fluids, including respiratory and genitourinary fluids, breast milk, and blood. Fetal infection can cause death or severe generalized disease, leading to anemia, hepatic damage, mental retardation, microcephaly, and deafness.

71. A viral infection of the liver transmitted in a manner similar to human immunodeficiency virus infection is called _____. An effective vaccination is available for its prevention.

72. _____ is a viral infection transmitted primarily by sexual contact. Active infection of the genital tract at the time of labor often requires cesarean birth.

MULTIPLE CHOICE: Circle the one correct option and state the rationale for the option chosen.

73. When measuring the BP to ensure consistency and facilitate early detection of BP changes consistent with gestational hypertension, the nurse should:
    A. Place the woman in a supine position.
    B. Allow the woman to rest for at least 15 minutes before measuring her BP.
    C. Use the same arm for all BP measurements.
    D. Use a proper-size cuff that covers at least 50% of the woman's upper arm.

74. When caring for a woman with mild preeclampsia, it is critical that the nurse be alert for signs of progression to severe preeclampsia. Progression to severe preeclampsia is indicated by which one of the following assessment findings?
    A. Proteinuria of 5 grams in a 24-hour collection.
    B. Dependent edema in the ankles and feet at bedtime
    C. Deep tendon reflexes 2; ankle clonus absent
    D. Blood pressure of 154/94 and 156/100 mm Hg 6 hours apart

75. A woman's preeclampsia has advanced to the severe stage. She is admitted to the hospital, and her primary health care provider has ordered an infusion of magnesium sulfate to be started. In implementing this order, the nurse:
    A. Prepares a solution of 20 g of magnesium sulfate in 100 ml of 5% glucose in water.
    B. Monitors maternal vital signs, fetal heart rate patterns, and uterine contractions every hour.
    C. Expects the maintenance dosage to be approximately 4 g/hour.
    D. Reports a respiratory rate of 12 breaths or less per minute to the primary health care provider immediately.

76. The primary expected outcome for care associated with the administration of magnesium sulfate is met if the woman:
    A. Exhibits a decrease in both systolic and diastolic BP.
    B. Experiences no seizures.
    C. States that she feels more relaxed and calm.
    D. Urinates more frequently, resulting in a decrease in pathologic edema.

77. A primigravida at 10 weeks of gestation reports slight vaginal spotting without passage of tissue and mild uterine cramping. When examined, no cervical dilation is noted. The nurse caring for this woman:

   A. Anticipates that the woman will be sent home and placed on bed rest with instructions to avoid stress or orgasm.

   B. Prepares the woman for a dilation and curettage.

   C. Notifies a grief counselor to assist the woman with the imminent loss of her fetus.

   D. Tells the woman that the doctor will most likely perform a cerclage to help her maintain her pregnancy.

78. A woman is admitted through the emergency department with a medical diagnosis of ruptured ectopic pregnancy. The primary nursing diagnosis at this time is:

   A. Acute pain related to irritation of the peritoneum with blood.

   B. Risk for infection related to tissue trauma.

   C. Deficient fluid volume related to blood loss associated with rupture of the uterine tube.

   D. Anticipatory grieving related to unexpected pregnancy outcome.

79. A woman diagnosed with an ectopic pregnancy is given an intramuscular injection of methotrexate. The nurse tells the woman that:

   A. Methotrexate is an analgesic that relieves the dull abdominal pain that she is experiencing.

   B. She should avoid alcohol until her primary care provider tells her that the treatment is complete.

   C. Follow-up blood tests are required for at least 6 months after the injection of the methotrexate.

   D. She should continue to take her prenatal vitamins to promote healing.

80. A pregnant woman at 32 weeks of gestation comes to the emergency department because she has begun to experience bright red vaginal bleeding. She reports that she is experiencing no pain. The admission nurse suspects:

   A. Abruptio placentae.

   B. Disseminated intravascular coagulation.

   C. Placenta previa.

   D. Preterm labor.

81. A pregnant woman at 38 weeks of gestation diagnosed with marginal placenta previa has just given birth to a healthy newborn boy. The nurse recognizes that the immediate focus for the care of this woman is:

   A. Preventing hemorrhage.

   B. Relieving pain.

   C. Preventing infection.

   D. Fostering attachment of the woman with her new son.

CRITICAL THINKING EXERCISES

1. Jean (2-1-0-0-1) is at 30 weeks of gestation and has been diagnosed with mild preeclampsia. The treatment plan includes home care with restricted activity, bathroom privileges and out of bed twice a day for meals, appropriate nutrition, and stress reduction. She and her husband are very anxious about the diagnosis and are also concerned about how they will manage the care of their active 3-year-old daughter, Anne.

   A. *INDICATE* the signs and symptoms that would have been present to indicate this diagnosis.

B. *LIST* three priority nursing diagnoses for Jean and her family.

C. *DESCRIBE* how you would help this couple organize their home care routine.

D. *SPECIFY* what you would teach them with regard to assessment of Jean's status and signs of worsening preeclampsia.

E. *DESCRIBE* the instructions that you would give Jean regarding her nutrient and fluid intake.

F. *DISCUSS* the measures that Jean can use to cope with the activity restriction requirement of her treatment plan.

2. Ellen, a pregnant woman at 37 weeks of gestation, is admitted to the hospital with a diagnosis of severe preeclampsia.

A. *INDICATE* the signs and symptoms that would have been present to indicate this diagnosis.

B. *LIST* three priority nursing diagnoses for Ellen.

C. *SPECIFY* the precautionary measures that should be taken to protect Ellen and her fetus from injury.

D. Ellen's physician orders magnesium sulfate to be infused at 4 g in 20 minutes as a loading dose, followed by a maintenance intravenous infusion of 2 g/hour.

1) *IDENTIFY* the guidelines that must be followed when administering magnesium sulfate intravenous piggy-back.

2) *EXPLAIN* the expected therapeutic effect of magnesium sulfate to Ellen and her family.

3) *LIST* the maternal-fetal assessments that should be done on a regular basis during the infusion of magnesium sulfate.

4) *IDENTIFY* the signs of magnesium sulfate toxicity.

5) *STATE* the interventions that must be instituted immediately if magnesium sulfate toxicity occurs.

E. Despite all prevention efforts, Ellen has a convulsion.

   1) *SPECIFY* the nursing measures that should be implemented at the onset of the convulsion and immediately afterward.

   2) *LIST* the problems that can occur as a result of the convulsion that Ellen has experienced.

F. Ellen successfully gave birth vaginally despite her high risk status. DESCRIBE Ellen's care management during the first 48 hours of her postpartum recovery period.

3. Marie, an 18-year-old primigravida, is diagnosed with hyperemesis gravidarum. She is admitted to the high risk antepartal unit.

A. *IDENTIFY* the predisposing and etiologic factors related to Marie's health problem.

B. *LIST* the physiologic and psychosocial factors of which the nurse should be aware when assessing Marie on her admission.

C. *STATE* two priority nursing diagnoses related to Marie's health problem.

D. *OUTLINE* the nursing care measures appropriate for Marie.

4. At times pregnant women require abdominal surgery.

   A. *IDENTIFY* the factors that can complicate diagnosis of and surgical treatment for abdominal problems during pregnancy.

   B. *IDENTIFY* the most common condition necessitating abdominal surgery during pregnancy. INDICATE the clinical manifestations that the pregnant woman would exhibit.

   FILL IN THE BLANKS: Insert the term that corresponds to each of the following.

   C. Preoperative care for a pregnant woman differs from that for a nonpregnant woman in one significant aspect (i.e., the presence of the _____). General preoperative observations and ongoing care are the same as for any surgery, with the addition of continuous _____ and _____ monitoring. Intraoperatively fetal oxygenation is improved by placing the woman on an operative table with a(n) _____ to avoid maternal _____. Continuous _____ and _____ monitoring must take place during the surgical procedure and in the postoperative period if intrauterine pregnancy continues.

   D. *IDENTIFY* the nursing considerations and topics for teaching related to the discharge planning process of the pregnant woman who has undergone abdominal surgery.

5. Andrea is admitted to the hospital, where a diagnosis of acute ruptured ectopic pregnancy in her fallopian tube is made.

A. *STATE* the risk factors associated with ectopic pregnancy.

B. *DESCRIBE* the findings most likely experienced and exhibited by Andrea as her ectopic pregnancy progressed and then ruptured.

C. *IDENTIFY* the other health care problems that share the same or similar clinical manifestations as ectopic pregnancy.

FILL IN THE BLANKS: Insert the term that corresponds to each of the following.

D. The major care management problem in ectopic pregnancy when the tube ruptures is _____.

E. _____ therapy is used as a nonsurgical treatment approach for hemodynamically stable women. This therapy causes _____ of the ectopic pregnancy if the mass is _____ and measures less than _____ in diameter by ultrasound.

F. *IDENTIFY* two priority nursing diagnoses appropriate for Andrea.

G. *OUTLINE* the nursing measures required during the preoperative and postoperative periods.

6. Janet is 10 weeks pregnant. She comes to the clinic and states that she has been experiencing slight bleeding with mild cramping for about 4 hours. No tissue has been passed, and pelvic examination reveals that the cervical os is closed. Her fundal height is consistent with a 10-week pregnancy.

A. *INDICATE* the most likely basis for Janet's signs and symptoms.

B. *OUTLINE* the expected care management of Janet's problem.

7. Denise, a primigravida, calls the clinic. She is crying while she tells the nurse that she has noted "a lot of bleeding" and she is sure that she is losing her baby.

A. *IDENTIFY* the questions that the nurse should ask Denise to obtain a more definitive picture of the bleeding that she is experiencing.

B. On the basis of the data collected, Denise is admitted to the hospital for further evaluation. Her signs and symptoms progress, and medical diagnosis of incomplete miscarriage is made. DESCRIBE the assessment findings that indicate the diagnosis of incomplete miscarriage.

C. *STATE* the nursing diagnosis that takes priority at this time.

D. *OUTLINE* the nursing measures that are appropriate for the priority nursing diagnosis you identified and the expected medical management of Denise's health problem.

E. *SPECIFY* the instructions that Denise should receive before her discharge from the hospital.

F. *LIST* the nursing measures appropriate for the nursing diagnosis of anticipatory grieving related to unexpected outcome of pregnancy.

8. Mary has been diagnosed with hydatidiform mole (complete).

A. *IDENTIFY* the typical signs and symptoms that Mary would most likely exhibit to establish this diagnosis.

B. *SPECIFY* the posttreatment instructions that the nurse must stress when discussing follow-up management with Mary.

FILL IN THE BLANKS: Insert the term that corresponds to each of the following.

C. A major concern associated with hydatidiform mole is the development of _____, which is indicated by a rising _____ titer and enlarging _____.

9. Two pregnant women are admitted to the labor unit with vaginal bleeding. Sara is at 29 weeks of gestation and is diagnosed with marginal placenta previa. Jane is at 34 weeks of gestation and is diagnosed with a moderate (grade II) premature separation of the placenta (abruptio placentae).

A. *COMPARE* the clinical picture that each of these women is likely to exhibit during assessment.

Sara   **Jane**

B. *CONTRAST* the care management approach required by each of the women as it relates to her diagnosis and the typical medical management.

Sara   **Jane**

C. *INDICATE* the considerations that must be given top priority following birth for each of these women.

Sara   **Jane**

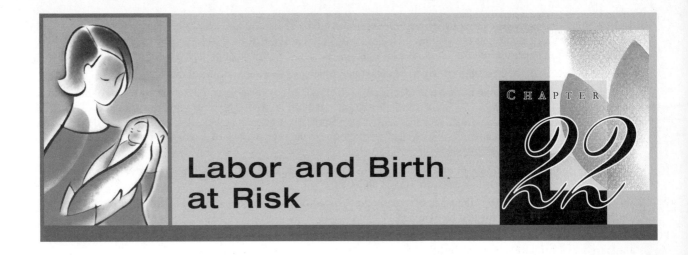

Labor and Birth at Risk

CHAPTER 22

CHAPTER REVIEW ACTIVITIES

FILL IN THE BLANKS: Insert the term that corresponds to each of the following.

Labor and Birth at Risk

1. _____ is any birth that occurs before the completion of 37 weeks of pregnancy.

2. _____ is defined as cervical changes and uterine contractions occurring between 20 and 37 weeks of pregnancy.

3. Preterm birth describes _____, whereas low birth weight describes only _____.

4. Low birth weight can be caused by _____, or _____, a condition of fetal growth not necessarily correlated with initiation of labor.

5. _____ can be used to predict who might experience preterm labor. The one most commonly used is _____.

6. _____ is a glycoprotein found in plasma and produced during fetal life. Its presence during the _____ trimesters may be related to _____, which is thought to be one cause of spontaneous preterm labor.

7. _____ is another possible predictor of preterm labor.

8. _____ is the rupture of the amniotic sac and leakage of amniotic fluid, beginning at least 1 hour before the onset of labor at any gestational age.

9. _____ is the rupture of the amniotic sac and leakage of fluid before 37 weeks of gestation. _____ often precedes this rupture, but the etiology remains unknown. _____ is an intraamniotic infection of the chorion and amnion that is potentially life threatening for the fetus and the woman.

10. _____ or _____, is defined as a long, difficult, or abnormal labor and is caused by various conditions associated with the _____.

11. _____ is described as abnormal uterine contractions that prevent the normal progress of _____, _____ (_____ powers), or _____ (_____ powers).

12. _____, or primary dysfunctional labor, often is experienced by an anxious first-time mother who is having _____ and _____ contractions that are ineffective in causing _____ or _____ to progress. These contractions usually occur in the _____ phase of the first stage of labor. _____ is usually prescribed for the management of this type of dysfunctional labor.

13. _____, or secondary uterine inertia, usually occurs when a woman initially makes normal progress into the active phase of labor and then uterine contractions become _____ and _____ or they _____.

14. _____ results from obstruction of the birth passage by an anatomic abnormality other than that involving the bony pelvis. The obstruction may result from _____, _____, _____, and a full _____ or _____.

15. _____ may be caused by anomalies, excessive fetal size and malpresentation, malposition, or multifetal pregnancy. _____, also called _____, is related to excessive fetal size. The most common fetal malposition is persistent _____. _____ is the most common form of malpresentation.

16. _____ is the gestation of twins, triplets, quadruplets, or more than four infants.

17. Six abnormal labor patterns have been identified and classified by Friedman (1989) according to the nature of _____ and _____. These patterns are _____, _____, _____, _____, _____, and _____. _____ is defined as a labor that lasts less than 3 hours from the onset of contractions to the time of birth. It can result from _____ that are _____ in intensity.

18. _____ is an attempt to turn the fetus from a breech or shoulder presentation to a vertex presentation for birth by exerting gentle, constant pressure on the abdomen.

19. A(n) _____ is the allowance of a reasonable period of spontaneous active labor so the safety of a vaginal birth for the mother and fetus can be assessed.

20. _____ is the chemical or mechanical initiation of uterine contractions before their spontaneous onset for the purpose of bringing about the birth.

21. _____ is a rating system used to evaluate the inducibility of the cervix. The five characteristics assessed are _____, _____, _____, _____, and _____. If the score is low, various hormones called _____ can be applied to the cervix to soften and thin or _____ the cervix.

22. _____ is the artificial rupture of the membranes. It can be used to _____ labor when the cervix is ripe or to _____ labor if the progress begins to slow.

23. _____ is the stimulation of uterine contractions after labor has started spontaneously but when progress is unsatisfactory. Common methods include _____ infusion and _____.

24. A(n) _____ is one in which an instrument with two curved blades is used to assist the birth of the fetal head.

25. _____ or _____ is a birth method involving the attachment of a vacuum cup to the fetal head using negative pressure.

26. _____ is the birth of the fetus through a transabdominal incision of the uterus.

27. A(n) _____ or _____ pregnancy is one that extends beyond the end of week 42 of gestation.

28. _____ is an uncommon obstetric emergency in which the head of the fetus is born but the anterior shoulder cannot pass under the pubic arch. Two major causes are _____ and _____.

29. _____ occurs when the cord lies below the presenting part of the fetus. Contributing factors to its occurrence include a(n) _____, _____, _____, or _____. When present, the woman is assisted into a position such as _____, _____, or _____. In these positions gravity keeps pressure of the _____ off the cord.

30. _____ or _____ occurs when a foreign substance enters the maternal circulation. The foreign substance that initiates the condition is presumed to be present in _____.

TRUE OR FALSE: Circle T if true or F if false for each of the following statements. Correct the false statements.

T   F   31. Spontaneous preterm births account for only one-fourth of all preterm births in the United States.

T   F   32. Preterm birth rates continue to rise.

T   F   33. Preterm birth is more dangerous than low birth weight because the shortened gestational time results in immature body systems.

T   F   34. The rate of preterm births among Caucasian women is nearly double the rate of African-American women in the United States.

T   F   35. Risk-scoring systems are excellent predictors of women who will go into labor prematurely.

T   F   36. Fetal fibronectin testing is more likely to predict women who will not go into preterm labor than women who will go into preterm labor.

T   F   37. Early recognition of preterm labor is essential in order to implement interventions to reduce neonatal morbidity and mortality.

T   F   38. Research evidence confirms that bed rest is highly effective in preventing preterm birth.

T   F   39. It is now thought that the best reasons to use tocolytics are to gain the time needed to administer antenatal glucocorticoids and to transfer the mother before birth to a hospital equipped to care for her preterm infant.

T   F   40. Dysfunctional labor can occur as a result of maternal factors such as fluid and electrolyte imbalance.

T   F   41. The most common type of uterine dysfunction is hypotonic uterine dysfunction.

T   F   42. A breech presentation is most common in term pregnancies.

T   F   43. Since 1980 the rate of multiple births has been increasing.

T   F   44. A diagnosis of secondary arrest of active labor is made when there has been no change in cervical dilation for 2 hours or more for both nulliparous and multiparous women.

T   F   45. Ripening of the cervix with a prostaglandin preparation usually results in a higher success rate for induction of labor.

T   F   46. Prepidil gel is inserted into the posterior fornix of the vagina.

T   F   47. Oxytocin is discontinued immediately, and the primary health care provider is notified if uterine hyperstimulation or a nonreassuring fetal heart rate (FHR) occurs during labor stimulation.

T   F   48. Research has consistently proven that the one-on-one support provided by a doula reduces the risk for cesarean birth for laboring women who receive this support.

T   F   49. The incidence of postterm pregnancy in the United States is approximately 25%.

T   F   50. Assisting the laboring woman into a hands-and-knees position can help resolve shoulder dystocia.

T   F   51. The maternal mortality rate for anaphylactoid syndrome of pregnancy is about 40%.

52. *IDENTIFY* two factors for each of the following risk categories for preterm labor and birth.

Demographic risks

Medical risks predating this pregnancy

Medical risks in current pregnancy

Behavioral and environmental risks

53. *EXPLAIN* why bed rest might be more harmful than helpful as a component of preterm labor care management.

MATCHING: Match the description of medications used as part of the management of preterm labor in Column I with the appropriate medication listed in Column II.

COLUMN I

_____ 54. Beta-adrenergic agonist often administered intravenously and the only drug approved by the Food and Drug Administration for the purpose of suppressing uterine contractions

_____ 55. Antenatal glucocorticoid used to accelerate fetal lung maturity when there is risk for preterm birth

_____ 56. Beta-adrenergic agonist often administered subcutaneously with a syringe or pump

_____ 57. Calcium channel blocker that relaxes smooth muscles, including those of the contracting uterus, administered orally

_____ 58. Classification of drugs used to suppress uterine activity

_____ 59. Central nervous system depressant used during preterm labor for its ability to relax smooth muscles; administered intravenously

_____ 60. Nonsteroidal antiinflammatory medication that relaxes smooth muscles as a result of prostaglandin inhibition; administered rectally or orally

COLUMN II

A. Tocolytic

B. Betamethasone

C. Ritodrine (Yutopar)

D. Terbutaline (Brethine)

E. Magnesium sulfate

F. Nifedipine (Procardia)

G. Indomethacin

MATCHING: Match the description of medications used for the management of cervical ripening and uterine stimulation in Column I with the medication listed in Column II.

COLUMN I

_____ 61. Tocolytic medication administered subcutaneously to suppress hyperstimulation of the uterus

_____ 62. Classification of hormones that can be used to ripen the cervix and/or stimulate uterine contractions

_____ 63. Cervical ripening agent in the form of a vaginal insert that is placed in the posterior fornix of the vagina

_____ 64. Cervical ripening agent in the form of a gel that is inserted into the cervical canal just below the internal os

_____ 65. Pituitary hormone used to stimulate uterine contractions in the augmentation or induction of labor

_____ 66. Cervical ripening agent used in the form of a tablet that can be administered orally, but more commonly intravaginally

COLUMN II

A. Oxytocin (Pitocin)

B. Misoprostol (Cytotec)

C. Dinoprostone (Cervidil)

D. Dinoprostone (Prepidil)

E. Terbutaline (Brethine)

F. Prostaglandin

67. *DESCRIBE* the five factors that cause labor to be long, difficult, or abnormal. Explain how they interrelate.

68. *EXPLAIN* the treatment approach of therapeutic rest.

69. Angela (1-0-0-0-0) is experiencing hypertonic uterine dysfunction, Bernice (3-1-0-1-1) is experiencing hypotonic uterine dysfunction, and Gloria (2-0-0-1-0) is having difficulty bearing down effectively. *COMPLETE* the following table by contrasting each woman's labor in terms of causes and precipitating factors, maternal-fetal effects, changes in pattern of progress, and care management.

	Angela (Hypertonic)	Bernice (Hypotonic)	Gloria (Inadequate Expulsion)
Causes/Precipitating factors			
Maternal-fetal effects			
Changes in progress of labor			
Care management			

70. Nurses caring for women during labor must always be alert for clinical manifestations of anaphylactoid syndrome of pregnancy (amniotic fluid embolism).

A. *IDENTIFY* the factors that increase a woman's risk for this life-threatening complication.

B. *LIST* the signs of anaphylactoid syndrome of pregnancy (amniotic fluid embolism) in each of the following categories for which the nurse must be alert when assessing pregnant women.

Respiratory distress

Circulatory collapse

Hemorrhage

C. *OUTLINE* the recommended care management of a woman experiencing anaphylactoid syndrome of pregnancy (amniotic fluid embolism).

71. *IDENTIFY* four indications for oxytocin induction and four contraindications to the use of oxytocin to stimulate the onset of labor.

Indications

Contraindications

MULTIPLE CHOICE: Circle the one correct option and state the rationale for the option chosen.

72. When assessing a woman during pregnancy, the nurse needs to be alert for signs that indicate risk for preterm labor and birth. Which of the following factors exhibited by a pregnant woman is associated with preterm labor and birth?

    A. Age of 30

    B. Obstetric history of 3-2-0-0-2

    C. Children 2 and 4 years of age

    D. Current treatment for second bladder infection in 4 months

73. A woman calls the prenatal clinic to report that she has been experiencing uterine contractions for the past hour at a frequency of every 8 to 10 minutes. One action the nurse tells this woman to take is to:

    A. Lie down on her side.

    B. Count contractions for 2 more hours.

    C. Reduce fluid intake.

    D. Report to the clinic for evaluation as soon as someone can bring her.

74. Bed rest for prevention of preterm birth is least likely to result in:

    A. Bone demineralization.

    B. Weight gain.

    C. Fatigue.

    D. Anxiety and depression.

75. A woman's labor is being suppressed using intravenous magnesium sulfate. Which of the following measures should be implemented during the infusion?

    A. Limit fluid intake to 2000 ml or less per day

    B. Assess FHR for tachycardia

    C. Ensure that calcium gluconate is available in case toxicity occurs

    D. Assist woman into a comfortable semirecumbent position

76. The physician has ordered that dinoprostone (Cervidil) be administered to ripen a pregnant woman's cervix in preparation for an induction of her labor. In fulfilling this order, the nurse:

    A. Inserts the dinoprostone into the cervical canal just below the internal os.

    B. Tells the woman to remain in bed for at least 15 minutes.

    C. Calls the woman's physician if she reports a history of asthma.

    D. Removes the dinoprostone if the woman begins to experience uterine contractions.

77. A nulliparous woman experiencing a postterm pregnancy is admitted for labor induction. Assessment reveals a Bishop score of 9. The nurse:

    A. Calls the woman's primary health care provider to order a cervical ripening agent.

    B. Mixes 20 U of oxytocin (Pitocin) in 500 ml of 5% glucose in water.

    C. Piggybacks the oxytocin solution into the port nearest the drip chamber of the primary intravenous tubing.

    D. Begins the infusion at a rate of 0.5 to 2 mU/min, as determined by the induction protocol.

78. A woman's labor is being induced. The nurse assesses the woman's status, that of her fetus, and the labor process itself just before an infusion increment of 2 mU/min. The nurse discontinues the infusion and notifies the woman's primary health care provider if which of the following had been noted during the assessment?

    A. Frequency of uterine contractions: Every 1½ minutes

    B. Variability of FHR: Present

    C. Deceleration pattern: Early decelerations noted with several contractions

    D. Intensity of uterine contractions at their peak: 80 to 85 mm Hg

79. A laboring woman's vaginal examination reveals the following: 3 cm, 50%, LSA, 0. The nurse caring for this woman:

    A. Places the ultrasound transducer in the left lower quadrant of the woman's abdomen.

    B. Recognizes that passage of meconium is a definitive sign of fetal distress.

    C. Expects the progress of fetal descent to be slower than usual.

    D. Assists the woman into a knee-chest position for each contraction.

CRITICAL THINKING EXERCISES

1. Imagine that you are a nurse-midwife working at an inner city women's health clinic. You are concerned about the rate of preterm labor and birth among the pregnant women who come to your clinic for care. *OUTLINE* a preterm labor and birth prevention program that you would implement at your clinic to reduce the rate of preterm labor and birth.

2. Sara, a primiparous woman (2-0-1-0-1) at 22 weeks of gestation, comes to the clinic for her scheduled prenatal visit. She is anxious because her last labor began at 26 weeks and she is worried that this will happen again. "I had no warning the last time. Is there anything I can do this time to have my baby later or at least know that labor is starting so I can let you know?"

    A. *IDENTIFY* the signs of preterm labor that the nurse-midwife should teach Sara.

    B. *EXPLAIN* how the nurse-midwife could help Sara implement a plan to reduce her risk for preterm labor.

C. About 3 weeks later, Sara calls the clinic and tells her nurse-midwife that she has been having uterine contractions about every 9 minutes or so for the last hour. *DESCRIBE* what the nurse-midwife should tell Sara to do.

D. Conservative measures do not work, and Sara's uterine contractions progress. She is admitted for possible tocolytic therapy. *SPECIFY* the criteria that Sara must meet before tocolysis can be safely instituted.

E. Sara is started on a tocolysis regimen that involves the intravenous administration of magnesium sulfate. *OUTLINE* the nursing care measures that must be implemented during the infusion to ensure the safety of Sara and her fetus.

F. The nurse is preparing to give Sara a dose of betamethasone as ordered by the physician.

1) *STATE* the purpose of this medication.

2) *EXPLAIN* the procedure that the nurse should follow in fulfilling this order.

3. Debra had been experiencing signs of preterm labor. After a period of hospitalization her labor was successfully suppressed, and she was discharged to be cared for at home. Debra is receiving terbutaline via a subcutaneous pump. She records her uterine activity twice a day with an ambulatory tokodynamometer device. Debra is on activity restriction with only bathroom privileges.

A. *IDENTIFY* two nursing diagnoses that would be appropriate related to Debra's home care regimen for preterm labor suppression.

B. *OUTLINE* what the nurse should teach Debra regarding the care and maintenance of the terbutaline subcutaneous pump that is being used.

C. *IDENTIFY* the side effects of terbutaline that the nurse should teach Debra before discharge.

D. *DESCRIBE* the instructions that Debra should be given regarding home uterine activity monitoring.

E. Debra has two children who are 5 and 8 years old. *SPECIFY* the suggestions that you would give to help Debra and her children cope with the activity restriction requirement ordered by Debra's primary health care provider.

4. Denise, a primigravida, has reached the second stage of her labor with her fetus at zero station and positioned LOP. She is experiencing intense low back pain. Denise did not attend any childbirth classes and is having difficulty pushing effectively. No anesthesia has been used.

A. *IDENTIFY* the factors that can have a negative effect on the secondary powers of labor (bearing-down efforts).

B. *DESCRIBE* how you would help Denise use her expulsive forces to facilitate the descent and birth of her baby.

C. *SPECIFY* the positions that would be recommended based on the position of the presenting part of Denise's fetus.

5. Anne, a primigravida, attended Lamaze classes with her husband, Mark. They were looking forward to working together during the labor and birth of their baby. Because of fetal distress, an emergency low-segment cesarean section with a transverse uterine incision was performed after 18 hours of labor. Even though Anne and her son are in stable condition and she is glad that "everything turned out okay for my son," she expresses a sense of failure, stating, "I couldn't manage to give birth to my son in the normal way, and now I never will!"

A. *LIST* the preoperative nursing measures that should have been implemented to prepare Anne physically and emotionally for the unexpected cesarean birth.

B. *SPECIFY* the assessment measures that are critical when Anne is in the recovery room following the birth.

C. *STATE* the postoperative nursing care measures that Anne requires.

6. A vaginal examination reveals that Marie's fetus is RSA. *SPECIFY* the considerations that the nurse should keep in mind when providing care for Marie.

7. Angela (2-0-0-1-0) is at 42 weeks of gestation and has been admitted for induction of her labor.

A. Assessment of Angela at admission included determination of her Bishop score. *STATE* the purpose of the Bishop score and *IDENTIFY* the factors that are evaluated.

B. Angela's score was 5. *INTERPRET* this result in terms of the planned induction of her labor.

C. Angela's primary health care provider ordered that dinoprostone be inserted. *STATE* the purpose of the dinoprostone, method of application, and potential side effects that can occur.

D. During induction of her labor, Angela's primary health care provider performs an amniotomy. *SPECIFY* the nursing responsibilities before, during, and after this procedure.

E. *INDICATE* which of the following actions reflect appropriate care (A) for Angela during the induction of her labor with intravenous oxytocin. If the action is not appropriate (NA), state what the correct action would be.

1) _____ Assist Angela into a lateral or upright position.
2) _____ Apply an external electronic fetal monitor and obtain a 15- to 20-minute baseline strip of FHR and pattern.
3) _____ Explain to Angela what to expect and techniques to be used.
4) _____ Prepare a primary line with an isotonic electrolyte solution.
5) _____ Attach the secondary line of dilute oxytocin (10 U in 1000 ml) to the distal port (farthest from the venipuncture site) of the primary intravenous line.
6) _____ Begin infusion at 4 mU/min.
7) _____ Increase oxytocin by 1 to 2 mU/min at 5- to 10-minute intervals after the initial dose until the desired pattern of contractions has been achieved.
8) _____ Stop increasing the dosage and maintain the level of oxytocin when contractions occur every 2 to 3 minutes, last 40 to 90 seconds, and reach an intrauterine pressure between 40 and 90 mm Hg if internal monitoring is being used.
9) _____ Monitor maternal blood pressure and pulse every 15 minutes and after every increment.

10) _____ Monitor FHR pattern and uterine activity every 15 minutes and with every increment.

11) _____ Limit intravenous intake to 1500 ml/8 hours.

F. *STATE* the major side effects of oxytocin for which the nurse must be alert when managing Angela's labor.

8. Lora is a 37-year-old nulliparous woman beginning her 42nd week of pregnancy. She and her primary health care provider have decided on a conservative "watchful waiting" approach because she and her fetus are not experiencing distress.

A. In helping Lora make this decision, the risks she and her fetus face as a result of a postterm pregnancy were explained. *IDENTIFY* the risks that Lora should have considered in making her decision.

B. *STATE* the clinical manifestations that Lora is likely to experience as her pregnancy continues.

C. *STATE* one nursing diagnosis appropriate for Lora's current situation.

D. *OUTLINE* the typical care management measures that should be implemented to ensure the safety of Lora and her fetus.

E. *SPECIFY* the instructions that the nurse should give to Lora regarding her self-care as she awaits the onset of labor.

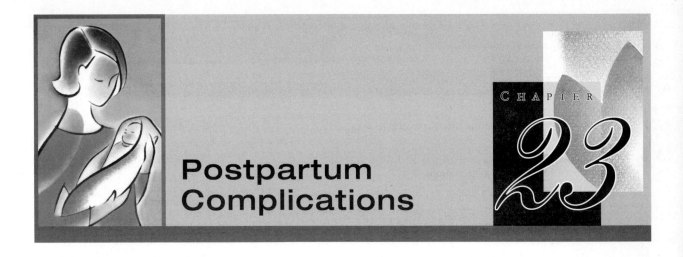

Postpartum Complications

CHAPTER REVIEW ACTIVITIES

FILL IN THE BLANKS: Insert the term that corresponds to each of the following.

Physical Complications Related to Childbirth

1. _____ is the loss of more than 500 ml of blood after vaginal birth and more than 1000 ml after cesarean birth. Additional criteria that might be used are a decrease in _____ of 10% or more between admission for labor and postpartum or a need for _____ . The leading cause is _____.

2. _____ or _____ occurs more than 24 hours but less than 6 weeks postpartum.

3. _____, _____, or _____ occurs within 24 hours of birth.

4. Marked hypotonia of the uterus is called _____.

5. A pelvic _____ is the collection of blood in vulvar, vaginal, or retroperitoneal tissue as a result of blood vessel damage. _____ are the most common. _____ are usually associated with a forceps-assisted birth, performance of an episiotomy, or status as a primigravida. The woman often complains of persistent _____ or _____ pain or a feeling of pressure in the _____.

6. _____ refers to the turning of the uterus inside out. The primary presenting signs of its presence are _____, _____, and _____. Contributing factors include _____ of the placenta, manual extraction of the _____, _____ umbilical cord, uterine _____, _____, and abnormally adherent _____.

7. _____ is the delayed return of the enlarged puerperal corpus to normal size and function.

8. _____ is an emergency situation in which profuse blood loss (hemorrhage) can result in severely compromised perfusion of body organs. Death can occur.

9. A(n) _____ is suspected when bleeding is continuous and there is no identifiable cause. _____ is an autoimmune disorder in which antiplatelet antibodies decrease the life span of the platelets. _____ is a type of hemophilia and is probably the most common of all types of hereditary bleeding disorders.

10. A(n) _____ is the formation of a blood clot or clots inside a blood vessel and is caused by _____ or partial _____ of the vessel. _____ involves the superficial saphenous venous system. In _____ involvement varies but can extend from the foot to the iliofemoral region. _____ occurs when part of a blood clot dislodges and is carried to the pulmonary artery, where it occludes the vessel and obstructs blood flow to the lungs.

11. _____ or _____ refers to any clinical infection of the genital canal that occurs within 28 days after miscarriage, induced abortion, or childbirth. The first symptom is usually a(n) _____ of 38° C or higher on _____ days of the first _____ postpartum days (not counting the first 24 hours).

12. _____ is the most common cause of postpartum infection. It usually begins at the _____ site.

13. _____ is an infection of the breast affecting approximately 1% to 10% of women soon after childbirth, most of whom are _____. This infection is almost always _____ and develops well after the _____ has been established.

14. _____ is a variation of the normal placement of the uterus, the most common type of which is _____ or retroversion.

15. Downward displacement of the uterus is known as _____. This dropping down of the uterus can range from mild to complete.

16. _____ is a protrusion of the bladder downward into the vagina. It develops when supporting structures in the vesicovaginal septum are injured.

17. _____ is the herniation of the anterior rectal wall through the relaxed or ruptured vaginal fascia and rectovaginal septum.

18. Uncontrollable leakage of urine is known as _____. When it occurs as a result of sudden increases in intraabdominal pressure associated with sneezing, coughing, or laughing, it is called _____.

19. A(n) _____ is an abnormal communication (opening) between one hollow viscus (organ) and another or from one hollow viscus to the outside. A communication between the bladder and the genital tract is called a(n) _____, and one between the rectum and the vaginal tract is called a(n) _____.

20. A(n) _____ is a device that can be placed in the vagina to support the uterus and hold it in the correct position.

21. Surgical repair of a cystocele is called _____, whereas _____ is the surgical repair of a rectocele.

TRUE OR FALSE: Circle T if true or F if false for each of the following statements. Correct the false statements.

T   F   22. Early PPH usually occurs as a result of uterine atony.

T   F   23. When a woman hemorrhages, changes in her baseline vital sign values might not be reliable indicators of shock in the immediate postpartum period because of the physiologic adaptations that occurred during pregnancy.

T   F   24. Dark red blood is a characteristic finding when deep lacerations of the cervix bleed.

T   F   25. Methergine is the oxytocic of choice for PPH if the woman is also experiencing preeclampsia.

T   F   26. Prostaglandin F2α (carboprost tromethamine, Hemabate) should be used with caution or not at all if the postpartum woman has asthma.

T   F   27. Placental retention because of poor separation is very common in postdate pregnancies.

T   F   28. Placenta percreta refers to a placenta that perforates the uterus.

T   F   29. Uterine inversion occurs most frequently in primiparous women with abruptio placentae.

T   F   30. The woman with a third- or fourth-degree laceration should not be given rectal suppositories or enemas to facilitate bowel elimination.

T   F   31. A major complication of blood replacement therapy is a hemolytic reaction.

T   F   32. Aspirin or aspirin-containing analgesics can be used safely if a woman is receiving heparin because aspirin enhances its effect.

T   F   33. The most effective and cost-saving treatment method for postpartum infection is prophylactic antibiotic therapy for 1 week postpartum.

T   F   34. Signs and symptoms of mastitis usually appear in the second to fourth postpartum week.

T   F   35. Lactation must be suppressed once mastitis has been diagnosed.

T   F   36. The most common type of uterine displacement is retroversion.

T   F   37. Symptoms of pelvic relaxation most often appear during the perimenopausal period as a result of decreasing ovarian hormone secretion.

T   F   38. Good hygiene of the genital area is critical when a pessary is being used.

T   F   39. An anterior and posterior colporrhaphy is performed to repair a uterine prolapse surgically.

40. *LIST* the factors that increase the risk for each of the following complications associated with childbirth.

Lacerations of the genital tract

Pelvic hematomas

Retained placenta

Inversion of the uterus

Subinvolution of the uterus

41. Hemorrhagic shock is an obstetric emergency. *LIST* the clinical manifestations indicative of hemorrhagic shock.

42. *STATE* the twofold focus of medical management of hemorrhagic shock.

43. *IDENTIFY* four priority nursing interventions for hemorrhagic shock.

44. *STATE* the standard of care for bleeding emergencies.

TRUE OR FALSE: Circle T if true or F if false for each of the following statements. Correct the false statements.

Postpartum Depression and Mood Disorders

T   F   45. Instructions regarding postpartum depression should be given to both the patient and her family.

T   F   46. Women who feel close to their husbands report fewer depressive symptoms.

T   F   47. Postpartum depression with psychotic features occurs in 1 to 2 per 1000 live births.

T   F   48. Once a woman has had postpartum depression with psychotic features, there is little risk that it will occur again with a subsequent pregnancy.

T   F   49. Women with postpartum depression might experience suicidal ideation and obsessional thoughts regarding violence to their newborns.

T   F   50. Women with postpartum depression are rarely treated with antidepressant medications.

T   F   51. Breastfeeding is contraindicated in a woman taking a psychotropic medication for depression.

FILL IN THE BLANKS: Insert the term that corresponds to each of the following.

52. Postpartum depression has a major impact on the health and well-being of the postpartum woman, her newborn, and her entire family. The definition of postpartum depression without psychotic features is a(n) _____ and _____ with _____ and _____. The incidence is from _____ to _____ of new mothers. These symptoms rarely disappear without outside help. A distinguishing feature of postpartum depression is _____. A prominent feature of postpartum depression is _____ of the infant, often caused by abnormal _____.

53. *STATE* the predisposing factors for postpartum depression.

54. *LIST* several of the clinical manifestations that are exhibited by women experiencing postpartum depression.

55. A common nursing diagnosis for postpartum depression is risk for impaired parenting related to limited ability of the depressed mother to interact with and care for her infant. *IDENTIFY* the nursing measures appropriate for this nursing diagnosis.

56. *CITE* measures and activities that can be used to prevent postpartum depression.

FILL IN THE BLANKS: Insert the term that corresponds to each of the following.

57. Postpartum psychosis is a syndrome most often characterized by _____, _____, and thoughts by the mother of _____. Symptoms of this syndrome often begin within _____ after birth, although the mean time to onset is _____ weeks and almost always within _____ weeks of the birth. Characteristically the woman begins to complain of _____, _____, and _____ and might have episodes of _____ and _____. Later _____, _____, _____, _____ statements, and _____ about the baby's well-being may be present. Delusions, when present, often are related to the _____, and in severe cases auditory hallucinations might command the mother to _____. A specific illness included in depression with psychotic features is _____, formerly called manic-depressive illness. This mood disorder is preceded or accompanied by _____ episodes and is characterized by _____, _____, or _____ moods.

58. *STATE* the focuses for care management of the woman with postpartum depression with psychotic features as they relate to the woman herself, her baby, and her family.

MULTIPLE CHOICE: Circle the one correct option and state the rationale for the option chosen.

59. Methylergonovine (Methergine) 0.2 mg is ordered to be administered intramuscularly for a profuse lochial flow with clots to a woman who gave birth vaginally 1 hour ago. Her fundus is boggy and does not firm after massage. She is still being treated for preeclampsia with intravenous magnesium sulfate, 1 g/hr. Her blood pressure, measured 5 minutes ago, was 155/98 mm Hg. In fulfilling this order, the nurse:
   A. Measures the woman's blood pressure again 5 minutes after administering the medication.
   B. Questions the order on the basis of the woman's hypertensive status.
   C. Recognizes that methylergonovine counteracts the uterine relaxation effects of the magnesium sulfate infusion that the woman is receiving.
   D. Tells the woman that the medication will lead to uterine cramping.

60. The nurse responsible for the care of postpartum women should recognize that the first sign of puerperal infection is most likely:
   A. Fever higher than 38° C after the first 24 hours following birth.
   B. Increased white blood cell count.
   C. Foul-smelling profuse lochia.
   D. Bradycardia.

61. The cesarean birth of a breastfeeding woman's infant occurred 2 days ago. Investigation of the pain, tenderness, and swelling in her left leg led to a medical diagnosis of deep vein thrombosis (DVT). Care management for this woman during the acute stage of the DVT involves:
   A. Explaining that she needs to stop breastfeeding until anticoagulation therapy has been completed.
   B. Administering warfarin orally.
   C. Placing the woman on bed rest with her left leg elevated.
   D. Fitting the woman with an elastic stocking so she can exercise her legs.

62. Which of the following measures is least effective in preventing postpartum depression?
   A. Sharing feelings and emotions with family members and her partner.
   B. Recognizing that emotional problems after having a baby are not unusual.
   C. Caring for the baby by herself to increase her level of self-confidence.
   D. Asking friends or family members to take care of the baby while she sleeps or has a "date" with her partner.

63. A priority question to ask a woman experiencing postpartum depression is:
   A. Have you thought about hurting yourself?
   B. Does it seem like your mind is filled with cobwebs?
   C. Have you been feeling insecure, fragile, or vulnerable?
   D. Does the responsibility of motherhood seem overwhelming?

1. Andrea is a multiparous woman (6-5-1-0-7) who gave birth to full-term twins vaginally 1 hour ago. Oxytocin (Pitocin) was used to augment her labor when hypotonic uterine contractions protracted the active stage of her labor. Special forceps were used to assist the birth of the second twin. Currently her vital signs are stable; her fundus is at the umbilicus, midline and firm; and her lochial flow is moderate to heavy, without clots.

   A. Early PPH is a major concern at this time. *STATE* the factors that have increased Andrea's risk for hemorrhage.

   B. *IDENTIFY* the priority nursing diagnosis at this time.

   C. During the second hour after birth the nurse notes that Andrea's perineal pad became saturated in 15 minutes and that a large amount of blood had accumulated on the bed under her buttocks. *DESCRIBE* the nurse's initial response to this finding. *STATE* the rationale for the action you described.

   D. The nurse prepares to administer 10 U of oxytocin intravenously as ordered by Andrea's physician. *EXPLAIN* the guidelines that the nurse should follow in fulfilling this order.

   E. During the assessment of Andrea, the nurse must be alert for signs of developing hypovolemic shock. *CITE* the signs that the nurse would be watching for.

F. *DESCRIBE* the measures that the nurse should use to support Andrea and her family in an effort to reduce their anxiety.

2. Nurses working on a postpartum unit must be constantly alert for signs and symptoms of puerperal infection in their patients.

   A. *LIST* the factors that can increase a postpartum woman's risk for puerperal infection.

   B. *IDENTIFY* the infection prevention measures that should be used when caring for postpartum women.

   C. *STATE* the typical clinical manifestations of endometritis for which the nurse should be alert when assessing postpartum women.

   D. *IDENTIFY* two nursing diagnoses that are appropriate for a woman diagnosed with endometritis.

   E. *DESCRIBE* the critical nursing measures essential in care management related to puerperal infection.

3. Sara, a primiparous breastfeeding mother at 2 weeks postpartum, calls her nurse-midwife to tell her that her right breast is painful and that she is not feeling well.

    A. *EXPLAIN* the assessment findings that the nurse-midwife should be alert for to indicate if Sara is experiencing mastitis.

    B. A medical diagnosis of mastitis of Sara's right breast is made. *STATE* two nursing diagnoses appropriate for this situation.

    C. *DESCRIBE* the treatment measures and health teaching that Sara needs regarding her infection and breastfeeding because she wishes to continue to breastfeed.

    D. *IDENTIFY* several behaviors that Sara should learn to prevent recurrence of mastitis.

4. Susan is a 36-year-old obese multiparous woman (4-3-0-1-3) who underwent a cesarean birth 2 days ago. A major complication of the postpartum period is the development of thromboembolic disease.

    A. *STATE* the risk factors for this complication that Susan presents.

B. When assessing Susan on the afternoon of her second postpartum day, the nurse notes signs indicative of DVT. *LIST* the signs that the nurse most likely observed.

C. A medical diagnosis of DVT is confirmed. *STATE* one nursing diagnosis appropriate for this situation.

D. *OUTLINE* the expected care management for Susan during the acute phase of DVT.

E. On discharge Susan will be taking warfarin for at least 3 months. *SPECIFY* the discharge instructions that Susan and her family should receive.

5. Teresa (6-5-0-1-5), a 60-year-old postmenopausal woman, has been diagnosed with a moderate uterine prolapse, accompanied by cystocele and rectocele.

A. *DESCRIBE* the signs and symptoms that Teresa most likely exhibited to establish this diagnosis.

B. *OUTLINE* the nursing care management approach recommended for Teresa's health problem.

C. Teresa will use a pessary during the day until a surgical repair can be accomplished. *SPECIFY* the instructions that you would give to Teresa regarding the use and care of a pessary.

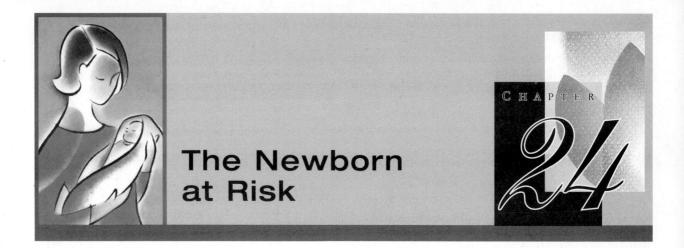

The Newborn at Risk

CHAPTER 24

CHAPTER REVIEW ACTIVITIES

TRUE OR FALSE: Circle T if true or F if false for each of the following statements. Correct the false statements.

T F 1. An extremely low-birth-weight infant is one whose weight at birth is 2000 g or less.

T F 2. Eight months after birth an infant born at 30 weeks of gestation is considered to be the corrected age of 5.5 months.

T F 3. The incidence of physical and emotional abuse is higher in infants who, because of preterm birth or illness, were separated from their parents for a time after birth.

T F 4. Preterm infants are at risk for polycythemia.

T F 5. Surfactant is administered intravenously to a preterm infant.

T F 6. Infants born before 36 weeks of gestation require exogenous surfactant administration to survive extrauterine life.

T F 7. Acrocyanosis is an assessment finding indicative of an underlying respiratory disorder.

T F 8. A preterm newborn's temperature should be monitored rectally to enhance accuracy.

T F 9. High risk infants usually have lower caloric, nutrient, and fluid requirements than those of the normal full-term newborn.

T F 10. Sucking on a pacifier during gavage feedings can facilitate the preterm newborn's transition to nipple feeding.

T F 11. The weight of most postmature infants is appropriate for gestational age.

T F 12. When meconium is present in the amniotic fluid at birth, the infant should be suctioned below the vocal cords before he or she takes his or her first breath.

T F 13. Preterm infants can better tolerate hypoglycemia than term infants.

T F 14. The presentation of the fetus can affect the type and location of birth injuries.

T F 15. A common clinical manifestation of Erb-Duchenne paralysis in the newborn is absence of the Moro reflex on the affected side.

T F 16. Neonatal spinal cord injuries are almost always a result of a birth complicated by shoulder dystocia.

T F 17. The woman infected with toxoplasmosis during pregnancy has a 90% chance of transmitting the infection to her fetus.

T F 18. Newborns infected with toxoplasmosis in utero are at risk for developing severe psychomotor problems or mental retardation.

T F 19. A major mode of transmission of gonorrhea to the fetus or newborn is via passage from an infected mother through her placenta to the fetus.

T   F   20. Maternal infection with syphilis is most dangerous to the fetus during the first trimester, when organogenesis takes place.

T   F   21. Penicillin is the antibiotic of choice for treating syphilis.

T   F   22. Infants born to mothers who had chickenpox 5 days before birth should be given varicella-zoster immune globulin at birth.

T   F   23. Women positive for the hepatitis B virus should not breastfeed their newborns.

T   F   24. Newborns infected with cytomegalovirus must begin receiving penicillin therapy within 24 hours of birth.

T   F   25. Snuffles is a common assessment finding exhibited by infants infected with herpes simplex virus (HSV).

T   F   26. The most common organism causing early onset neonatal sepsis is *Escherichia coli*.

T   F   27. Hepatitis B during pregnancy is associated with an increased risk for intrauterine growth retardation.

T   F   28. To prevent a chlamydial infection of the eyes, silver nitrate should be instilled over the cornea of the newborn's eyes immediately after birth.

T   F   29. Infants diagnosed with fetal alcohol syndrome (FAS) might develop learning, speech, and behavioral problems.

T   F   30. Maternal heroin use, especially during the first trimester, results in a high rate of congenital anomalies.

T   F   31. Marijuana use during pregnancy might result in a higher incidence of intrauterine growth restriction.

T   F   32. Newborns exposed to cocaine in utero begin a process of withdrawal within 24 hours of birth.

T   F   33. ABO incompatibility is more common than Rh incompatibility but causes less severe problems in the affected infant.

T   F   34. At birth, an indirect Coombs' test is performed on the newborn's cord blood to determine if the fetus has produced antibodies to his or her mother's blood.

T   F   35. Major congenital defects are the leading cause of death among infants in the United States.

T   F   36. The etiology for congenital heart defect is readily identified in the majority of diagnosed infants.

37. *EXPLAIN* the purpose of administering exogenous surfactant to the preterm newborn.

38. *DESCRIBE* kangaroo care.

39. The preterm infant is vulnerable to a number of complications related to immaturity of body systems. *COMPLETE* the following table by identifying the potential problems and the physiologic basis for each of the functions listed.

Physiologic Function	Potential Problems	Physiologic Basis
Respiratory function		
Cardiovascular function		
Maintenance of body temperature		
Central nervous system function		
Maintenance of adequate nutrition		
Maintenance of renal function		
Maintenance of hematologic status		
Resistance to infection		

40. *STATE* the infections represented by each letter in the acronym **"TORCH."**

  T

  O

  R

  C

  H

41. Sepsis is one of the most significant causes of neonatal morbidity and mortality.

  A. When caring for newborns, nurses must be alert for factors that increase the newborn's risk for sepsis. *IDENTIFY* the major risk factors that, if present, should alert the nurse to the increased potential for infection in the neonate.

  B. Early diagnosis is critical for successful treatment. *LIST* the signs that a neonate might exhibit indicating that sepsis is present.

  C. *DESCRIBE* two effective nursing measures for each of the following categories.

Prevention	**Cure**	**Rehabilitation**

42. *DESCRIBE* the physiologic basis for ABO incompatibility.

MATCHING: Match the description in Column I with the appropriate complication associated with oxygen therapy in Column II.

COLUMN I

_____ 43. Disorder of developing blood vessels in the eye often associated with oxygen tensions that are too high for the level of retinal maturity, resulting initially in vasoconstriction and continuing problems after the oxygen is discontinued

_____ 44. Acute inflammatory disease of the gastrointestinal mucosa commonly complicated by perforation

_____ 45. Result of the fetal shunt between the pulmonary artery and the aorta failing to constrict after birth or reopening after constriction has occurred

_____ 46. Chronic pulmonary iatrogenic condition caused by barotrauma from pressure ventilation oxygen toxicity

_____ 47. One of the most common types of brain injury encountered in the neonatal period and among the most severe in regard to both short-term and long-term outcomes

COLUMN II

A. Chronic lung disease (formerly bronchopulmonary dysplasia)

B. Retinopathy of prematurity

C. Patent ductus arteriosus

D. Periventricular-intraventricular hemorrhage

E. Necrotizing enterocolitis

FILL IN THE BLANKS: Insert the term that corresponds to each of the following.

48. Respiratory distress syndrome (RDS) is a lung disorder usually associated with preterm birth.
    A. RDS is caused by a lack of _____, which leads to progressive _____, loss of _____, and a(n) _____ imbalance, with uneven distribution of _____.
    B. Clinical signs of RDS include _____, _____, _____, _____, _____, _____ or _____ acidosis and _____ and _____. These respiratory symptoms usually occur immediately after _____. Physical examination reveals _____, _____, _____, and occasionally _____.
    C. RDS is usually self-limiting, with respiratory symptoms abating after _____ hours.
    D. Treatment for RDS is supportive. It involves establishing and maintaining adequate _____ and _____, administrating _____, and maintaining a(n) _____ environment.

49. A small brain present in a normally formed head is termed _____.

50. _____ results when the urinary meatus opens below the glans penis or anywhere along the ventral surface of the penis, scrotum, or peritoneum. _____ results when the urethral meatus opens on the dorsal surface of the penis. Abnormal development of the bladder, abdominal wall, and pubic symphysis that causes the bladder, urethra, and ureteral orifices to be exposed is called _____.

51. Enlargement of the ventricles of the brain, usually as a result of an imbalance between production and absorption of cerebrospinal fluid (CSF), characterized by a bulging anterior fontanel, an abnormal increase in the circumference of the head, and an increasing CSF pressure, is termed _____.

52. _____, a type of congenital disorder, can result in ventricular septal defects and tetralogy of Fallot.

53. _____, a common form of clubfoot, is characterized by plantar flexion, in which the toes are lower than the heel.

54. The most common congenital anomaly of the nose requiring emergency surgery after birth is _____. It consists of a bony or membranous septum between the nose and the pharynx.

55. _____ is a form of spina bifida cystica (a neural tube defect) in which an external sac containing the meninges and spinal fluid protrudes through a defect in the vertebral column.

56. _____ is a covered defect of the umbilical ring into which varying amounts of the abdominal organs can herniate. It is covered with a peritoneal sac. Herniation of the bowel through a defect in the abdominal wall to the right of the umbilical cord is termed _____. No membrane covers the contents.

57. _____ is the term denoting when the passageway from the mouth to the stomach ends in a blind pouch or narrows into a thick cord; thus a continuous passageway to the stomach is not present. An abnormal connection between this passageway and the trachea is called a(n) _____.

58. _____ is a type of neural tube defect characterized by the absence of both cerebral hemispheres and the overlying skull. It is incompatible with life.

59. _____ is a disorder characterized by displacement of the abdominal organs into the thoracic cavity.

60. _____ is a form of spina bifida cystica (a neural tube defect) in which an external sac containing the meninges, spinal fluid, and nerves protrudes through a defect in the vertebral column.

MULTIPLE CHOICE: Circle the one correct option and state the rationale for the option chosen.

61. Preterm infants are at increased risk for developing respiratory distress. The nurse should assess for signs that indicate that the newborn is having difficulty breathing. A sign of respiratory distress is:
   A. Use of abdominal muscles to breathe.
   B. Respiratory rate of 40 breaths/min or higher.
   C. Periodic breathing pattern.
   D. Suprasternal retraction.

62. When caring for a preterm infant at 30 weeks of gestation, the nurse should recognize that the newborn's priority nursing diagnosis is:
   A. Risk for infection related to decreased immune response.
   B. Impaired gas exchange related to deficiency of surfactant.
   C. Ineffective thermoregulation related to immature thermoregulation center.
   D. Imbalanced nutrition: less than body requirements related to ineffective suck and swallow.

63. A nurse is preparing to insert a gavage tube and feed a preterm newborn. As part of the protocol for this procedure, the nurse:
   A. Determines the length of tubing to be inserted by measuring from tip of nose to lobe of ear to midpoint between xiphoid process and umbilicus.
   B. Coats the tube with water-soluble lubricant to ease passage.
   C. Inserts tube through the nose as the preferred route for most infants.
   D. Checks placement of tube by injecting 2 to 3 ml of sterile water into the tube and listening for gurgling with a stethoscope.

64. The care management of a newborn whose mother is human immunodeficiency virus (HIV) positive most likely includes:
   A. Isolating the newborn in a special nursery.
   B. Cleansing of skin with soap, water, and alcohol before invasive procedures such as vitamin K administration.
   C. Wearing gloves for routine care measures such as feeding.
   D. Initiating zidovudine treatment once the newborn's HIV status has been determined.

65. An Rh-negative woman (2-2-0-0-2) has just given birth to an Rh-positive baby boy. The direct and indirect Coombs' test results are both negative. The nurse:
    A. Prepares to administer Rh$_o$(D) immunoglobulin (RhoGAM) to the newborn within 24 hours of his birth.
    B. Observes the newborn closely for signs of pathologic jaundice.
    C. Recognizes that RhoGAM is not needed because both Coombs' test results are negative.
    D. Administers RhoGAM intramuscularly to the mother within 72 hours of her baby's birth.

66. A newborn female has been diagnosed with myelomeningocele. Which of the following is an important nursing measure to protect the newborn from injury and further complications during the preoperative period?
    A. Maintaining the newborn in a lateral or prone position
    B. Telling the parents that they cannot hold their newborn
    C. Covering the sac with Vaseline gauze to keep it moist and intact
    D. Placing a collection bag over the genitalia to collect urine

CRITICAL THINKING EXERCISES

1. Baby girl Jane has been receiving oxygen therapy. Her health care providers are preparing to begin the process of weaning her from the oxygen.

    A. *DESCRIBE* signs indicating that Jane is ready to be weaned from oxygen therapy.

    B. *OUTLINE* the guidelines that should be followed when weaning Jane from oxygen therapy.

2. The neonatal intensive care unit (NICU) is a stressful environment for preterm infants and their families.

    A. *IDENTIFY* the common sources of stress facing infants and their families in an intensive care environment.

    Infant stressors   **Family stressors**

B. Nurses working in the NICU must be aware of infant cues and adjust stimuli accordingly. *LIST* infant cues that indicate overstimulation and those that indicate a relaxed state.

Overstimulation

Relaxed state

C. *IDENTIFY* specific measures that can be used to protect infants from overstimulation yet provide appropriate stimulation to meet their developmental and emotional needs.

D. *SPECIFY* the guidelines that should be followed regarding infant positioning.

E. *DESCRIBE* the nursing measures that should be used to support the parents of an infant who is being cared for in an NICU.

3. Marion is beginning her 43rd week of pregnancy.

A. *SUPPORT THIS STATEMENT:* Perinatal mortality is significantly higher in the postmature fetus and neonate.

B *STATE* the assessment findings typical of a postmature infant.

C. *DISCUSS* the two major complications that can be experienced by a postmature infant.

4. Baby girl Susan was born 2 hours ago. Her mother tested positive for HBsAg antibodies as a result of infection with hepatitis B virus.

A. *DESCRIBE* the protocol that should be followed in providing care for Susan.

B. Susan's mother asks the nurse if she can breastfeed her baby daughter. *DISCUSS* the nurse's response to this mother's question.

5. Baby boy Andrew is a full-term newborn who was just born by spontaneous vaginal delivery. Genital herpes (HSV) recurred in his mother, and her membranes ruptured before the onset of labor.

A. *IDENTIFY* the four modes of transmission of HSV to the newborn. *INDICATE* the mode most likely to have transmitted the infection to Andrew.

B. *LIST* the clinical signs that Andrew would exhibit as evidence of a disseminated and localized HSV infection.

C. *DESCRIBE* the recommended nursing measures related to each of the following.

Management after birth before discharge

Vidarabine or acyclovir therapy

6. Baby girl Mary is 1 day old. Her mother is HIV positive but received no treatment during pregnancy.

A. *DISCUSS* Mary's potential for development of HIV infection.

B. *IDENTIFY* the modes of transmission of HIV to Mary.

C. *NAME* the opportunistic and secondary infections, if contracted by Mary, that would strongly suggest that she is infected with HIV.

D. *DESCRIBE* the care measures recommended for Mary.

E. Mary's mother wishes to breastfeed Mary because she has read that it can prevent infection and help her to bond with her infant. *DISCUSS* the nurse's response to this mother's request.

7. Jane, a newborn, has been diagnosed with FAS as a result of moderate-to–sometimes heavy binge drinking by her mother throughout pregnancy.

A. *DESCRIBE* the characteristics that Jane most likely exhibited to establish the diagnosis of FAS.

B. *STATE* three long-term effects that Jane could experience as she gets older.

C. *DESCRIBE* two nursing measures that could be effective in promoting Jane's growth and development.

8. Maternal substance abuse can be harmful to fetal and newborn health status as well as growth and development.

   A. *DESCRIBE* the assessment findings associated with newborn withdrawal from each of the following substances.

   Heroin

   Methadone

   B. Susan has just been born. Her mother used cocaine during pregnancy. *IDENTIFY* the effects that Susan might exhibit as a result of exposure to cocaine while in utero.

9. Tony is a 2-hour-old newborn. It is suspected that his mother abused drugs during pregnancy.

   A. *LIST* the signs associated with neonatal abstinence syndrome that the nurse should look for when assessing Tony.

   B. Tony begins to exhibit signs confirming that his mother used heroin during pregnancy. *CITE* two nursing diagnoses that are appropriate for Tony.

   C. *OUTLINE* the care management that Tony and his mother require.

10. Angela, who is Rh negative, had a miscarriage at 13 weeks of gestation, which resulted in what she said was just a heavier-than-usual menstrual period. Six months later she became pregnant again.

   A. *DESCRIBE* the physiologic basis for Rh incompatibility and the occurrence of sensitization.

   B. An indirect Coombs' test is positive. *STATE* the meaning of this finding.

   C. *INDICATE* whether Angela is a candidate for RhoGAM. *SUPPORT* your answer.

   D. *DESCRIBE* RhoGAM and its use.

   E. Angela's fetus is at risk for erythroblastosis fetalis and hydrops fetalis. *EXPLAIN* each of these conditions.

   Erythroblastosis fetalis

   Hydrops fetalis

F. *DESCRIBE* the treatment approaches that can be used to prevent intrauterine fetal death and early neonatal death for Angela's baby.

11. Baby girl Jennifer was born with spina bifida cystica, myelomeningocele. *DESCRIBE* the measures that the nurse should use to manage Jennifer's care and help her parents cope with this congenital anomaly.

12. Baby boy Thomas was just born. He is exhibiting signs that the nurse-midwife and the neonatologist believe are consistent with a diaphragmatic hernia.

A. *IDENTIFY* the clinical manifestations that Thomas most likely exhibited to cause his health care providers to suspect diaphragmatic hernia.

B. *STATE* the priority nursing diagnosis for Thomas.

C. *OUTLINE* the essential care measures during the immediate postbirth period.

13. Baby girl Denise was born with a cleft lip and palate.

    A. *STATE* three nursing diagnoses faced by Denise and her parents. *DISCUSS* the rationale for each nursing diagnosis stated.

    B. *OUTLINE* several nursing measures that need to be implemented to ensure Denise's well-being until surgical repair can be accomplished.

14. Anita gave birth to a baby boy who died shortly thereafter as a result of multiple congenital anomalies, including anencephaly. She and her husband, Bill, are provided with the opportunity to see their baby.

    A. *DISCUSS* how the nurse can help Anita and Bill make a decision about seeing their baby that is right for them.

    B. Anita and Bill decide to see their baby. *SPECIFY* the measures that the nurse can use to make the time Anita and Bill spend with their baby as easy as possible and provide them with an experience to facilitate the grieving process.

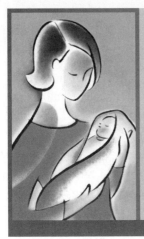

Answer Key

CHAPTER 1: 21ST CENTURY MATERNITY NURSING: CULTURALLY COMPETENT, FAMILY AND COMMUNITY FOCUSED

Chapter Review Activities

1. C, 2. H, 3. D, 4. F, 5. A, 6. G, 7. B, 8. E, 9. J, 10. M, 11. L, 12. K, 13. N, 14. I

15. Maternity Nursing

16. Evidence-based practice

17. Telehealth

18. Ethnocentrism

19. Acculturation

20. Assimilation

21. Cultural relativism

22. Cultural context

23. Cultural knowledge

24. Cultural competence

25. Family dynamics: negotiation, boundaries, channels

26. Family systems theory

27. Family life cycle (developmental) theory

28. Family stress theory; internal, external

29. aggregates

30. Vulnerable populations; adolescent, older, incarcerated, homeless

31. A, 32. B, 33. D, 34. C

35. T, 36. T, 37. F, 38. T, 39. F, 40. T, 41. F, 42. T, 43. F, 44. T, 45. T, 46. F, 47. F, 48. F, 49. T, 50. T, 51. T, 52. T, 53. T, 54. F, 55. T, 56. T

57. *Identify factors related to infant mortality:* limited maternal education, young maternal age, unmarried, poverty, lack of prenatal care, poor nutrition, smoking, alcohol and drug use, poor maternal health status.

58. *State and describe three major changes in health care of women and their infants:* nurse-midwives, family-centered care, LDR/LDRPs, early discharge, neonatal security systems

59. *List barriers to prenatal care in United States:* lack of insurance with resultant inability to pay, lack of transportation, dependent child care, minority status, young maternal age, homelessness, lack of providers for low-income women

60. *Family theories:* see Family Theories section for a description of family theory.

61. *Discuss how to consider products of culture when providing care:*

    A. *Communication:* consider language; need for a translator; dialect, style, and volume of speech; meaning of touch and gestures.

    B. *Space:* include feelings of territoriality (varies); comfort zone must be established in terms of touch, proximity to others, handling of possessions; patient must be in control of personal space to ensure a sense of autonomy and security.

    C. *Time:* consider past, present, and future orientations and how these could affect meeting appointments and health care practices, beliefs, and goals.

    D. *Family roles:* include parents' role; roles for grandparents; and father's participation in pregnancy, labor, birth, and child care.

62. *Identify factors that influence woman's and family's adherence to cultural beliefs and practices:* mention individual subculture within the primary group, degree of acculturation, income level, and amount of contact with older generations.

63. *Indicators to assess community health and well-being:* see Box 1-9, which lists each category of indicators.

64. *Cite the problems faced by migrant laborers and families:* see Women and the Migrant Work Force subsection; include such problems as financial instability; child labor; poor housing and education; cultural barriers; limited access to services; hazardous work conditions; domestic violence; and health problems such as diabetes, hypertension, asthma, malnutrition, TB, substance abuse, and infection.

65. *Three characteristics of refugees that increase their vulnerability:* see characteristics listed in the Refugees and Immigrants subsection; focus on cultural and language barriers and on significant physical and emotional problems, including the experience of violence.

Critical Thinking Exercises

1. *High-technology care will not reduce rate of preterm birth and LBW infants:* see sections that cover the following topics:
   - Factors associated with LBW and IMR
   - Factors that escalate rate of high risk pregnancy
   - High-tech care: what it can and cannot do

2. *Proposed changes with rationale:* should reflect efforts toward improving access to care, using research-based approaches and standards to guide care, and creating health care services that address the factors associated with poor pregnancy outcomes.

3. *Self-management approaches proposed:* should emphasize health teaching regarding nutrition and stress management; anticipatory guidance during pregnancy and parenting; facilitated decision making by providing information regarding the pros and cons of care choices available such as nurse-midwives, doulas, birth settings, and length of stay; and referral to self-help groups.

4. *Imagine that you are a nurse working in a multicultural prenatal clinic:* consider the components of communication, space, time, roles; identify the degree to which each woman and family adheres to cultural beliefs and practices; do not stereotype.

5. *Pamela, a Native-American woman who is pregnant:*
   A. *Questions to ask:* see questions listed in the Cultural Considerations section.
   B. *Communication approach to use:* see Childbearing Beliefs and Practices section; include concepts of communication patterns, space, time, and family roles.
   C. *Identify Native-American beliefs and practices:* determine her individual beliefs and practices—do not stereotype.

6. *Hispanic family—recent birth of twin girls:*
   A. *Process of providing care in a cultural context:* Cultural Considerations box.
   B. *Describe cultural beliefs and practices:* see Childbearing Beliefs and Paractices section.

7. *Refugee couple from Bosnia—prenatal care:*
   - Consider the process of working with an interpreter, as outlined in Box 1-7; be sure to show respect for this couple by addressing the questions and comments to them and not to the interpreter.
   - Consult Chapter 3 for information regarding the stressors faced by refugees and the health care needs they present.
   - Research Bosnia: cultural and religious beliefs and practices and current political turmoil that led this couple to come to the United States.

8. *Home care nurse must become familiar with neighborhoods and their resources:*
   A. *Walking survey:* use observational skills during a walking tour through a community
   B. *Use of findings:* see Box 1-9, which discusses each of the components of the survey. Describe how each of these components could reflect the strengths and problems of a community; try using the survey to assess your community and the community in which your college is located.

CHAPTER 2: ASSESSMENT AND HEALTH PROMOTION

Chapter Review Activities

1. *Preconception Care:* see Preconception Counseling section and Box 2-1 to formulate answer.
   A. *Describe preconception care:* helps couples avoid unintended pregnancy and guides risk management so harmful behaviors can be changed to those that promote well-being because the first trimester is critical for fetal development (woman might not even know she is pregnant).
   B. *List purposes:* identify and treat problems so they do not recur; minimize fetal malformation; use behavior modification and risk reduction.
   C. *Components:* health promotion, risk factor assessment, interventions.
   D. *Individuals who should participate:* all women of childbearing age; women who have had problems with a previous pregnancy; men who plan a pregnancy with their partner.

2. *Identify reasons for seeking health care:* preconception care and counseling, pregnancy, well-woman care, fertility control, infertility treatment, menstrual problems, perimenopause.

3. F, 4. T, 5. T, 6. T, 7. T, 8. F, 9. F, 10. F, 11. T, 12. T, 13. T, 14. F, 15. T, 16. F, 17. F, 18. T, 19. F, 20. T, 21. F, 22. F, 23. F 24. T, 25. T, 26. F, 27. F, 28. F, 29. T, 30. T

31. *Components of well-woman care:* these include health assessment, age-appropriate screening, and health promotion and illness prevention activities such as attention to health risks and support from health care provider; using holistic approach that considers culture, religion, age, personal differences; and ensuring that access to care is facilitated by addressing barriers.

32. *Barriers to seeking health care:* see Barriers to Seeking Health Care section; address financial, cultural, and gender issues.

33. *Impact of illicit drugs on the maternal-fetal unit:* see specific subsection for each drug; consider effects of cocaine, heroin, marijuana.

34. *See* Cycle of Violence subsection—answer should include the three phases of the cycle of violence: repeated, increasing tension, battery; calm and remorse; honeymoon.

35. Intimate partner violence, wife battering, spouse abuse, domestic, family violence, physical, sexual, psychologic, economic; pregnancy

36. Rape, penile penetration, sex organ, labia; sexual assault, touches, kisses, hugs, petting, intercourse, sexual

37. *List consequences of STIs:* infertility, ectopic pregnancy, neonatal morbidity and mortality, genital cancers, AIDS, death

38. *Identify risks for gynecologic cancers:* see Gynecologic Conditions Affecting Pregnancy section; several risk factors for cervical, endometrial, and ovarian cancers are identified.

39. *Characteristics of women in battering relationships:* blaming for not being a good partner, history of violence in family of origin, social isolation, low self-esteem.

40. Mons pubis

41. Labia majora

42. Labia minora

43. Prepuce

44. Frenulum

45. Fourchette

46. Clitoris

47. Vestibule

48. Perineum

49. Vagina, rugae, Skene's, Bartholin

50. Fornices

51. Uterus, cul-de-sac of Douglas

52. Corpus

53. Isthmus

54. Fundus

55. Endometrium

56. Myometrium

57. Uterine (fallopian) tubes

58. Ovaries, ovulation, estrogen, progesterone, androgen

59. Cervix, endocervical, internal os, external os, squamocolumnar, Pap

60. Breasts

61. Tail of Spence

62. Nipple

63. Areola

64. Montgomery's tubercles

65. Acini

66. Lactiferous sinuses (ampullae)

67. *Label illustrations:*

A. *External female genitalia:* A. prepuce; B. labia minora; C. hymen; D. orifice of vagina; E. vestibule; F. fourchette; G. anus; H. perineal body; I. opening of Bartholin gland; J. labia majora; K. orifice of urethra; L. clitoris; M. mons pubis

B. *Perineal body:* A. posterior fornix; B. buttocks; C. rectum; D. anus; E. perineal body; F. vagina; G. urethra; H. symphysis pubis; I. bladder; J. anterior fornix; K. uterus; L. cul de sac of Douglas

C. *Cross section of uterus, adnexa, and upper vagina:* A. fundus; B. body (corpus) of uterus; C. endometrium; D. myometrium; E. internal os of the cervix; F. external os of the cervix; G. vagina; H. endocervical canal; I. fornix of vagina; J. cardinal ligament; K. uterine blood vessels; L. broad ligament; M. ovary; N. fimbriae; O. infundibulum of uterine tube; P. ampulla; Q. ovarian ligament; R. isthmus of uterine tube; S. interstitial portion of uterine tube

D. *Female breast (sagittal section):* A. clavicle; B. intercostal muscle; C. pectoralis major; D. alveolus; E. ductule; F. duct; G. lactiferous duct; H. lactiferous sinus; I. nipple pore; J. suspensory ligament of Cooper; K. sixth rib; L. second rib. *Female breast (anterior dissection):* A. acini cluster; B. lactiferous (milk) ducts; C. lactiferous sinus ampulla; D. nipple pore; E. areola; F. Montgomery's tubercle

E. *Female pelvis:* A. seventh lumbar vertebra; B. iliac crest; C. sacral promontory; D. sacrum; E. acetabulum; F. obturator foramen; G. subpubic arch under symphysis pubis; H. ischium; I. pubis; J. ilium; K. sacroiliac joint

68. Label illustrations:

A. *Label diagram of menstrual cycle:* A. gonadotropin-releasing hormone; B. FSH; C. LH; D. follicular phase; E. luteal phase; F. graafian follicle; G. ovulation; H. corpus luteum; I. estrogen; J. progesterone; K. menstruation; L. proliferative phase; M. secretory phase; N. ischemic phase; O. hypothalamic-pituitary cycle; P. ovarian cycle; Q. endometrial cycle

B. *Hormones of menstrual cycle:* see Endometrial Cycle, Hypothalamic-Pituitary Cycle, Ovarian

Cycle, and Prostaglandin sections for a description of each hormone.

69. *Description of pelvic examination:* each component of the examination is fully described in a separate subsection of the Pelvic Examination section.

70. *Guidelines for performing a Pap test:* see Procedure box—Papanicolaou (Pap) Test for preparation guidelines related to douching, use of vaginal preparations, intercourse, and menstruation.

71. *Breast self-examination technique:* A. –, B. –, C. +, D. +, E. +, F. –, G. –, H. +, I. +

72. A is correct; all women including their partners, not just specific groups, should participate in preconception care 1 year before planning to get pregnant.

73. C is correct; smoking is associated with preterm birth, not with postterm pregnancies.

74. C is correct; self-examination should not be used for self-diagnosis but rather for detecting early changes and seeking guidance of a health care provider if changes are noted.

75. C is correct; women should not tub bathe, use vaginal medications or contraceptives, or douche for 24 hours before the test.

76. A is correct; all women should be screened because abuse can happen to any woman; abuse often escalates during pregnancy. The most commonly injured sites are head, neck, chest, abdomen, breasts, and upper extremities. If abuse is suspected, the nurse must assess further to encourage disclosure and then assist the woman to take action and formulate a plan.

Critical Thinking Exercises

1. *Process of preconception counseling:*
   - Explain importance of preparing for pregnancy and how critical it is to be in good health and follow good health habits in the first trimester even before you know that you are pregnant.
   - Implement the components of preconception care.
   - Include George in counseling and care.

2. *Describe approach for well-woman care with woman who is anxious and embarrassed:*
   - Support and reassure from the first contact so she will feel comfortable coming for care in the future; serious concerns may surface.
   - Coordinate her care—ensure that all appropriate services are provided, assessment completed, and health guidance given; consider that this might be her only contact with the health care system.
   - Interview with sensitivity and do a careful, respectful examination because she might be embarrassed by her signs and symptoms.

3. *Pregnant woman who smokes:*
   - Discuss impact of smoking on pregnancy, using statistics, illustrations, research, and case studies to convince woman of the harmful effects that her habit has on her, her pregnancy, and her baby before and after it is born; see Smoking subsection of Substance Use and Abuse section.
   - Help her change her behavior by referring her to smoking cessation programs; use motivation of pregnancy to at least limit, if not stop, smoking completely; see Substance Use Cessation subsection of Anticipatory Guidance for Health Promotion, Prevention section.

4. *Health promotion and illness prevention class for a group of young adult women:*
   A. Content outline: see individual subsections for nutrition, exercise, and health risk prevention in Anticipatory Guidance for Health Promotion and Prevention sections; consider forming support groups for women who wish to change behaviors using the concept of a "buddy system" to facilitate positive, long-lasting change.
   B. *Meaning of safer sex:* discuss meaning of risky behavior, consequences of infections and how to prevent them
   C. *Measures to protect self from violence and injury:* inform woman regarding protective and legal services, including resources and hotlines; facilitate access; promote assertiveness; refer to self-defense courses and support or self-help groups; educate to develop independence; see Health Protection section.

5. *Woman experiencing stress:*
   A. *Identify effects of stress:* see Stress subsection of Health Risk section.
   B. *Stress management techniques:*
      - Identify sources of stress and measures that can be used to reduce the stress from these sources.
      - Discuss stress relievers, time management skills, relaxation exercises, use of biofeedback and guided imagery, role playing.
      - See Stress Management subsection in Anticipatory Guidance for Health Promotion and Prevention sections.

6. *Conducting a health history interview of a female patient:*
   A. *Writing questions to use:* use Health History outline in the Health Assessment section as a guide for question areas; questions should be open-ended, clear, and concise and should progress from the general to the specific.
   B. *Communication variations:* See Cultural Considerations box.

7. *Teaching self-examination techniques:* because each technique involves cognitive, psychomotor, and affective learning, a variety of methodologies must be used, including discussion of techniques (when and how often to do it, why it should be done, what is normal and abnormal, who to call if changes are noted, what will happen to determine basis of the change, and feelings regarding performance), literature, demonstration and redemonstration, videos and illustrations, breast models, and guest speakers (women who have used the techniques successfully for early detection and prompt treatment).

   A. *Breast self-examination:* see Patient Instructions for Self-Management box—Breast Self-Examination for full explanation of the technique.

   B. *Vulvar (genital) self-examination (VSE):* see VSE subsection of the Pelvic Examination section for a full explanation of the technique.

8. *Culturally sensitive approach to women's health care:*

   • Approach woman in a respectful and calm manner.

   • Consider modifications in the examination to maintain her modesty.

   • Incorporate communication variations such as conversational style, pacing, space, eye contact, touch, time orientation.

   • Take time to learn about woman's cultural beliefs and practices regarding well-woman care.

9. *Screening for abuse when providing well-woman care:* see Abused Women subsection of Women with Special Needs section.

   A. *Adjusting the environment:* provide for comfort and privacy; assess woman alone without her partner or adult children present.

   B. *Abuse indicators:* indications of abuse and areas of the body most commonly injured include head, neck, chest, abdomen, breasts, and upper extremities; note location and patterns of bruises and burns and specific somatic complaints.

   C. *Questions to ask:* Fig. 2-11 lists four questions that *ALL* women should be asked.

   D. *Approach if abuse is confirmed:*

   • Acknowledge the abuse and affirm that it is unacceptable and common; tell her that you are concerned and that she does not deserve it.

   • Communicate that it can recur; discuss the cycle of violence and inform her that help is available. Empower woman to use the help available to her and her children.

   • Help her formulate an escape plan.

10. *Assisting with a pelvic examination:* see Procedure box—Assisting with Pelvic Examination and Pelvic Examination section.

   A. Woman should be taught about what is going to occur as part of the examination and assisted to change clothes and get into the position required for the examination; inform and support woman during the examination and provide privacy; assist with cleansing, getting into an upright position, and dressing after the examination; discuss any questions and concerns that woman might have related to the examination.

   B. Assist with preparing and supporting the patient, preparing equipment, and taking care of specimens.

CHAPTER 3: COMMON CONCERNS

Chapter Review Activities

1. Amenorrhea

2. Dysmenorrhea

3. Primary

4. Estrogen and progesterone

5. Secondary dysmenorrhea; a few days before menses

6. Premenstrual syndrome, symptoms occur in the luteal phase and resolve within a few days of the onset of menstruation, symptom-free period occurs in the follicular phase, symptoms are recurrent, symptoms have a negative effect on woman's life, other diagnoses have been excluded

7. Endometriosis; proliferative, secretory, menstruation, inflammatory, fibrosis, adhesions

8. Dysmenorrhea, dyspareunia, infertility; diarrhea, pain with defecation, constipation; fertility

9. Oligomenorrhea; oral contraceptive pills

10. Metrorrhagia

11. Menorrhagia

12. Dysfunctional uterine bleeding, anovulation, luteinizing hormone, progesterone, corpus luteum; menarche, menopause

13. T, 14. T, 15. T, 16. F, 17. F, 18. F, 19. T, 20. T, 21. F, 22. T, 23. F, 24. F, 25. T, 26. T, 27. F, 28. T, 29. F, 30. F, 31. F, 32. T, 33. F

34. *Complete table related to STIs and vaginal infections:* see Infection section for specific subsection for each infection listed on the table.

35. Uterine tubes, uterus, ovaries, peritoneal

36. *C. trachomatis,* one half; vagina, endocervix, upper genital tract; menses, infectious agent, abortion, pelvic surgery, childbirth

37. Ectopic pregnancy, infertility, chronic pelvic pain, dyspareunia, pyosalpinx, tuboovarian abscess, pelvic adhesions

38. Pain, fever, chills, nausea and vomiting, increased vaginal discharge, symptoms of urinary tract infection, irregular bleeding

39. Prevention, education to avoid STIs, preventing lower genital tract infections from ascending to the upper genital tract

40. *Risk factors for hepatitis B:* ethnic background, place of employment and type of job, types of contacts with other persons such as family and friends, multiple sex partners, and intravenous drug use

41. *HIV in women:* see HIV Infection section

    A. *Mode of transmission:* exchange of body fluids

    B. *Signs and symptoms during seroconversion:* viremic, influenza-type responses such as fever, headache, night sweats, malaise, lymphadenopathy, myalgia, nausea, diarrhea, weight loss, sore throat, and rash

    C. *Risk behaviors:* IV drug use, high risk sex partner, multiple sex partners, history of multiple STIs

    D. *Management:* education, expert multidisciplinary care with a holistic focus, referrals (psychologic, legal, financial), measures to prevent infection and maintain resistance, prophylactic medication; see Management subsection

42. *State two precautions for Standard Precautions and Precautions for Invasive Procedures:* see Box 3-4, which describes several precautions for each category.

43. *Risk factors for breast cancer:* see Box 3-5 for a full list.

44. A is correct; decreasing the ingestion of red meats and switching from a high-fat to a low-fat diet have been associated with symptom relief; asparagus and cranberry juice have a natural diuretic effect that can reduce edema and related discomforts; simple refined sugars, not complex carbohydrates, and salt should be avoided for 7 to 10 days before menstruation to reduce fluid retention.

45. D is correct; alcohol, tobacco, and caffeine can worsen symptoms, whereas exercise can provide relief, as can peaches and watermelon, both of which have a natural diuretic effect; current research suggests that vitamin B_6 is not an effective form of treatment.

46. C is correct; women taking danazol often experience masculinizing changes; it is taken orally for 3 to 6 months; ovulation might not be fully suppressed and thus birth control is essential because this medication is teratogenic.

47. C is correct; dysfunctional uterine bleeding is most commonly associated with anovulatory cycles in women at the extremes of their reproductive years (puberty, perimenopause); it can also occur when women secrete low levels of progesterone; it is associated with obesity.

48. A is correct; because these infections are often asymptomatic, they can go undetected and untreated, causing more severe damage, including ascent of the pathogen into the uterus and pelvis, resulting in PID and infertility. Many effective treatment measures are available, including for chlamydia.

49. B is correct; A indicates candidiasis; C indicates HSV 2; D indicates trichomoniasis.

50. B is correct; metronidazole is used to treat bacterial vaginosis and trichomoniasis; penicillin is effective in the treatment of syphilis; acyclovir is used to treat HSV-2.

51. D is the correct answer; recurrent infections commonly involve only local symptoms that are less severe; stress reduction, healthy lifestyle practices, and acyclovir can reduce recurrence rate; viral shedding can occur before lesions appear.

52. D is correct; fibroadenomas are generally small, unilateral, firm, nontender, movable lumps in the upper outer quadrant; borders are discrete and well defined; discharge is not associated with this breast disorder.

Critical Thinking Exercises

1. *Woman with hypogonadotropic amenorrhea* (see Hypogonadotropic Amenorrhea section):

    A. *Risk factors exhibited:* athletic competition subjectively scored, inappropriate fat-to-lean ratio, nutritional deficits related to need to maintain body size, stress, rigorous exercise, need to wear body-revealing clothing, prepubertal body shape for success

    B. *Nursing diagnosis:* risk for disturbed body image or anxiety related to delayed onset of menstruation and development of secondary sexual characteristics

    C. *Expected outcomes:* Maria will:

      • Verbalize understanding of basis for delayed onset of pubertal changes.

      • Participate in a therapeutic regimen that favors age-appropriate physical development.

    D. *Care management:*

      • Use stress reduction measures.

      • Reduce exercise or gain weight through good nutrition to alter fat-to-lean ratio.

      • Involve family and coach in treatment plan.

      • Discuss risk for osteoporosis.

      • Begin hormone treatment or calcium supplementation if needed.

2. *Woman experiencing dysmenorrhea* (see Dysmenorrhea—Primary subsection of Menstrual Problems section):

    A. *Nursing diagnosis:* consider the areas of pain and altered role performance as the focus for nursing management of this woman's primary dysmenorrhea; use assessment findings to determine which takes precedence.

B. *Self-care measures:* discuss basis of problem and explain that it usually diminishes with age; suggest nonpharmacologic measures such as exercise, relaxation techniques, good nutrition, heating pad; pharmacologic measures such as nonsteroidal anti-inflammatory drugs and oral contraceptives can be ordered.

3. *Woman with PMS—nursing approach* (see PMS section):

A. *Typical signs and symptoms:* clinical manifestations are usually related to the effects of fluid retention, behavioral and emotional changes, cravings, headache, fatigue and energy level, and backache.

B. *Nursing diagnoses:* nursing diagnoses might include acute pain, activity intolerance, disturbed sleep pattern, constipation or diarrhea, ineffective role performance; use assessment findings to determine those that would apply to a particular woman, including those that are a priority.

C. *Nursing approach:*
   • Obtain a detailed history and encourage woman to keep a diary of her physical and emotional manifestations (what occurs, when, circumstances) from one cycle to another.
   • Individualize plan based on this woman's experiences.
   • Discuss nutrition, exercise, and lifestyle and career measures.
   • Refer to appropriate support group or to counseling, if needed.
   • Discuss pharmacologic approaches available.

4. *Woman with endometriosis* (see Endometriosis section):

A. *Clinical manifestations:* dysmenorrhea, pelvic pain and heaviness, thigh pain, gastrointestinal symptoms, dyspareunia, metrorrhagia, menorrhagia

B. *Pathophysiology of the disorder:* growth of endometrial tissue is outside the uterus, mainly in the pelvis; implants respond to cyclical changes in hormones; bleeding leads to inflammatory response and formation of scar tissue, adhesions, and fibrosis.

C. *Pharmacologic management:* each pharmacologic approach is discussed in the Management subsection; oral contraceptives (create a pseudopregnancy and shrink implants), gonadotropin-releasing hormone antagonists, and androgenic synthetic steroids create a pseudomenopause.

D. *Support measures:* educate regarding basis for clinical manifestations, discuss treatment options for relief, both pharmacologic and nonpharmacologic; refer to support groups and counseling as needed; work with the couple together and separately; review options for pregnancy, because infertility can be an outcome.

5. *Woman with pelvic inflammatory disease (PID)* (see Pelvic Inflammatory Disease section):

A. *Nursing management plan:*
   • **Position and activity:** recommend bed rest in the semi-Fowler's position to keep pelvis in the dependent position; elevate legs slightly to prevent pulling on pelvis, which would increase discomfort.
   • **Comfort measures:** use analgesics, back rub, hygiene, relaxation techniques, diversional activities.
   • **Support measures:** provide time for woman to discuss feelings and include partner in care as appropriate; help woman deal with effects of the PID and the potential long-term effects; use a nonjudgmental, empathetic approach.
   • **Health education:** teach how to comply with treatment regimens, including taking medications properly, refraining from intercourse until fully healed, and using contraceptives and safer sex measures.

B. *Self-management during recovery phase:* see Patient Instructions for Self-Management box—Prevention of Genital Tract Infections.

6. *Measures to prevent transmission of hepatitis B virus* (see Hepatitis B subsection of Virally Transmitted STI section): teach immunoprophylaxis for household members and sexual contacts, high level of personal hygiene, careful disposal of items contaminated with blood or body fluids including saliva, safer sex measures.

7. *Woman concerned regarding possible exposure to HIV:*

A. *Risky behaviors:* mention exposure to infected body fluids, including semen and blood; discuss sexual practices and partners and possible intravenous drug use.

B. *Testing procedure:* see HIV Testing and Counseling subsection for full description of testing protocol, counseling required, and legal implications; nurse should witness an informed consent, tell woman how long it will take for results to be available, consider ethical issues of confidentiality and privacy, and use a nonjudgmental, empathetic approach.

C. *Counseling protocol:* counseling should occur before and after testing and be done by the same person; counseling should take place in a private area with no interruptions.

D. *Instruction following a negative test result* (see Prevention subsection of STI section): use Sonya's risky behaviors as a basis for discussing prevention measures, including safer sex practices; discuss the impact that HIV infection could have on her health and her fetus should she become pregnant.

8. *Woman diagnosed with HSV 2* (see HSV—Management section):

   A. *Measures to relieve pain and prevent secondary infection:*

      - Use appropriate antiviral medications.
      - Cleanse lesions twice a day with saline; use a warm sitz bath with baking soda.
      - Keep dry with cool hair dryer or pat dry; use hydrogen peroxide, Burow's solution.
      - Wear cotton underwear, loose clothing.
      - Use oral analgesics; limit use of topicals to decrease discomfort.
      - Follow healthy diet and lifestyle to enhance healing.

   B. *Preventing and reducing recurrence:*

      - Educate regarding cause, signs and symptoms of recurrence, transmission, treatment, precipitating factors for reactivation of the virus.
      - Keep diary to identify stressors, recurrences, helpful measures.
      - Use stress reduction measures; avoid heat, sun, hot baths; use a lubricant during intercourse to reduce friction.

9. *Woman with a lump in her left breast* (see Cancer of Breast section):

   A. *Diagnostic protocol:* include clinical examination of the breast by health care provider, mammography, needle aspiration and localization biopsy, laboratory testing (complete blood count, liver enzymes, serum calcium, alkaline phosphatase).

   B. *Preoperative care measures:* answer should emphasize education and support, including a visit from a woman who has had the same procedure; implement typical preoperative physical care measures; immediate postoperative care measures: answer should emphasize establishing physiologic stability, taking care not to take blood pressure, perform a venipuncture, or give parenteral medications in the affected arm; care for dressing and drains, being alert for signs of hemorrhage (check drainage container and area under the patient for excessive bleeding).

   C. *Self-management instructions for home:* see Patient Instructions for Self-Management box—Post-Mastectomy for identification of areas for health teaching to prepare woman to care for herself at home.

   D. *Support measures:*

      - Help woman and her partner deal with her change in appearance and self-concept; encourage open communication with nurse and one another; meet with woman and partner together and separately.

   - Refer to community resources, including Reach For Recovery.
   - Discuss follow-up treatments that might be required, including chemotherapy and radiation.
   - Discuss reconstructive surgery and use of prosthesis, as appropriate, for this woman.

CHAPTER 4: CONTRACEPTION, ABORTION, AND INFERTILITY

Chapter Review Activities

1. T, 2. T, 3. F, 4. F, 5. T, 6. F, 7. T, 8. T, 9. F, 10. F, 11. F, 12. T, 13. T, 14. F

15. *Characteristics of ideal contraceptive:* safe, easily available, economical, acceptable, simple to use, promptly reversible

16. *Meaning of "BRAIDED":* benefits, risks, alternatives, inquiries, decisions, explanations, documentation

17. *Fill in the Blanks:*

    A. Irregular menstrual periods

    B. 5, 22

    C. Ovulation-detection, cervical mucus, amount, consistency

    D. Basal body temperature (BBT), cervical mucus, increased libido, midcycle spotting, mittelschmerz, pelvic fullness, or tenderness, vulvar fullness

    E. Luteinizing hormone (LH), 12 to 24

18. *Label as C correct or I incorrect:*

    A. C; B. C; C. I; D. C; E. I; F. I

19. *Label as C correct or I incorrect:*

    A. C; B. C; C. C; D. C; E. I; F. I; G. I; H. C

20. *Cite four factors for seeking an abortion:* preserve life and health of the mother, genetic disorder of fetus, rape or incest, pregnant woman's request.

21. T, 22. T, 23. F, 24. T, 25. T, 26. T, 27. F

28. *Couple makes first visit to fertility clinic* (see Infertility section and subsections):

    A. *Identify and describe components for normal fertility:* include normal male and female reproductive tract, hormonal support for gametogenesis, timing of intercourse, adequate sperm and ova, patent tubal system for passage of sperm and ova.

    B. *Support statement that assessment for infertility must involve both partners:* see Box 4-6, which outlines findings favorable for fertility indicating male and female factors; cite statistics that reveal that a female factor causes 50%, a male factor causes 35%, and unexplained factors cause 15%.

29. *Pharmacologic measures to treat infertility:* Table 4-4 reviews medications used in the treatment of infertility.

30. *Alternative reproductive technologies:*

　A. *Definitions of each type:* see Table 4-5.

　B. *Issues:* see Box 4-5, which identifies religious and cultural considerations related to the use of alternative reproductive technologies.

31. A is correct; oral contraception provides no protection from sexually transmitted infections (STIs); therefore a condom and spermicide are still recommended to prevent transmission; B, C, and D reflect appropriate actions and recognition of adverse reactions.

32. B is correct; cervical mucus is thickened, thereby inhibiting sperm penetration; ovulation and the development of the endometrium are also inhibited; there is no protection from STIs; the overall effectiveness rate is nearly 100% if used correctly.

33. B is correct; spinnbarkeit refers to the stretching capability of cervical mucus at ovulation to facilitate passage of sperm; there is an LH surge before ovulation; BBT rises in response to increased progesterone after ovulation; cervical mucus becomes thinner and more abundant with ovulation.

34. B is correct; danazol is used to create pseudomenopause when a woman has endometriosis—its use causes the implants to atrophy and shrink, thereby increasing the chance that a woman will be fertile after treatment has been completed; she should not attempt to get pregnant during treatment because danazol is teratogenic.

Critical Thinking Exercises

1. *Discuss approach to use when woman seeks information about birth control:*

　• *Level of knowledge regarding how her body works and different methods:* determine her and/or her partner's preferences for and objections to specific measures; fully discuss methods preferred or not known to the woman and/or her partner

　• *Sex practices:* beliefs and preferences, number of partners, frequency of coitus:

　　— Level of contraceptive involvement: comfort with touching genitalia, myths and misconceptions, religious and cultural factors

　　— Health status as determined during a thorough health history interview, physical examination, and laboratory testing as appropriate

2. *Woman choosing to use a combination estrogen-progestin oral contraceptive:*

　A. *Mode of action:* suppression of hypothalamus and anterior pituitary, altered maturation of the endometrium, and thickened cervical mucus.

　B. *Advantages of use:* easy to take at same time of day, not directly related to sex act, improved sexual response, regular predictable menses with decreased blood loss, decreased dysmenorrhea and premenstrual syndrome, protection from endometrial and possibly ovarian cancer, reduced incidence of benign breast disease, protection against functional ovarian cysts, decreased risk for ectopic pregnancy.

　C. *Contraindications:* history of thromboembolic disorders, cerebrovascular or coronary artery disease, breast cancer, estrogen-dependent tumors, pregnancy, impaired liver function/tumor, smoker older than 35 years, lactation less than 6 weeks postpartum, headaches with focal neurologic symptoms, hypertension, with blood pressure higher than 160/100 mm Hg, diabetes mellitus with vascular disease.

　D. *Signs and symptoms requiring woman to stop taking oral contraceptive pill (OCP) and notify her health care provider:* see Signs of Potential Complications box—Oral Contraceptives for full explanation of "ACHES."

　E. *Specify patient instructions:*

　　• Follow specific directions on package insert in terms of taking the pill and what to do if one or more are missed.

　　• Use own pills, not someone else's, because OCPs vary.

　　• Discuss side effects and complications.

　　• Check effect of other medications being taken on the effectiveness of the OCP.

　　• Stress importance of using STI protection and alternative method for the first cycle on the OCP.

3. *Woman using a cervical cap:* discuss proper size and fit, when to insert and length of time it can and should stay in place, how to insert and check placement, use of spermicide, and no use during menses.

4. *Instructions following insertion of intrauterine device (IUD):* see Signs of Potential Complications box—Intrauterine Devices; teach woman how and when to check the string (after menses, at ovulation, and before coitus); inform woman when the IUD needs to be replaced.

5. *Couple contemplating sterilization* (see Sterilization section):

　A. *Decision-making approach:* nurse acts as a facilitator to help couple explore the pros and cons of sterilization itself and the methods available; nurse also provides information about each method.

　B. *Preoperative and postoperative care measures and instructions:*

　　• **Preoperative period:** complete holistic health assessment in terms of history, physical examination, and laboratory tests; discuss preparatory instructions, witness an informed consent.

- **Postoperative period:** discuss prevention and early detection of bleeding and infection; self-care measures in terms of hygiene, comfort, reduction of swelling with ice packs, scrotal support, moderate activity restriction for 2 or 3 days.
- **Caution that sterility is not immediate:** an alternative method must be used until sperm count is zero for two consecutive semen analyses; STI protection must be considered as appropriate.

6. *Couple using symptothermal method of contraception:*

   A. *List components:* BBT, cervical mucus, secondary cycle phase-related symptoms

   B. *Measuring BBT:* see Contraception subsection and Fig. 4-3; *evaluating cervical mucus characteristics:* see Patient Instructions for Self-Management box—Cervical Mucus Characteristics.

7. *Couple undergoing testing for infertility:*

   A. *Assessment of the man and woman:* see Assessment subsection of Care Management section and Boxes 4-3 and 4-4 for identification of factors that influence fertility and should be the basis for assessment.

   B. *Procedure for semen analysis:* see Semen Analysis subsection of Assessment of Male Infertility section; emphasize need to abstain for 2 to 5 days before the collection; not to use a spermicide; to bring the specimen to the laboratory within 2 hours of collection, making sure to use a clean container; and not to expose the specimen to excessive heat or cold.

   C. *Semen characteristics:* see Box 4-7 for a full list of expected characteristics in terms of liquification, volume, pH, density, morphology.

   D. *Nursing support measures:* see Psychosocial subsection of Care Management section; help the couple express feelings and openly discuss sexuality issues; help the couple with the decision-making process; facilitate the grieving process when they determine that biologic children are not in their future; refer to support groups or adoption agencies as appropriate.

CHAPTER 5: GENETICS, CONCEPTION, AND FETAL DEVELOPMENT

Chapter Review Activities

1. Ovum, ovarian follicle; cilia; 24

2. Sperm, 4 to 6, 2 to 3; capacitation; ampulla; zona reaction

3. Nuclei, diploid; zygote; 3, morula; blastocyst, implanted, 6 to 10; decidua; chorionic villi, trophoblast; basalis

4. *Functions of yolk sac, amniotic and fluid membranes, umbilical cord, placenta:* see individual subsections for each structure in the Development of the Embryo section.

5. Fetal circulation—shunts: see Fetal Circulatory System subsection in the Fetal Maturation section; Fig. 5-12; discuss ductus venosus (liver bypass), ductus arteriosus (lung bypass), and foramen ovale (shunt between the atria; lung bypass).

6. T, 7. F, 8. T, 9. T, 10. F, 11. F, 12. T, 13. F, 14. F, 15. T, 16. F, 17. T, 18. T, 19. F, 20. F, 21. T, 22. F

23. *Genetic counseling* (see Genetics section for a discussion of each section of this question):

   A. *Estimation of risk:* use mendelian principles for disorders caused by a specific factor that segregates during cell division (unifactorial inheritance); estimation of risk for multifactorial inheritance is much less accurate.

   Interpretation of risk: explanation of risk to the couple without giving advice about what to do; couple makes decision, not the health care provider.

   B. *Nurse's role in genetic counseling:* clarify information and provide follow-up care, which includes providing emotional support and referring the couple to agencies and support groups related to their specific genetic disorder.

   C. *Ethical considerations:* considerations revolve around the issues of stem cell research, pregnancy termination as an option, autonomy, privacy, confidentiality, and use of the human genome.

24. *Complete table related to primary germ layers:* see Primary Germ Layers subsection of the Embryo and Fetus section for identification of tissues and organs that develop from each layer.

25. *Factors that determine risk for inheritable disorder* (see Genetics section): health status of family members, abnormal reproductive outcomes, history of maternal disorders, drug exposures, illnesses, advanced maternal and paternal age, and ethnic origin.

26. *Explain each type of inheritance and give example:*

- **Unifactorial inheritance:** inheritable characteristic is controlled by a single gene, recessive or dominant.
- **Multifactorial inheritance:** congenital disorder results from a combination of genetic and environmental factors.
- **X-linked inheritance:** transmission of abnormal genes on the X chromosome; both males and females can be affected; abnormality tends to be less severe in females because they also have a normal gene on their second X chromosome.

27. A is correct; autosomal dominant inheritance is unrelated to exposure to teratogens; each pregnancy has

the same potential for expression of the disorder. There is no reduction in risk if one child is already affected by the disorder; if the gene is inherited, it is always expressed.

28. D is correct; there is a 25% chance that females will be carriers; if males inherit the X chromosome with the defective gene, the disorder will be expressed and they can transmit the gene to female offspring; females are affected if they receive the defective gene from both parents.

29. D is correct; cystic fibrosis, as an inborn error of metabolism, follows an autosomal recessive pattern of inheritance; two defective genes (one from each parent) are required for the disorder to be expressed. She does not have the disorder, and the father does not have the defective gene; therefore none of their children will have the disorder, but there will be a 50% chance that they will be carriers of the defective gene.

30. D is correct; feeling movement is called quickening; the gender of a baby is determined at conception; the heart begins to pump blood by the third week, and a beat can be heard with ultrasound by the eighth week of gestation.

Critical Thinking Exercises

1. *Questions from prenatal patients to nurse-midwives:*

    A. *Progress of fetal development at 2 months, 5 months, and 7 months:* see Table 5-1 to formulate answer; use of illustrations and life-size models facilitates learning.

    B. *Survival after 35 weeks of gestation:* discuss how the respiratory system develops, including the critical factor of surfactant production; describe how surfactant helps the newborn to breathe.

    C. *Fetal sensory perception:* discuss sensory capability of the fetus using Sensory Awareness subsection of the Fetal Maturation section; fetus can hear sounds such as parents' voices and can respond to light touch.

    D. *Sex determination:* discuss function of the X and Y chromosomes; inform mother that sex of fetus becomes recognizable around 12 weeks of gestation.

    E. *Multiple gestation—twins:* discuss monozygotic (identical) and dizygotic (fraternal) twinning and how each occurs; emphasize that fraternal-type twinning tends to occur in families.

2. *Couple facing a genetic disorder:*

    A. *Process to determine genetic risk:* Tay-Sachs is an autosomal recessive disorder that follows a unifactorial inheritance pattern; Mr. G. needs to be tested because he must also be a carrier to produce a child with the disorder; emphasize nurse's role in terms of emotional support, facilitation of the decision-making process, and interpretation of diagnostic test results and how can they influence future childbearing decisions.

    B. *Inheritance possibility when both parents carry a recessive gene:* because both parents are carriers of a recessive gene, there is a one-in-four chance that the child will be normal, two-in-four chance that the child will be a carrier, as they are, and one-in-four chance that the child will have the disorder. This inheritance pattern is the same for every pregnancy; there is no reduction or increase in risk from one pregnancy to another.

    C. *Decision-making process for this couple:* discuss nature of this disorder, extent of risk and consequences if the child inherits the disorder, options available related to pregnancy, use of amniocentesis to determine whether child is affected, choice to continue with the pregnancy or have an abortion, use of reproductive technology, adoption, or childlessness; couple must ultimately make their own informed decision.

CHAPTER 6: ANATOMY AND PHYSIOLOGY OF PREGNANCY

Chapter Review Activities

1. Gravidity
2. Parity
3. Gravida
4. Nulligravida
5. Nullipara
6. Primigravida
7. Primipara
8. Multigravida
9. Multipara
10. Viability
11. Preterm
12. Term
13. Postterm, postdate
14. Human chorionic gonadotropin (hCG)
15. C, 16. P, 17. K, 18. T, 19. S, 20. U, 21. J, 22. N, 23. V, 24. B, 25. G, 26. A, 27. O, 28. I, 29. Q, 30. E, 31. M, 32. W, 33. F, 34. H, 35. D, 36. R, 37. L

38. *Complete table related to signs and symptoms of pregnancy:* presumptive, probable, positive; see Table 6-2 for identification of signs and symptoms in each category along with time of occurrence and possible causes other than pregnancy for the categories of presumptive and probable.

39. *Use of four-digit and five-digit system of obstetric history:*

    A. 3-2-0-1; 3-1-1-0-1

    B. 4-2-1-2; 4-2-0-1-2

    C. 4-2-1-3; 4-1-1-1-3

40. T, 41. T, 42. F, 43. T, 44. F, 45. T, 46. F, 47. F, 48. F, 49. T, 50. T, 51. F, 52. T, 53. T, 54. F

55. *Changes in vital signs as pregnancy progresses:* see relevant subsection of General Body Systems.

 - **Blood pressure:** see Table 6-4; blood pressure decreases in the second trimester by 5 to 10 mm Hg and returns to prepregnancy levels during the third trimester

 - **Heart rate and patterns:** pulse increases by 10 to 15 beats/min, and murmurs and palpitations can occur.

 - **Respiratory rate and patterns:** see Table 6-5; breathing becomes more thoracic in nature, and volume is deeper, with no change or only a slight increase in rate; some shortness of breath might be experienced in the second half of pregnancy as the diaphragm is pushed up by the enlarging uterus until lightening occurs.

 - **Temperature:** baseline temperature increases slightly because of increase in BMR and effects of the increase in progesterone secretion; women can experience heat intolerance as a result.

56. *Mean arterial pressure calculation:* see Box 6-2 to formulate answer; results are 91, 81, 90, 110.

57. *Specify value changes in selected laboratory tests:* see appropriate section; see Table 6-3 for each laboratory test result change listed.

58. *Expected adaptations in elimination:*

 - **Renal:** see Renal System subsection; slowed passage of urine and dilation of ureters as a result of progesterone increase possibility of urinary tract infections; bladder irritability, nocturia, urinary frequency and urgency (first and third trimesters after lightening).

 - **Bowel:** see Esophagus, Stomach, Intestines subsection; constipation and hemorrhoids; progesterone decreases peristalsis, and enlarging uterus displaces intestines.

59. *Changes in endocrine function and secretions of hormones:* see Endocrine System subsection for full description of each hormone and how its level changes with pregnancy.

60. A is correct; hCG indicates a positive pregnancy test result and is a probable sign of pregnancy; breast tenderness and morning sickness are presumptive signs; fetal heart sounds are a positive sign of pregnancy.

61. D is correct; gravida (total number of pregnancies including the present one = 5); para (term birth of daughter at 39 weeks) = 1; stillbirth at 32 weeks and triplets at 30 weeks = 2; miscarriage at 8 weeks = 1; total number of living children = 4.

62. C is correct; although little change occurs in respiratory rate, breathing becomes more thoracic in nature with the upward displacement of the diaphragm;

women normally experience a greater awareness of their breathing and might even complain of dyspnea at rest as pregnancy progresses. Supine hypotension syndrome, with a decrease in systolic pressure as much as 30 mm Hg, occurs as a result of vena cava and aorta compression by the uterus when the woman is in a supine position. Baseline pulse rate increases by 10 to 15 beats/min; systolic and diastolic blood pressures decrease by approximately 5 to 10 mm Hg beginning in the second trimester of pregnancy, returning to prepregnancy levels by the third trimester.

63. D is correct; recording cycle information assists with accuracy of diagnosis. C reflects the most common error of performing this test too soon; the test will need to be repeated in 1 week if the result is negative. A first-voided morning specimen should be used because it is most concentrated and apt to have the largest amount of hCG; anticonvulsants, tranquilizers, and diuretics can result in inaccurate results.

64. B is correct; friability refers to cervical fragility, resulting in slight bleeding when scraped or touched; Chadwick's sign refers to a deep bluish color of the cervix and vagina as a result of increased circulation; Hegar's sign refers to softening and compressibility of the lower uterine segment.

Critical Thinking Exercises

1. *Responses to patient's concerns and questions:*

 A. *Spotting after intercourse:* discuss cervical and vaginal friability and fragility and increased vascularity, which make the vagina and cervix softer and more delicate; thus spotting after intercourse is expected; caution that any bleeding should be reported so it can be evaluated as to cause.

 B. *Use of a home pregnancy test:* see Pregnancy Tests section; emphasize the importance of following directions carefully because each test brand is a little different; use first-voided morning specimen for most concentrated urine; and notify health care provider for an appointment regardless of the test result.

 C. *Vaginal and bladder infections:* discuss impact of increased vaginal secretions, which are more alkaline, and stasis of urine, which contains nutrients and has a higher pH; review prevention measures at this time.

 D. *Breast changes with pregnancy:* discuss changes in breasts such as enlargement of Montgomery's tubercles and development of lactation structures, resulting in larger breasts that are tender during the first trimester; tell her that she might notice bilateral changes in consistency and presence of lumpiness when she does a breast self-examination.

 E. *Effect of pregnant woman's position:* discuss supine hypotensive syndrome, which is caused by compression of the vena cava and abdominal aorta when the woman is in a supine position; cardiac output decreases and blood pressure falls; lateral position for rest is best.

F. *Nosebleeds:* tell her that estrogen increases the vascularity of the upper respiratory tract and causes edema, congestion, and hyperemia of the tissue, making nosebleeds more common.

G. *Ankle edema:* explain to her that the swelling of her ankles is a result of the pressure of her enlarging uterus and the dependent position of her legs when sitting; the iliac veins and inferior vena cava increase venous pressure and decrease blood flow; elevating legs and exercising them help decrease edema; caution her never to take someone else's medications or to self-medicate.

H. *Posture change and low back pain:* lordosis occurs as a result of the enlarging uterus, which decreases abdominal muscle tone, and the increased mobility of the pelvic joints tilting the pelvic forward; this results in lower back pain, a change in posture, and shifting forward of the center of gravity.

I. *Braxton-Hicks:* the woman is describing false labor contractions because they diminish when she increases her activity level; these contractions facilitate blood flow and promote oxygen delivery to the fetus; compare these contractions with true labor contractions.

J. *Shortness of breath during pregnancy:* explain that what she is experiencing is a result of increased sensitivity of her respiratory center to carbon dioxide and the elevation of the diaphragm by the enlarging uterus; assess the woman for signs of pulmonary edema to be sure that the shortness of breath she is experiencing is physiologic rather than pathologic in nature.

2. *Blood pressure protocol:* consider the effect of maternal age, activity level, health status, level of stress, arm used, and position; protocol should emphasize consistency in arm used and patient position and use of the proper size of cuff. Provide time for the woman to relax before the blood pressure is assessed; repeat if the reading is inconsistent with the woman's baseline level or is abnormal.

CHAPTER 7: NURSING CARE OF THE FAMILY DURING PREGNANCY

Chapter Review Activities

1. Presumptive; probable; positive

2. Nägele's, estimated date of birth, 3 months, 7 days, last menstrual period; trimesters

3. Supine hypotension; pallor, dizziness, faintness, breathlessness, tachycardia, nausea, clammy skin (sweating)

4. Fundal height; pinch

5. Fetal movement, fetal heart rate (FHR) and rhythm, maternal or fetal symptoms; gestational age

6. Developmental, accepting the pregnancy, identifying with the role of mother, reordering relationships with her mother and her partner, establishing a relationship with the unborn child, preparing for the birth experience

7. Biologic fact of pregnancy, "I am pregnant"; growing fetus as distinct from herself, person to nurture; "I am going to have a baby"; birth, parenting; "I am going to be a mother"

8. Emotional lability; ambivalence

9. Announcement; moratorium; focusing; couvade

10. Birth plan

11. Prescriptions; proscriptions; taboos

12. Neural tube defects, Down syndrome, other chromosomal abnormalities; 16 to 18; maternal serum alpha-fetoprotein, human chorionic gonadotropin, unconjugated estriol, inhibin-A

13. Head, breasts, abdomen, genitalia; sexual assault

14. *Calculating expected date of birth:* use Nägele's rule by subtracting 3 months, adding 7 days, and adjusting the year to the first day of the last menstrual period:

A. February 12, 2011

B. October 21, 2010

C. April 11, 2011

15. *Cultural beliefs and practices:* see Cultural Influences subsection of Variations in Prenatal Care section.

A. *Describe how cultural beliefs affect participation in prenatal care:* consider the following factors: beliefs that conflict with typical prenatal practices, lack of money and transportation, communication difficulties, concern regarding modesty and gender of health care provider, fear of invasive procedures, view of pregnancy as healthy whereas health care providers imply illness, view of pregnancy problems as a normal part of pregnancy.

B. *Prescriptions and proscriptions:* see specific subsections for emotional response, clothing, physical activity and rest, sexual activity, and diet.

16. *Completing table regarding components of initial and follow-up visits:* see subsections for the Initial Visit and Follow-up Visits in the Care Management—Assessment and Nursing Diagnoses section; content of each component is fully described.

17. *Components of fetal assessment:* measurement of fundal height, gestational age determination, health status of fetus, including FHR and pattern, fetal movements, and unusual or abnormal maternal or fetal signs and symptoms; see specific subsections for each component in the Follow-up Visits section.

18. *Nurse's responsibility for identifying complications during pregnancy:*

A. *List signs of potential complications:* see Signs of Potential Complications box, which lists signs according to the first trimester and second and third trimesters.

B. *Nursing approach when discussing signs of complications with pregnant woman and her family:*

- Inform as to what the signs are, possible cause, when and to whom to report.
- Present the signs verbally and in written form.
- Provide time to answer questions and discuss concerns; make follow-up phone calls.
- Gather full information of signs that are reported; use this information as the basis for action.
- Document all assessments, actions, and responses.

19. T, 20. T, 21. T, 22. T, 23. F, 24. F, 25. F, 26. F, 27. T, 28. F, 29. T, 30. F, 31. F, 32. F, 33. T, 34. T, 35. F, 36. T, 37. T, 38. T, 39. T

40. *Protocol for fundal measurement:* consider woman's position, type of measuring tape used (paper, non-stretchable), measurement method (Fig. 7-7), and conditions of the examination such as empty bladder and condition of uterus (relaxed or contracted).

41. *Factors used to estimate gestational age:* include menstrual history, contraceptive history, pregnancy test result, and specific findings related to the maternal-fetal unit (e.g., time of appearance of the specific signs of pregnancy).

42. *Prevention of injury during pregnancy:*

A. *Principles of body mechanics:* see Fig. 7-12 and Patient Instructions for Self-Management box—Posture and Body Mechanics.

B. *Safety guidelines with rationale:* see Patient Instructions for Self-Management box—Safety during Pregnancy and the prevention measures identified in each subsection of Education for Self-Management section.

43. *Contraindications for breastfeeding:* include deep-seated aversion to breastfeeding by the mother or her partner; need to take certain medications or use illicit drugs; medical complications such as positive HIV infection.

44. B is correct; A and C are probable signs, and D is a positive sign diagnostic of pregnancy.

45. A is correct; use Nägele's rule by subtracting 3 months and adding 7 days and 1 year to the first day of the last menstrual period, which in this case is September 10, 2010. The estimated date of birth (EDB) is June 17, 2011.

46. D is correct; supine hypotension related to compression of aorta and vena cava is being experienced; the first action is to remove the cause of the problem by turning the woman on her side; this should alleviate the symptoms being experienced, including nausea; assessment of vital signs can occur after the woman's position is changed.

47. A is correct; intake of at least 2 to 3 L/day is recommended; B, C, and D are accepted methods of preventing urinary tract infections, along with frequent regular urination, good genital hygiene, and not wearing tight-fitting jeans for long periods.

Critical Thinking Exercises

1. *Health history interview* (see Initial Visit subsection of Assessment and Nursing Diagnoses section):

A. *Purpose of health history interview:*

- Establish a therapeutic relationship with the woman and those who come with her.
- Have planned time for purposeful communication to gather baseline data related to woman's subjective appraisal of her health status and to gather objective information based on nurse's observation of the woman's affect, posture, body language, skin color, and other physical and emotional signs.

B. *Components:* obtain reason for seeking care, current pregnancy, OB/GYN history, medical history, nutritional history, drug and herbal therapy use, family history, social and experiential history, history of abuse, review of systems.

C. *Write two questions for each component:* be sure that questions reflect the principles of effective questioning; consider the need to plan in follow-up questions to clarify and gather further information when a problem is identified; each question should be clear, understandable, and open-ended, with only one piece of information targeted.

2. *Care of woman at initial visit who is anxious and unsure about prenatal care:* answer should emphasize:

- Establishing a therapeutic trusting relationship that will make the woman comfortable about coming for further prenatal care.
- Teaching the woman about the importance of prenatal care for her own health and that of her baby.
- Involving her boyfriend in the care process so he will encourage her participation in prenatal care.
- Following guidelines for health history interview, physical examination, and laboratory tests; ensuring her privacy and comfort during the examination and teaching her about how her body is changing.
- Evaluating desire for this pregnancy and the need for community agency support.

3. *Couple during the first trimester—concerns and questions:*

A. *Accuracy of EDB:* reliability depends on the accuracy of the date of first day of her last menstrual period and the regularity of her menstrual cycles; birth can normally occur 1 to 2 weeks before or after the calculated EDB.

B. *Kegel exercises:* pelvic muscle exercises to maintain pelvic muscle tone and ability to support organs; see Kegel Exercises subsection of Education for Self-Management section and Teaching Guidelines box—Kegel Exercises in Chapter 2.

C. *Effect of pregnancy on sexuality:* see Patient Instructions for Self-Management box—Sexuality in Pregnancy; emphasize that intercourse is safe as long as pregnancy is progressing in a healthy manner; sexual expression should be in tune with the woman's changing needs and emotions; inform them that spotting can occur afterward because of cervical and vaginal changes with pregnancy and that changes in positions and activities might be helpful as pregnancy progresses and the woman's body changes.

D. *Morning sickness:* see Table 7-2 (First Trimester section); fully assess what she is experiencing; then discuss why it happens, how long it will last, and what relief measures are available.

4. *Physical activity and exercise in pregnancy:* see Physical Activity subsection of the Education for Self-Management section and Patient Instructions for Self-Management box—Exercise Tips for Pregnant Women; assess her usual exercise patterns and consider their safety; discuss precautions and guidelines to follow for safe yet effective exercise; emphasize that moderate physical activity and exercise during pregnancy are good for her and for her baby and will prepare her for the work of labor and birth.

5. *Nursing diagnosis, expected outcome, and nursing measures for pregnant women in various situations:*

A. *Risk for infection of urinary tract related to lack of knowledge regarding changes in renal system during pregnancy:* woman should drink at least 3 L of fluid each day and empty bladder at first urge; nursing measures: increase fluid intake, use acid ash-forming fluids such as cranberry juice, void frequently, perform adequate perineal hygiene, use side-lying position when resting to enhance renal perfusion and urine formation.

B. *Acute pain in lower back related to neuromuscular changes associated with pregnancy at 23 weeks of gestation:* woman experiences lessening of lower back pain following implementation of suggested relief measures; nursing measures should include explanation of the basis for lower back pain and relief measures, including back rubs, pelvic rock, and posture changes (see Table 7-2 and Fig. 7-11); in addition, encourage woman to change her footwear for better stability and safety.

C. *Anxiety related to lack of knowledge concerning the process of labor and birth and appropriate measures they can use to cope with the pain and discomfort:* couple will enroll in childbirth classes in the seventh month of pregnancy; nursing measures should include overview of childbirth process, current measures used to relieve pain, both nonpharmacologic and pharmacologic, and role of the coach; make a referral to childbirth classes; assist with preparation of birth plan; discuss childbirth options and prebirth preparations.

6. *Supine hypotension syndrome:* see Emergency box—Supine Hypotension:

A. *Explanation of assessment findings:* supine hypotension.

B. *Immediate action:* turn on side and keep her in this position until vital signs stabilize and signs and symptoms diminish.

7. *Woman in the third trimester—questions and concerns:*

A. *Nipple condition for breastfeeding:* perform pinch test to see if nipples evert; if they do not, the woman can use a nipple shell inside her bra to help the nipples protrude; no special exercises are recommended because they might stimulate preterm labor in susceptible women; keep nipples and areola clean.

B. *Ankle edema:* see Table 7-2 (Third Trimester section); discuss basis for the edema and encourage use of leg, ankle, and foot exercises and elevation of legs periodically during the day (Fig. 7-15); emphasize importance of fluid intake.

C. *Leg cramps:* see Table 7-2 (Third Trimester section); discuss the cause; then demonstrate relief measures such as pressing weight onto the foot while standing or dorsiflexing the foot while lying in bed; avoid toe pointing.

8. *Concerns regarding preterm labor and birth:*

A. *Signs of preterm labor:* see section on Recognizing Preterm Labor.

B. *Action if signs are noted:* empty bladder, drink three to four glasses of water for hydration, lie on side, and continue to assess contractions for 1 more hour; if contractions do not diminish, the primary health care provider should be notified.

9. *Sibling preparation:* to formulate answer, use Sibling Adaptation section, Box 7-2, and Fig. 7-2, which provide tips for sibling preparation; emphasize importance of considering each child's developmental level; prepare children for prenatal events, time during hospitalization, and arrival home of the new baby; refer to sibling classes and encourage sibling visitation after birth.

10. *Woman experiencing emotional lability:* see Maternal Adaptation section and Table 7-2 (First Trimester section); discuss hormonal and metabolic basis of the mood swings; describe what a woman is experiencing during the first trimester, including ambivalent feelings regarding female role, sexuality, timing of pregnancy, and changes in her life; identify measures man can use to help both himself and pregnant partner cope.

11. *Home birth:* see Home Birth subsection of Birth Setting Choices section; answer should include preparation of the home, including obtaining supplies and equipment, arranging for medical backup and transportation in the event of an emergency, and choosing and preparing those who will be attending the birth.

CHAPTER 8: MATERNAL AND FETAL NUTRITION

Chapter Review Activities

1. Healthful diet; folic acid (folate), neural tube

2. Intrauterine growth restriction; small-for–gestational age, preterm

3. Age, activity level, current weight, number of fetuses, alteration in health; energy, 340 kcal, 462 kcal

4. Pregnant adolescents, poor women, women who adhere to unusual diets

5. Iron deficiency anemia; 60-120 mg of ferrous iron daily

6. Lactose intolerance

7. Pica, clay, dirt, laundry starch, cornstarch, ice, baking powder, soda; craving

8. OB/GYN effects on nutrition, medical history, usual maternal diet, herbal supplements; anthropometric, height, weight; body mass index (BMI)

9. Vegetables, fruits, legumes, nuts, seeds, grains; semi-vegetarian; lacto-ovo vegetarians; vegans, strict vegetarians

10. Pyrosis

11. *Complete nutrient table:* use Table 8-1 and specific subsections for each nutrient to complete this table.

12. *Indicators of nutritional risks:* Box 8-3 lists many indicators of nutritional risks during pregnancy.

13. *Guidelines to follow when planning menu with a vegan:* see Vegetarian Diets subsection of Cultural Influences section; consider that this woman's diet is deficient in vitamin B_{12} (needs supplementation or fortified foods) and is low in iron, calcium, zinc, vitamin B_6, and perhaps calories; foods need to be combined to ensure that all amino acids are provided.

14. *Signs of good and inadequate nutrition:* see Table 8-4 for full list of signs in terms of specific body functions and areas.

15. *Nursing measures for specific nursing diagnoses:* see appropriate subsection in Coping with Nutrition-Related Discomforts of Pregnancy section:

A. *Imbalanced nutrition:* less than body requirements related to inadequate intake associated with nausea and vomiting: see Nausea and Vomiting subsection for identification of relief measures.

B. *Constipation related to decreased intestinal motility associated with increased progesterone level during pregnancy:* see Constipation subsection; measures include fluid and roughage intake, exercise and activity, and regular time for elimination.

16. *Calculation of BMI and determination of weight gain pattern:* see Weight Gain subsection of Nutrient Needs during Pregnancy section and use the formula weight (in kg) ÷ height (in m²) to determine the BMI of each woman. All women should gain approximately 1 to 2.5 kg in the first trimester; weight gain per week is recommended for the second and third trimesters.

- **June:** BMI—22, normal; total 11.5 to 16 kg; 0.4 kg/week

- **Alice:** BMI—34, obese; total at least 7 kg; 0.3 kg/week

- **Ann:** BMI—16, underweight; total 12.5 to 18 kg; 0.5 kg/week

17. T, 18. F, 19. F, 20. T, 21. T, 22. F, 23. T, 24. T, 25. F, 26. F, 27. T, 28. F, 29. T, 30. F, 31. F, 32. T

33. *Nutrition guidelines for lactation:* adequate calcium intake, at least 1800 kcal/day; adequate fluid intake; avoid tobacco, alcohol, and excessive caffeine.

34. *Factors that increase nutrient need during pregnancy:* growth and development of uterine-placental-fetal unit, expansion of maternal blood volume and RBCs, mammary changes, increased basal metabolic rate.

35. D is correct; bran, tea, coffee, milk, oxalates, and egg yolks all decrease iron absorption; tomatoes and strawberries contain vitamin C, which enhances iron absorption; meats contain heme iron, which enhances absorption; ideally iron is best absorbed on an empty stomach and should be taken between, not with, meals, if possible.

36. B is correct; BMI indicates that the woman is at normal weight; total gain should be 11.5 to 16 kg, representing a gain of 0.4 kg/week and 1.6 kg/month during second and third trimesters.

37. C is correct; small, frequent meals are better tolerated than large meals, which can distend the stomach. Hunger can worsen nausea; therefore meals should not be skipped; dry, starchy foods should be eaten in the morning and at other times during the day when nausea occurs; fried, fatty, and spicy foods should be avoided; a bedtime snack is recommended.

38. C is correct; green leafy vegetables are a good source of folic acid, as are whole-grain and fortified cereals, oranges, asparagus, liver, and artichokes; A, B, and

D are not good sources of folic acid, although they do supply other important nutrients for pregnancy.

39. A is correct; only two to three servings of meat, poultry, fish, dry beans, eggs, and nut group during pregnancy; B, C, and D are all appropriate for pregnancy; orange juice contains vitamin C, which enhances iron absorption.

Critical Thinking Exercises

1. *Nutrition and weight gain concerns:*

   A. *Concern regarding amount of recommended weight gain:*

      - Identify components of maternal weight gain.

      - Discuss impact of maternal weight gain on fetal growth and development and the association among poor maternal weight gain, intrauterine growth rate, low birth weight, preterm birth, and infant mortality.

      - Discuss total and pattern of weight gain for a woman with a normal 20 BMI.

   B. *Eating for two during pregnancy:*

      - Emphasize quality food that meets nutrient requirements, not the quantity of food.

      - Discuss expected weight gain total and pattern for a normal 22 BMI; appropriate intake of nutrients will reflect this pattern.

      - State that excessive weight gain during pregnancy might be difficult to lose after pregnancy and could lead to chronic obesity.

   C. *Vitamin supplementation during pregnancy:* determine what woman takes and how much; compare with recommendations for pregnancy; discuss potential problems with toxicity, especially with overuse of fat-soluble vitamins.

   D. *Heartburn:* recommend relief measures—small, frequent meals; fluid between, not with, meals; avoid spicy, fatty foods; remain upright after meals.

   E. *Weight reduction diets during pregnancy:*

      - BMI indicates overweight status; she should gain approximately 7 to 11.5 kg during pregnancy.

      - Discuss hazards of inadequate calories during pregnancy in terms of growth and development of fetus (LBW) and pregnancy-related structures and effects of ketoacidosis.

      - Discuss quality foods; use this time to develop good nutrition habits that can be used during the postpartum period as part of a sensible weight reduction plan.

      - Discuss importance of exercise and activity during pregnancy.

   F. *Reduction of water intake:* discuss importance of fluid to meet demands of pregnancy-related changes, regulate temperature, prevent constipation and urinary tract infections; consider possible association between preterm labor and dehydration.

   G. *Lactose intolerance:* discuss basis for problem; reduce lactose intake by using nondairy sources of calcium and calcium supplements; take lactase supplements.

   H. *Weight loss with lactation:* discuss weight loss patterns with lactation; emphasize that fat stores from pregnancy are used as part of the lactation process with a resultant weight loss; the increased need for nutrients, calories, and fluids is used up during the process of lactation.

2. *Taking iron supplements effectively:* see Iron subsection of Nutrient Needs section, Counseling about Iron Supplementation subsection of the Care Management section, and Table 8-1 for iron food sources.

   - Discuss importance of iron—why she and her baby need it.

   - Emphasize importance of vitamin C for iron absorption; discuss food sources for both vitamin C and iron.

   - Discuss ways to take iron supplements to enhance absorption and minimize side effects, including gastrointestinal upset and constipation.

   - Identify foods that can decrease iron absorption if consumed at the same time.

3. *Native-American woman meeting nutritional needs:*

   A. *Counseling approach:*

      - Assess her current nutritional status and habits; obtain a diet history.

      - Analyze current patterns as a basis for menu planning.

      - Discuss weight gain pattern for an underweight woman; her BMI is 16.5.

      - Use a variety of teaching methods; keep woman actively involved in the process, especially because she has already expressed interest and motivation.

      - Emphasize importance of good nutrition for herself and her newborn.

   B. *Menu plan:* use Table 8-5 for specific Native-American–type foods and Fig. 8-3 to determine number of servings of required nutrients when planning the 1-day menu. Be sure to distribute nutrients throughout the day in meals and nutrition snacks.

CHAPTER 9: LABOR AND BIRTH PROCESSES

Chapter Review Activities

1. Membrane-filled spaces, sutures
2. Overlapping, bones
3. Part of the fetus, inlet; cephalic, breech, shoulder
4. First felt by the examiner's finger, vaginal; occiput, sacrum, scapula
5. Flexed, occiput
6. Long axis (spine) of the fetus, long axis (spine) of the mother; spines are parallel, spines are at right angles (perpendicular)
7. Fetal body parts to each other; flexion
8. Transverse; anteroposterior; flexion
9. Presenting part, quadrants, pelvis
10. Largest transverse (biparietal), pelvic brim (inlet), true pelvis, ischial spines, zero
11. Presenting part, ischial spines; centimeters, ischial spines, descent
12. Shortening, thinning, cervix, first, percentages; 0%, 100%
13. Enlargement, widening, cervical opening (os), cervical canal; centimeters, 1 cm, 10 cm
14. Dropping, presenting part (usually the head), true pelvis, 2 weeks, onset of true labor
15. Brownish or blood-tinged cervical mucus, mucous plug (operculum), ripens
16. Turns and adjustments, birth canal; cardinal movements, engagement, descent, flexion, internal rotation, extension, external rotation (restitution), expulsion
17. *Identify and describe signs of prodromal labor:* see Signs Preceding Labor subsection of the Process of Labor section and Box 9-1 for a description of the signs and symptoms to teach this woman to alert her that the onset of labor is approaching.
18. *Identify and describe five factors affecting progress of labor:* see separate subsection for each of the five factors (i.e., passenger, passage, powers, position of the mother, and psychologic responses of the mother).
19. *Events of each state of labor:* see Stages of Labor subsection of the Process of Labor section:
    - **First stage:** cervical stage with effacement and dilation
    - **Second stage:** birth stage with birth of fetus
    - **Third stage:** placental stage with separation and expulsion of the placenta
    - **Fourth stage:** recovery stage with maternal stabilization after birth

20. *Label illustrations:*
    - **Fetal skull:** A. Mentum (chin); B. Occipitofrontal diameter; C. Frontal bone (sinciput) ; D. Suboccipitobregmatic diameter; E. Parietal bone (vertex); F. Occipitomental diameter; G. Occiput; H. Sagittal suture; I. Lambdoid suture; J. Posterior fontanel; K. Biparietal diameter; L. Coronal suture; M. Frontal suture and bone; N. Anterior fontanel (bregma)
    - **Maternal pelvis:** A. Symphysis pubis; B. Anteroposterior diameter; C. Transverse diameter; D. Sacral promontory; E. Sacrum; F. Sacroiliac joint; G. Ischial spine; H. Pubic bone; I. Sacrotuberous ligament; J. Pubic arch; K. Ischial tuberosity; L. Coccyx; M. Sacroiliac joint
21. *Presentation, presenting part, position, lie, and attitude for each illustration:*
    A. Cephalic, occiput, LOA, longitudinal, flexion
    B. Cephalic, occiput, LOT, longitudinal, flexion
    C. Cephalic, occiput, LOP, longitudinal, flexion
    D. Cephalic, occiput, ROA, longitudinal, flexion
    E. Cephalic, occiput, ROT, longitudinal, flexion
    F. Cephalic, occiput, ROP, longitudinal, flexion
    G. Cephalic, mentum, LMA, longitudinal, extension
    H. Cephalic, mentum, RMP, longitudinal, extension
    I. Cephalic, mentum, RMA, longitudinal, extension
    J. Breech, sacrum, LSA, longitudinal, flexion
    K. Breech, sacrum, LSP, longitudinal, flexion
    L. Shoulder, scapula, SCA, transverse, flexion
22. *Three factors that affect fetal circulation:*
    - Maternal position, blood pressure, cardiac output
    - Uterine contractions
    - Umbilical cord blood flow
23. F, 24. T, 25. F, 26. F, 27. T, 28. T, 29. F, 30. T, 31. F, 32. F, 33. T, 34. T, 35. F, 36. T
37. B is correct; attitude is extension of head and neck as indicated by the mentum (chin) as the presenting part; the lie is longitudinal as indicated by the cephalic presentation.
38. C is correct; systolic blood pressure increases with uterine contractions in the first stage, whereas both systolic and diastolic blood pressure increase during contractions in the second stage; white blood cell count can increase as high as 25,000/mm^3; gastric motility decreases and can lead to nausea and vomiting, especially during the transition phase of the first stage of labor.
39. A is correct; the first stage can last up to 20 hours for the primigravid woman; the second stage lasts an average of 50 minutes or longer and up to 2 to 3 hours, especially in nulliparous labors or if an epidural has been used; the third stage lasts 3 to 5 minutes; the fourth stage lasts approximately 1 to 2 hours.

40. D is correct; quickening refers to the woman's first perception of fetal movement at 16 to 20 weeks of gestation; urinary frequency, lightening, and weight loss of 0.5 to 1 kg occur to signal that the onset of labor is near; backache, stronger Braxton Hicks contractions, and bloody show are also noted.

Critical Thinking Exercises

1. *Analysis of vaginal examination:*
   - **Exam I:** ROP (right occiput posterior), cephalic (vertex) presentation, longitudinal lie, flexed attitude; −1, station at 1 cm above the ischial spines; 50% effaced; 3 cm dilated
   - **Exam II:** RMA (right mentum anterior), cephalic (face) presentation, longitudinal lie, extended attitude; 0, station at the ischial spines; 25% effaced; 2 cm dilated
   - **Exam III:** LST (left sacrum transverse), breech presentation, longitudinal lie, flexed attitude; 1, station at 1 cm below the ischial spines; 75% effaced; 6 cm dilated
   - **Exam IV:** OA (occiput anterior), cephalic (vertex) presentation, longitudinal lie, flexed attitude; 3, station at 3 cm below the ischial spines near or on the perineum; 100% (fully effaced); 10 cm (fully dilated).

2. *Woman with questions or concerns regarding the process of labor:*
   A. *Onset of labor:* see Onset of Labor subsection of the Process of Labor section; interaction of fetal and maternal hormonal changes, uterine distention, increasing intrauterine pressure, aging of placenta, fetal fibronectin.
   B. *Signs of prodromal labor:* see Box 9-1, in which signs preceding labor are identified; lightening, urinary frequency, backache, Braxton Hicks contractions, weight loss, energy surge, bloody show, and possible rupture of the membranes are signs that the woman notes; health care provider notes cervical changes in terms of ripening, dilation, and effacement.
   C. *Duration of labor:* see Stages of Labor subsection for approximate times; give woman ranges but not absolutes, especially since this is her first labor; use this time to discuss her role in facilitating the progress of labor.
   D. *Position changes during labor:*
      - Emphasize that the position of the woman is one of the five P's of labor.
      - Discuss each position and describe its effect in terms of facilitating the progress of labor (Fig. 9-12).
      - Demonstrate each position and have her practice them with her partner.

   - Emphasize beneficial effects of ambulation and changing positions on fetus, circulation, comfort, and progress.

CHAPTER 10: MANAGEMENT OF DISCOMFORT

Chapter Review Activities

1. Visceral; cervical, ischemia; lower portion, lumbar, thighs
2. Somatic; perineal, perineal tissue, peritoneum, utero-cervical
3. Referred, abdominal wall, lumbosacral area of the back, iliac crests, gluteal area, thighs, lower back
4. Gate-control; massage, stroking, music, imagery, breathing, relaxation
5. Endorphins
6. Dick-Read, Lamaze, Bradley
7. Distraction, perception of pain; slow-paced, half
8. Shallow, twice
9. Cleansing breath
10. Transition; hyperventilation, respiratory alkalosis, lightheadedness, dizziness, tingling of fingers, circumoral numbness; breathe into a paper bag or cupped hand; carbon dioxide, bicarbonate
11. Effleurage, counterpressure, gate-control
12. *Factors influencing response to pain:* culture, anxiety and fear, previous experience with pain and with childbirth, childbirth preparation activities, comfort measures, secretion of endorphins, support, history of substance abuse, history of sexual abuse, pain tolerance and perception.
13. *Theoretic basis of effectiveness of massage, stroking, music, and imagery in reducing pain sensation:* discuss the gate-control theory of pain; see Factors Influencing Pain Response section.
14. B, 15. F, 16. H, 17. A, 18. G, 19. L, 20. D, 21. I, 22. K, 23. C, 24. E, 25. J
26. *Complete table related to types of regional anesthetics:* see appropriate subsections for local infiltration, pudendal block, spinal block and anesthesia, and epidural block in the Pharmacologic Management of Discomfort section.
27. *Systemic analgesics:* see Systemic Analgesia subsection of Pharmacologic Management of Discomfort:
   A. *Factors influencing effect of systemic analgesics on fetus:* maternal dosage, pharmacokinetics of the specific drug, route, time when administered during labor.
   B. *Fetal effects of systemic analgesics:* central nervous system (CNS) depression as a result of the direct effect of the drug when it crosses the placenta and/or the indirect effect of maternal hypotension and hypoventilation resulting from the action of the drug on maternal function; CNS

depression slows the fetal heart rate, decreases variability, and leads to respiratory depression and hypoxia.

28. *Examples of opioid agonist analgesic, opioid agonist-antagonist analgesic, analgesic potentiator, and opioid antagonist, and how each is used in childbirth:* see Medication Guides and specific subsections for each classification in Pharmacologic Management of Discomfort section.

29. T, 30. T, 31. T, 32. F, 33. T, 34. F, 35. T, 36. F, 37. T, 38. F, 39. T, 40. T

41. *Advantage of intravenous (IV) administration of systemic analgesics:* the IV route of administration is preferred because the onset of analgesia is faster and more reliable and predictable; smaller dosages can be used.

42. B is correct; Narcan is an opioid antagonist; Stadol is an opioid agonist-antagonist analgesic; Sublimaze is an opioid agonist analgesic.

43. D is correct; onset of effect is within 30 seconds of IV injection; a 25-mg dose is appropriate for IV administration; this medication is a potent opioid agonist analgesic; thus respiratory depression is a concern.

44. A is correct; position with a curved back separates the vertebrae and facilitates administration of the anesthetic; alternating lateral positions after administration will prevent supine hypotension and enhance distribution of the medication; ambulation is unsafe because of weakness and numbness of the legs; because the dura is not punctured, there is no leakage of cerebrospinal fluid, which could cause a spinal headache.

Critical Thinking Exercises

1. *Explaining the basis of childbirth pain to expectant fathers:* explain the neurologic origins of pain (see subsection in Discomfort during Labor and Birth section); describe how women experience the pain and factors that influence the experience; explain types of pain, including somatic, visceral, and referred, that can occur during childbirth; discuss the measures that they can use to help the woman reduce and cope with the pain experienced.

2. *Working with a couple with unrealistic, incorrect views regarding pain and pain relief during labor:* see Care Management section:
   - Inform couple regarding basis of pain in childbirth and its potentially adverse effects on the maternal-fetal unit and the progress of labor; pain can inhibit labor as a result of the stress response, circulation can be altered, and the woman's ability to work with her labor can be inhibited.
   - Discuss a variety of nonpharmacologic and pharmacologic measures that can be used in labor and

their effects, including level of safety and benefit for the maternal-fetal unit and ability to enhance the progress of labor as a result of a decrease in maternal stress and tension.
   - Emphasize that mother and fetus will be thoroughly assessed before, during, and after any measure to ensure safety.

3. *Benefits of water therapy:*
   - Describe the beneficial effects of water therapy and how it can be used to facilitate the labor process through relaxation, relief of discomfort and tension, shortening of the duration of labor, and enhanced progress, thereby decreasing the possibility of cesarean birth; use research findings to substantiate these claims.
   - Describe the successful experiences of other clinical agencies that have implemented water therapy and how this has affected the number of births per year.
   - Use the favorable reports of women who now have a more positive view of their labor as a result of using water therapy and how this has influenced their opinion of the care they received at that agency; consider how this might affect what they tell other women of childbearing age who will decide about where they will give birth.

4. *Occurrence of hypotension after administration of epidural during labor* (see Emergency box—Maternal Hypotension with Decreased Placental Perfusion to formulate answer):
   A. *What is being experienced by this woman:* maternal hypotension related to the effects of epidural anesthesia decreases placental perfusion and results in an alteration in fetal oxygen level, as reflected in nonreassuring changes in FHR pattern.
   B. *Nursing diagnosis:* ineffective uteroplacental tissue perfusion related to maternal hypotension associated with epidural block.
   C. *Immediate nursing actions:* turn woman on side or put wedge under hip, maintain IV infusion, administer oxygen, elevate legs from hip, assess maternal-fetal unit for effectiveness of actions taken; notify primary health care provider for further instructions; document all assessment findings, actions taken, and patient responses.

5. *Woman who will receive an epidural block for childbirth:* see Epidural Block subsection of Pharmacologic Management of Discomfort section:
   A. *Assessment before induction of block:* include status of maternal-fetal unit, progress of labor in terms of phase, contraindications for use.
   B. *Preparation measures:* explain procedure to be used and expected effects; witness informed consent according to agency policy; hydrate

patient; and assess urinary output, including bladder condition.

C. *Positions for induction:* list lateral (modified Sims with back curved forward) or sitting with back curved forward to separate vertebrae; assist her into position and help her maintain position without movement during the induction.

D. *Nursing management during the epidural block:* assess response on maternal-fetal unit and progress of labor, maintain hydration, assist with bladder emptying and positioning of legs safely, change her position frequently from side to side, maintain site to prevent infection; consider anesthesia recovery in the postpartum period.

CHAPTER 11: FETAL ASSESSMENT DURING LABOR

Chapter Review Activities

1. Normal (reassuring), abnormal (nonreassuring); compromise, hypoxemia, hypoxia

2. Auscultation, fetoscope, ultrasound device

3. Electronic fetal monitoring; ultrasound transducer, tocotransducer; spiral electrode, intrauterine pressure catheter

4. Variable deceleration; amnioinfusion

5. Tocolytic; tocolysis; terbutaline

6. *Factors that affect fetal oxygen supply and expected characteristics of FHR and uterine activity* (see Fetal Response subsection in Basis for Monitoring section):

   A. *Factors that can reduce fetal oxygen supply:* list reduction in blood flow through maternal vessels, reduction in oxygen content of maternal blood, alterations in fetal circulation, and reduction in blood flow in placenta.

   B. *Characteristics of reassuring FHR pattern:* include baseline, 110 to 160 beats/min, no periodic changes, moderate baseline irritability, and accelerations with fetal movement.

   C. *Characteristics of normal uterine activity:* list frequency of contractions every 2 to 5 minutes, duration less than 90 seconds, moderate-to-strong intensity or intensity less than 100 mm Hg, rest period of at least 30 seconds, with average intrauterine pressure of 15 mm Hg or less.

7. *Characteristics of nonreassuring FHR patterns:* see Fetal Compromise subsection; characteristics are fully identified in terms of changes in rate, variability, and pattern associated with uterine contractions.

8. I, 9. H, 10. G, 11. J, 12. F, 13. C, 14. B, 15. D, 16. E, 17. A, 18. K

19. Maternal vital signs, 30 minutes, 15 minutes

20. Maternal vital signs, 15 minutes, 5 minutes

21. *Intermittent auscultation to assess fetus during labor:*
    - **Advantages:** high-touch/low-tech approach, natural method that facilitates activity, comfortable and noninvasive.
    - **Disadvantages:** inconvenient, time-consuming, increased anxiety of patient if nurse has difficulty locating point of maximal intensity, less information is determined about the FHR pattern.

22. *Outline guidelines to follow for intermittent auscultation:* see Intermittent Auscultation subsection of Monitoring Techniques section; specific guidelines/steps are described.

23. *Legal responsibilities related to fetal monitoring during childbirth:* see Legal Tip—Fetal Monitoring Standards in the Electronic Fetal Monitoring Pattern Recognition section; consider correct interpretation of FHR pattern as reassuring or nonreassuring; take appropriate action; evaluate response; notify primary health care provider appropriately and in a timely fashion; know the chain of command if a dispute in interpretation occurs; and document assessment findings, action, and response.

24. T, 25. F, 26. T, 27. F, 28. T, 29. T, 30. T, 31. F, 32. F, 33. T, 34. T, 35. T, 36. F, 37. T

38. *Emergency measures for nonreassuring patterns:* the concept of intrauterine resuscitation should be the major focus of the answer.

39. *Nursing measures for monitored woman and her family:* see Box 11-8 for guidelines related to teaching, assessing, and caring for the monitored woman and her family during labor.

40. *Documentation regarding fetal status on patient record and monitor strip:* see Documentation section under Care Management and Box 11-9.

41. D is correct; the resting pressure should be 15 mm Hg or less; A, B, and C are all findings within the expected ranges.

42. B is correct; Leopold maneuvers are used to locate the point of maximal intensity for correct placement of the ultrasound transducer; the tocotransducer, which assesses uterine contractions, is always placed over the fundus; reposition the ultrasound transducer every 2 hours and the tocotransducer every hour; it is not the nurse's role to apply a spiral electrode.

43. A is correct; the baseline rate should be 110 to 160 beats/min; accelerations should occur with fetal movement; no late deceleration pattern of any magnitude is reassuring, especially if it is repetitive.

44. C is correct; the FHR increases as the maternal core body temperature elevates; thus tachycardia is the pattern exhibited; it is often a clue of intrauterine infection because maternal fever is often the first sign.

45. B is correct; the pattern described is an early deceleration pattern, which is considered benign, reassuring,

and requiring no action other than documentation of the finding; it is associated with fetal head compression; changing a woman's position and notifying the physician are appropriate if nonreassuring signs such as late or variable decelerations have been occurring; prolapse of cord is associated with variable decelerations as a result of cord compression.

Critical Thinking Exercises

1. *Woman concerned about use of external monitoring to assess her fetus and labor:*

   • Discuss how fetus responds to labor and how the monitor will assess these responses.

   • Explain the advantages and purpose of monitoring.

   • Show her a monitor strip and explain what it reveals; tell her how she can use the strip to help her with her breathing techniques.

2. *Woman whose labor is being induced and external monitoring is being used* (use Table 11-2 to formulate answer):

   A. *Pattern described and causative factors:* late deceleration patterns are occurring as a result of uteroplacental insufficiency associated with intense uterine contractions, supine position, and placental changes (aging) related to postterm gestation.

   B. *Nursing interventions:* discontinue Pitocin to stop stimulation of uterine contractions; change to lateral position to enhance uteroplacental perfusion; administer oxygen via mask to increase available oxygen to fetus; assess response to actions; notify primary health care provider regarding assessment findings, actions taken, and patient response; document.

3. *Analysis of monitor tracings:*

   A. *Reassuring FHR pattern:* see Fetal Response subsection in Basis for Monitoring section; compare criteria of reassuring FHR pattern and normal uterine contractions with what is seen on the monitor tracing.

   B. *Late deceleration pattern with minimal variability:* see Fig. 11-11 *and* Box 11-4.

   C. *Bradycardia with moderate variability, average FHR of 90 beats/min:* see Fig. 11-8 and Table 11-3 to formulate answer.

   D. *Early deceleration:* recognize this as a reassuring pattern; see Fig. 11-10 and Box 11-3 to formulate answer.

   E. *Tachycardia with average FHR of 210 beats/min:* see Table 11-3 to formulate answer.

   F. *Variable deceleration pattern:* see Box 11-5 and Fig. 11-12 to formulate answer.

CHAPTER 12: NURSING CARE OF THE FAMILY DURING LABOR AND BIRTH

Chapter Review Activities

1. TL, 2. FL, 3. FL, 4. TL, 5. TL, 6. FL, 7. TL, 8. FL, 9. TL, 10. TL, 11. TL

12. Fetus is born; dilation, effacement, baby's birth, latent, descent, transition; 2

13. Baby is born, delivered; separation, fundus, discoid, globular (ovoid), gush of dark blood, lengthening, fullness

14. F, 15. I, 16. G, 17. B, 18. L, 19. A, 20. E, 21. J, 22. D, 23. C, 24. H, 25. K,

26. Uterine contractions

27. Increment

28. Acme

29. Decrement

30. Frequency

31. Intensity

32. Duration

33. Resting tone

34. Interval

35. Bearing down

36. *Assessment of uterine contractions:*

   A. *Label illustration:* A. Beginning of a contraction; B. Duration; C. Frequency; D. Relaxation (interval between contractions); E. Intensity; 1. Increment; 2. Acme; 3. Decrement

   B. *Method of assessment:* place hand on fundus and determine changes in tone for several contractions and rest periods; press finger into fundus at acme (peak) of contraction to determine intensity.

37. *Admission of woman in labor:* see Assessment and Nursing Diagnoses subsection of Care Management—First Stage of Labor section to formulate answer:

   A. *Information from prenatal record:* see Prenatal Data subsection; include such information as age; weight gain; health status and medical problems during pregnancy; past and present obstetric history (gravida, para), including outcomes and problems encountered; laboratory and diagnostic tests with results, estimated date of birth; baseline data from pregnancy, including vital signs and fetal heart rate.

   B. *Information regarding status of labor:* factors distinguishing false labor from true labor are uterine contractions (onset, characteristics), show, status of membranes, fetal movement, discomfort (location, characteristics), and any other signs and symptoms of labor experienced.

   C. *Information regarding current health status:* include health problems, respiratory status, allergies, character and time of last oral intake, and emotional status.

38. F, 39. F, 40. T, 41. F, 42. T, 43. F, 44. T, 45. T, 46. F, 47. F, 48. F, 49. F, 50. T, 51. F, 52. F, 53. F, 54. T

55. *Complete table related to labor stressors and support measures:* see Stress in Labor and Culture subsections of Assessment—First Stage of Labor section; see Supportive Care during Labor and Birth subsection in Plan of Care and Interventions within the First Stage of Labor section, Plan of Care—Labor and Birth section; include physical and emotional stressors and the changing nature of stressors as labor progresses; support measures identified should reflect the changing nature of the stressors; a couple's birth plan often identifies the type of support measures that they prefer.

56. *Signs of potential complications:* see Signs of Potential Complications box.

57. *Complete table related to labor positions:* see Box 12-4 and Ambulation and Positioning subsection of Plan of Care and Interventions within the First Stage of Labor section.

58. *Critical factors to include in physical assessment of maternal-fetal unit during labor:* see care paths for low-risk woman in first stage of labor and second and third stages of labor:
   - **Maternal factors:** Vital signs, uterine activity, cervical changes, show and bleeding, amniotic fluid, behavior, appearance, mood, energy level, bearing-down effort, and use of childbirth preparation methods.
   - **Fetal factors:** Fetal heart rate (FHR) pattern, activity level, progress in cardinal movements of labor, and passage of meconium.

59. *Laboratory and diagnostic tests during labor:* see Laboratory and Diagnostic Tests subsection of Assessment and Nursing Diagnoses—First Stage of Labor section; complete blood count, type, and Rh; analysis of urine and dipstick for protein, ketone, glucose; nitrazine and ferning tests of amniotic fluid; additional testing depends on condition of the maternal-fetal unit and requirements of state law, such as human immunodeficiency virus screening.

60. *Complete table regarding events, behaviors, and support measures during the second stage of labor:* see care path for woman during second stage of labor and Table 12-3.

61. *Factors influencing duration of second stage of labor:* include use of regional anesthesia such as epidural block; quality of bearing-down efforts and positions used; parity, size, presentation, and position of the fetus; maternal pelvic adequacy; and physical status of the mother, including level of energy.

62. *Recommended positions for second stage of labor and bearing-down efforts:* see Maternal Position and Bearing-Down Efforts subsections of Second Stage of Labor section and Fig. 12-15; describe squatting, side-lying, semisitting, standing, and hands-and-knees positions.

63. A is correct; although B, C, and D are all important questions, the first question should obtain information about whether the woman is in labor.

64. C is correct; pH of amniotic fluid is 6.5 or higher, ferning is noted when examining fluid with a microscope, and the fluid is relatively odorless; a strong odor is strongly suggestive of infection.

65. C is correct; O or occiput indicates a vertex presentation with the neck fully flexed and the occiput in the transverse section (T) of the woman's pelvis; the station is 2 cm below the ischial spines (2); the woman is entering the active phase of labor; the lie is longitudinal because the head (cephalic, vertex) is presenting.

66. B is correct; maternal blood pressure, pulse, and respirations should be assessed every 30 minutes; temperature should be assessed every 2 hours once the membranes rupture; vaginal examinations are performed as indicated by labor events and not on a regular basis.

67. B is correct; research has indicated that enemas are not needed during labor; according to research findings, A, C, and D have all been found to be beneficial and safe during pregnancy.

Critical Thinking Exercises

1. *Woman calls nurse thinking she is in labor* (see Teaching Guidelines box—How to Distinguish True Labor from False Labor and Box 12-1):
   A. *Nursing approach:* determine the status of her labor by asking her to describe what she is experiencing and comparing her description with the characteristics of false and true labor.
   B. *Write questions:* questions should be clear, concise, open-ended, and directed toward distinguishing her labor status and creating a basis for action.
   C. *Instructions for home care of woman in latent labor:* discuss comfort measures, distracting activities, measures to reduce anxiety, and measures to enhance labor progress; inform regarding assessment measures to use to determine progress of labor and signs of problems, when and whom to call, and when to come to the hospital; nurse can make follow-up phone call to determine how woman is progressing.

2. *Women in first stage of labor at various phases:*
   A. *Identify phase of labor for each woman:* see Table 12-1 to determine phase; Denise: active phase; Teresa: transition; Danielle: latent.
   B. *Describe behavior and appearance expected for each woman:* see Tables 12-1 and 12-3 for

descriptions; consider the phase of the woman's labor when formulating answer.

C. *Specify physical and emotional care required:* see care path for low-risk woman in first stage of labor and Tables 12-1, 12-2, and 12-3 for care measures required for each woman according to her phase of labor.

3. *Procedure for locating point of maximal impulse (PMI) before auscultation of FHR or application of ultrasound transducer:* realize that fetal presentation and position affect location of PMI of FHR (see Fig. 12-6) and that Leopold maneuvers facilitate location of this point; also realize that this point will change as the baby progresses through the birth canal.

4. *Actions and rationale when membranes rupture:* carry out immediate assessment of FHR and pattern for changes associated with cord compression and vaginal examination (status of cervix, check for cord prolapse), assess fluid (amount, characteristics); use strict infection control measures after rupture because risk for infection increases.

5. *Nursing diagnosis:* anxiety related to lack of knowledge and experience regarding the process of childbirth.

   • **Expected outcome:** couple will cooperate with measures to enhance progress of their labor as their anxiety level decreases.

   • **Nursing measures:** provide full, simple explanations about each aspect of labor and care measures as they occur, demonstrate and assist with simple breathing techniques and relaxation measures, use phases of labor to tailor health teaching (doing more during latent phase and then less as labor progresses), and model coaching and comfort measures that father of baby can perform.

6. *Couple surprised by changes in approaches to facilitate the labor process:*

   • Discuss advantages of the new approaches: internal locus of control (listening to her own body) and maternal position that applies principle of gravity facilitate the process of labor and can even shorten its duration, advantageous for both mother and fetus.

   • Assure couple that new bearing-down efforts are safer (better oxygenation) and more effective (less tiring while applying effective force to facilitate descent) and that new positions enhance uteroplacental circulation. Use illustrations, models, and even video to help couple learn techniques while woman is still in the latent phase of labor.

   • Demonstrate positions and help her practice them.

7. *Criteria of effective pushing:* see Bearing-Down Efforts subsection of Second Stage of Labor section; include cleansing breaths, open-glottis pushing with no breath holding longer than 5 to 7 seconds, catch breaths, strong expiratory grunt, and upright position.

8. *Second stage of labor with reluctance to bear down and give birth:* see Bearing-Down Efforts subsection:

   A. *Reasons for reluctance:* many are listed in this section; include not feeling ready to be a mother, waiting for someone to come, being embarrassed about pushing and what happens during bearing-down efforts, feeling fear for self and baby, giving up, and having previous negative experience.

   B. *Nursing intervention:* recognize her feeling, identify her reason for not continuing, address her concern, and help her continue.

9. *Are episiotomies needed?*—see Perineal Trauma Related to Childbirth section; compare episiotomies with spontaneous laceration in terms of tissue affected, long-term sequelae, healing, and discomfort; compare reasons given for performing episiotomies with what research has demonstrated to be true.

10. *Siblings at childbirth:* include research findings regarding effect of sibling participation on family and on the sibling; consider developmental readiness of child for this experience; use developmental principles to prepare the sibling for the experience; evaluate parental comfort with this childbirth option; and arrange for a support person to remain with the child during the entire childbirth process. See Siblings during Labor and Birth subsection to formulate your answer.

11. *Primipara exhibiting disinterest in newborn during the fourth stage of labor:* see Third Stage of Labor—Family-Newborn relationships subsection:

    A. *Factors accounting for this behavior:* included are exhaustion, discomfort, cultural beliefs, disappointment, difficult labor and birth, taking-in stage of recovery.

    B. *Nursing measures:* continue to assess response to newborn; provide time for close contact with newborn when mother is more comfortable and rested; provide for her needs and help her meet these needs during the taking-in stage in terms of comfort, rest, nutrition, and desire to review childbirth events.

CHAPTER 13: MATERNAL PHYSIOLOGIC CHANGES

Chapter Review Activities

1. T, 2. F, 3. F, 4. T, 5. T, 6. F, 7. T, 8. F, 9. T, 10. F, 11. T, 12. F, 13. T, 14. F

15. *Assessment of bladder for distention:* see Urethra and Bladder subsection of Urinary System section.

    A. *Reasons bladder distention is more likely to occur:* include birth-induced trauma to urethra and bladder, edematous urethra, increased bladder capacity, effect of conduction anesthesia, pelvic soreness, lacerations and episiotomy, and increased urine production as a result of diuresis.

B. *Problems associated with bladder distention:*
- **Early:** pushes uterus up and to the side, preventing uterus from contracting firmly and leading to excessive bleeding;
- **Later:** overdistention can lead to stasis of urine and urinary tract infection.

16. *Factors interfering with bowel elimination:* see Bowel Evacuation subsection of Gastrointestinal System section; include decreased muscle tone on the intestine, effect of progesterone, prelabor diarrhea, lack of oral intake and dehydration from labor, anticipated discomfort related to hemorrhoids and perineal trauma, and resistance to urge to defecate.

17. *Hypovolemic shock less likely to occur in postpartum woman:* see Blood Volume subsection of Cardiovascular System section; pregnancy-induced hypervolemia allows most women to tolerate considerable blood loss during childbirth; decreased size of maternal vascular bed occurs with delivery of placenta, stimulus for vasodilation is lost, and extravascular water stored during pregnancy is mobilized.

18. *Factors increasing risk for thromboembolism:* see Coagulation Factors subsection of Blood Components section; increase in clotting factors and fibrinogen levels during pregnancy continues into the postpartum period; hypercoagulable state plus vessel damage with childbirth and decreased activity level of postpartum period increase risk.

19. *Compare and contrast lochial and nonlochial bleeding:* use Table 13-1 to formulate answer.

20. D is correct; fundus should be at midline; deviation from midline might indicate a full bladder; bright-to–dark red uterine discharge refers to lochia rubra; edema and erythema are common shortly after repair of a wound; decreased abdominal muscle tone and enlarged uterus result in abdominal protrusion; separation of the abdominal muscle walls, diastasis rectus abdominis, is common during pregnancy and the postpartum period.

21. B is correct; the woman is describing the normal finding of postpartum diaphoresis, which is the body's attempt to excrete fluid retained during pregnancy; documentation is important but not the first nursing action; infection assessment and physician notification are not needed at this time.

22. D is correct; afterpains are most likely to occur in the following circumstances: multiparity, overdistention of the uterus (macrosomia, multifetal pregnancy), breastfeeding (endogenous oxytocin secretion), and administration of an oxytocic.

Critical Thinking Exercises

1. *Postpartum women's questions and concerns:*
   A. *Afterpains:* basis for afterpains includes the fact that this woman is breastfeeding; sucking of the infant stimulates the posterior pituitary gland to secrete oxytocin for the let-down reflex; but it also stimulates the uterus to contract, creating uterine cramps for the first few days postpartum.
   B. *How long uterus will be palpable through the abdomen:* after 1 week the uterus is in the true pelvis, and after the ninth day it is not palpable through the abdomen.
   C. *Stages and duration of lochia:* see Lochia subsection of Uterus section; discuss characteristics of rubra, serosa, and alba, including color, consistency, amount, odor, and duration.
   D. *Protruding abdomen:* see Abdominal section; enlarged uterus plus stretched abdominal muscles with diminished tone creates a still-pregnant appearance for the first few weeks after birth; by 6 weeks the abdominal wall will almost return to its prepregnant state; skin will regain most of its elasticity; striae will fade but remain; discuss exercise and a sensible weight loss program to facilitate return of tone and diminish protrusion.
   E. *Diaphoresis and diuresis:* see Postpartal Diuresis subsection of Urinary section; discuss normalcy of these processes to rid body of fluid retained during pregnancy.
   F. *Breastfeeding as a contraceptive method:* see Pituitary Hormones and Ovarian Function subsection of Endocrine System section; emphasize that breastfeeding is not a reliable method because return of ovulation is unpredictable and might precede mensturation; discuss appropriate contraceptive measures, taking care to avoid hormonally based methods until lactation is firmly established.
   G. *Lactation suppression in bottle-feeding woman:* see Nonbreastfeeding Mothers subsection of Breast section; breasts will fill with milk as estrogen and progesterone levels decrease; engorgement resolves spontaneously, and discomfort decreases within 24 to 36 hours; because milk is not removed, the cycle shuts down, and the milk is absorbed into the circulatory system; she will need to support her breasts with a snug bra, avoid warmth on breasts and expressing any of the milk, and use ice for comfort.
   H. *Sexuality during postpartum period of breastfeeding woman:* see Vagina and Perineum subsection of Reproductive System and Associated Structures section; discuss role of prolactin in suppressing estrogen secretion, thereby decreasing vaginal lubrication and resulting in vaginal dryness and dyspareunia; these effects persist until ovulation resumes; use water-soluble lubricant to decrease discomfort.

CHAPTER 14: NURSING CARE OF THE FAMILY DURING THE FOURTH TRIMESTER

Chapter Review Activities

1. Fourth stage of labor

2. Couplet care; mother and baby, single-room maternity

3. Oxytocic

4. Uterine atony; excessive bleeding (hemorrhage)

5. Sitz bath

6. Afterpains (afterbirth pains)

7. Splanchnic engorgement; orthostatic hypotension

8. Positive Homans' sign

9. Kegel

10. Engorgement

11. Rubella

12. Rh immune globulin; Kleihauer-Betke

13. *Reasons for breastfeeding in fourth stage of labor:* it takes advantage of the infant's alert state during the first period of reactivity, aids in contraction of the uterus to prevent hemorrhage, is a good opportunity to instruct the mother and assess breasts, facilitates the bonding and attachment process, and stimulates infant's bowel so bilirubin-containing meconium is passed.

14. *Measures to assist with voiding:* see Prevention of Bladder Distention subsection in Plan of Care and Interventions section; help her to assume an upright position on bedpan or in bathroom, listen to running water, put hands in warm water, pour water over perineum with peri bottle, stand in shower or sit in a sitz bath; put spirits of peppermint in bedpan, and provide analgesics.

15. *Measures to prevent thrombophlebitis:* see Ambulation subsection of Plan of Care and Interventions; have woman exercise legs with active ROM of knees, ankles, feet, and toes; ambulate; wear support hose; and keep well hydrated.

16. *Measures for bottle-feeding mother to suppress lactation and relieve discomfort of engorgement:* see Lactation Suppression subsection of Plan of Care and Interventions section; have woman wear supportive bra or breast binder continuously for at least the first 72 hours postpartum, avoid stimulating breasts (no warm water during shower, no infant sucking, no pumping or removal of milk from the breasts), apply ice packs or cabbage leaves intermittently to relieve soreness; use a mild analgesic.

17. *Two major interventions to prevent postpartum hemorrhage in early postpartum period:* see Prevention of Excessive Bleeding section:

    • Maintain uterine tone: massage fundus if boggy; expel clots when fundus is firm; administer oxytocic medications; have woman breastfeed.

    • Prevent bladder distention.

18. T, 19. F, 20. T, 21. F, 22. F, 23. F, 24. T, 25. F, 26. F, 27. T, 28. F

29. *Recovery room nurse report:* see Transfer from the Recovery Area subsection of the Fourth Stage of Labor section: outline essential information that should be reported regarding the condition of the woman and her new baby and the significant events and findings from her prenatal and childbirth periods.

30. *Infection control measures* (see Prevention of Infection subsection of Plan of Care and Interventions section

    A. *Measures to prevent transmission of infection from person to person:* include clean environment, handwashing, use of Standard Precautions, proper care and use of equipment.

    B. *Infection prevention measures to teach the woman:* teach avoidance of walking barefoot; use of handwashing; hygienic measures (general, breast, perineal); prevention of bladder infection; measures to enhance resistance to infection, including nutrition and rest.

31. *Signs of potential complications during the postpartum period:*

    • **Physiologic complications:** see Nursing Process box—Physiologic Postpartum Concerns and Table 14-1; signs are listed according to vital signs, energy level, uterus, lochia, perineum, legs, breasts, appetite, elimination, and rest.

    • **Psychosocial complications:** see Nursing Process box—Psychosocial Postpartum Concerns; problems identified relate to communication, self-esteem, mood, and support.

Critical Thinking Exercises

1. *Pain relief for the postpartum woman:* see Comfort subsection of Plan of Care and Interventions section; begin by assessing her pain and its characteristics (e.g., severity, type, location, relief measures tried and their effectiveness) as the basis for action; reassure the mother regarding the importance and safety of pain relief for her recovery; use a combination of nonpharmacologic and pharmacologic measures; if woman is breastfeeding, administer a systemic analgesic just before or just after breastfeeding; make sure that the analgesic is not contraindicated during lactation.

2. *Woman exhibiting signs of hemorrhage and shock:*

    A. *Criteria to determine if flow was excessive:* see Emergency box—Hypovolemic Shock and Prevention of Excessive Bleeding subsection of Plan of Care and Interventions section; note length of time that the pad was on and the degree to which it is saturated with lochia; check on the bed underneath the woman to determine if lochia has also pooled there.

    B. *Priority action:* assess fundus and massage if boggy; once firm, express clots if present; check bladder for distention and assist woman to empty if it is distended; administer oxytocics if ordered.

C. *Additional interventions:* see list of measures in the Emergency box—Hypovolemic Shock.

3. *Administering rubella vaccine to a postpartum woman:* see Health Promotion of Future Pregnancies and Children section; recheck titer results and order, determine if woman or any household member is immunocompromised, check allergies (duck eggs), inform her regarding side effects, and emphasize that she must not become pregnant for at least 2 to 3 months after the immunization.

4. *Administering* Rh immunoglobulin *(RhoGAM) to a postpartum woman:* check woman's and infant's Rh status and results of direct and indirect Coombs' test; obtain RhoGAM from blood bank, carefully checking all identification data before administration intramuscularly; mother must be Rh negative and infant Rh positive, and both Coombs' tests results must be negative.

5. *Sexual changes after pregnancy and childbirth:* see Sexual Activity/Contraception subsection of Discharge Teaching section and Patient Instructions for Self-Management box—Resumption of Sexual Intercourse; identify changes that might occur, discuss physical and emotional readiness of the woman, stress importance of open communication, discuss how to prevent discomfort in terms of position and lubrication, and emphasize the importance of using birth control, because the return of ovulation cannot be predicted accurately.

6. *Postpartum women:* nursing diagnosis, expected outcome, and management:

   A. *Nursing diagnosis:* risk for infection of episiotomy related to ineffective perineal hygiene measures.

   - **Expected outcome:** episiotomy will heal without infection.
   - **Management:** see Prevention of Infection subsection of Plan of Care and Interventions section and Box 14-4 for full identification of measures to enhance healing and prevent infection.

   B. *Nursing diagnosis:* constipation related to inactivity and lack of knowledge regarding measures to promote elimination during the postpartum period.

   - **Expected outcome:** patient will have bowel movement within 2 days.
   - **Management:** see Promotion of Normal Bladder and Bowel Patterns subsection; determine what she usually does to enhance bowel elimination; encourage activity, roughage, fluids; obtain order for a mild stool softener and laxative combination.

   C. *Nursing diagnosis:* acute pain related to episiotomy and hemorrhoids.

   - **Expected outcome:** patient will experience a reduction in pain following implementation of suggested relief measures.
   - **Management:** see Promotion of Comfort subsection and Box 14-4; emphasize nonpharmacologic relief measures such as perineal care, sitz bath, topicals, side-lying position when in bed, Kegel exercises, measures to enhance bowel and bladder elimination; use pharmacologic measures if local measures are ineffective.

7. *Postpartum woman with fundus above umbilicus and off midline:*

   A. *Most likely basis:* suspect bladder distention; confirm by palpating the bladder and asking the woman about the last time she voided.

   B. *Nursing action:* assist woman to empty bladder; measure amount voided and characteristics of the urine; palpate bladder and fundus again to determine response. Catheterization might be required if woman cannot empty bladder fully because a distended bladder can lead to hemorrhage and urinary tract infections.

8. *Resumption of physical activity after giving birth:* see Ambulation subsection of Plan of Care and Interventions section.

   - Assess postanesthesia recovery and physical stability.
   - Assist and supervise first few times out of bed because orthostatic hypotension can cause her to become dizzy and fall.
   - Show her where the call light is and what to do if she is alone and begins to feel dizzy or light-headed.

9. *Resumption of full oral intake after giving birth:* see Promotion of Nutrition subsection of Plan of Care and Interventions section; assess woman for physiologic stability (vital signs, fundus, lochia, perineum) before she resumes full diet; determine type of anesthesia used for birth (if general anesthesia, make sure that woman is fully alert and gag reflex has returned).

10. *Woman preparing for early discharge:*

   A. *Nurse's legal responsibility in terms of discharge:* nurse must assess woman, newborn, and family to confirm that criteria for discharge are fully met; if the criteria are not met, the nurse must notify the primary health care provider of the findings; document all assessment findings, actions, and responses.

   B. *Criteria for discharge—maternal, newborn, general:* see Box 14-2, which fully identifies the criteria that must be met before early discharge.

   C. *Outline essential content that must be taught before discharge:* see Discharge Teaching section; include information regarding self-care, signs of complications, sexual activity, prescribed medications, and routine mother and baby checkups; arranging for a follow-up telephone call and/or a home visit within 1 to 2 days of discharge is critical when early discharge occurs; give hotline telephone number and instructions on how to contact health care provider.

11. *Cultural beliefs:* see Cultural Considerations box—Postpartum Period and Family Planning.

   A. *Importance of using a culturally sensitive approach:* recognition of a woman's cultural beliefs and practices is essential so the designed plan of care meets her individual needs; such an approach demonstrates respect, caring, and concern.

   B. *Korean-American Women—heat and cold balance:* ask woman about the substances and practices that she identifies to be hot and cold; then intervene appropriately.

   C. *Muslim woman in postpartum period:* emphasize dietary modification and modesty.

CHAPTER 15: TRANSITION TO PARENTHOOD

Chapter Review Activities

1. *Complete table related to maternal adjustment:* see Parental Role After childbirth section.

2. *Attachment of newborn to parents and parents to newborn:* see Parental Attachment, Bonding, and Acquaintance section:

   A. *Define attachment and bonding:*

- **Attachment:** process by which a parent comes to love and accept a child and a child comes to love and accept a parent.

- **Bonding:** sensitive period in the first few minutes and hours after birth when parents must have close contact with their infants for optimal later development; definition has been modified to recognize the adaptability of human parents.

- Terms are often used interchangeably.

   B. *Conditions to facilitate attachment:* emotionally healthy parents, competent in communication and caregiving; parent and newborn fit in terms of state, temperament, and gender; proximity and time for interaction; positive feedback and mutually satisfying experience.

   C. *Describe acquaintance process:* parents use eye contact, touch, talking, and exploring to become acquainted and to get to know their newborn; claiming or identification in terms of likeness, difference, and uniqueness is part of this process.

   D. *Assessment of the progress of attachment:* see Tables 15-1 and 15-2 for specific facilitating and inhibiting behaviors that should be assessed; see Box 15-1 for specific attachment behaviors.

3. *Parental tasks:* see Parental Tasks and Responsibilities subsection of Parental Role after Childbirth section:

- Establish a place for the newborn within the family.

- Reconcile actual child with fantasy or dream child.

- Become skillful in care of infant.

- Recognize cues and needs and respond appropriately.

4. *Parent-infant contact:* see specific subsection for each form of contact in Parent-Infant Contact section:

- **Early contact:** important to provide time for parents to see, touch, and hold their baby as soon as possible after birth; stress to parents that attachment is an ongoing process that occurs over time; interference with this early contact because of maternal and/or newborn problems will not have long-term effects.

- **Extended contact:** family-centered care, mother-baby care, and use of LDR/LDRP rooms facilitate this type of contact; this is especially important for parents at risk for parenting inadequacies.

5. Mutuality

6. Acquaintance, eye contact, touching, talking, exploring

7. Claiming; likeness, differences, uniqueness

8. Entrainment, waving of arms, lifting of head, kicking of legs, dancing in tune

9. Biorhythmicity; loving care, alert, responsive, social interactions, learning

10. Reciprocity; synchrony

11. En face

12. Engrossment

13. *Complete table related to parent and infant facilitating and inhibiting behaviors as they relate to the process of attachment:* see Table 15-1, which covers infant behaviors affecting parent attachment, and Table 15-2, which covers parental behaviors affecting infant attachment, to complete the table.

14. *Factors that influence manner in which parents respond to the birth of their child:* see the information provided in the separate subsections for each of the factors in the Parental Responses section.

15. D is correct; A reflects the first phase of identifying likenesses; B reflects the second phase of identifying differences; C reflects a negative reaction of claiming the infant in terms of pain and discomfort; D reflects the third or final stage of identifying uniqueness.

16. B is correct; early close contact is recommended to initiate and enhance the attachment process.

17. A is correct; engrossment refers to a father's absorption, preoccupation, and interest in his infant; B represents the claiming process, phase I, identifying likeness; C represents reciprocity; D represents en face or face-to-face position with mutual gazing.

18. B is correct; taking-in is the first 1 to 2 days of recovery following birth; other behaviors exhibited include reliance on others to help her meet needs, excitation, and talkativeness.

19. C is correct; approximately 75% to 80% of women experience postpartum blues; new parents should be reassured that their skills as parents develop gradually and that they should seek help to develop these skills; postpartum blues, which are self-limiting and short lived, do not require psychotropic medications; support and care of the postpartum woman and her newborn by her partner and family are the most effective prevention and coping strategies; feelings of fatigue from childbirth and meeting demands of the newborn can accentuate feelings of depression.

Critical Thinking Exercises

1. *Teaching parents regarding communicating with their newborn:* see Communication between Parent and Infant section:

   A. *Communication techniques to interact with newborn:* discuss techniques related to touch, eye contact, voice, and odor; demonstrate techniques, have parents try them, and point out newborn's response in terms of quieting, alerting, making eye contact, and gazing; help parents interpret cues.

   B. *Manner in which baby communicates with them:* point out infant responses; discuss processes of entrainment, biorhythmicity, reciprocity, synchrony, and repertoire of behaviors.

2. *Woman following emergency cesarean birth disappointed with lack of immediate bonding time with newborn:*

   • Discuss concepts of early and extended contact.

   • Emphasize that the parent-infant attachment process occurs over time and is ongoing; her emotional bond with her baby will not be weaker.

   • Discuss adaptability of human parents in forming emotional relationship with their infant.

   • Help her to meet her own physical and emotional needs so she develops readiness to meet her newborn's needs.

   • Provide time and help her to get to know her baby, interact with her, and care for her; point out newborn characteristics, including how the newborn is responding to her efforts.

   • Show her how to communicate with her newborn and how her newborn communicates with her.

   • Arrange for follow-up after discharge to see how things are progressing in terms of her transition to the parenthood role.

3. *Sibling adjustment to the newborn:* see Sibling Adaptation section, which describes how siblings react to a newborn, and Box 15-3, which identifies strategies parents can use to help their other children

adapt; caution her that adjustment takes time and is very much related to the developmental level and experiences of the sibling.

4. *Parents unsure and anxious about caring for their newborn baby:* see Parental Attachment, Bonding, and Acquaintance section and Table 15-3:

   A. *Nursing diagnosis:* risk for impaired parent-infant attachment or risk for impaired parenting related to lack of knowledge and feelings of incompetence regarding infant care.

   B. *Nursing strategies can include:*

   • Performing a newborn assessment with the parents present, pointing out newborn characteristics, and encouraging parents to participate and ask questions.

   • Demonstrating newborn care skills and providing time for parents to practice and obtain feedback.

   • Providing extended contact with their newborn until discharge.

   • Making referrals for follow-up in the home with telephone contacts and home visits; referring to parenting classes and support groups.

   • Recommending books, magazines, and videos that discuss newborns and their characteristics and care.

5. *Parental disappointment with newborn's gender and appearance:* see Parental Tasks and Responsibilities section; foster attachment and claiming; help parents get acquainted with the infant and help them reconcile the real child with the fantasy child; discuss the basis for molding, caput, and forceps marks and how they will be resolved; be alert for problems with attachment and care so follow-up can be arranged.

6. *Grandparent adjustment:* see Grandparent Adaptation section; observe interaction between grandparents and parents, taking note of signs of effective interaction and signs of conflict; involve grandparents in teaching sessions as appropriate; spend time with grandparents to help them be supportive of the new family without "taking over" and informative without being critical; help the new parents recognize the unique role that grandparents can play as parenting role models, nurturers for the new generation, and providers of respite care for the parents.

7. *Postpartum woman experiencing postpartum blues:*

   • **Nursing diagnosis:** ineffective coping related to hormonal changes and increased responsibilities of the postpartum period.

   • **Expected outcome:** woman will report feeling more content with her new role following use of recommended coping strategies for postpartum blues.

   • **Nursing management:** see Patient Instructions for Self-Management box—Coping with Postpartum Blues; be sure to involve both Jane and her husband in teaching and developing a plan for coping with the blues; it is essential that this occur early to prevent development of postpartum depression.

CHAPTER 16: PHYSIOLOGIC AND BEHAVIORAL ADAPTATIONS OF THE NEWBORN

Chapter Review Activities

1. P, 2. N, 3. N, 4. P, 5. N, 6. N, 7. N, 8. N, 9. P, 10. N, 11. N, 12. N, 13. P, 14. N, 15. P, 16. N, 17. P, 18. N, 19. N, 20. N, 21. P, 22. N, 23. P

24. *Newborn—establishment of respirations:*

   A. *Factors initiating breathing after birth:* reflex triggered by such factors as pressure changes, chilling, noise, light, and other sensations associated with exposure to extrauterine life and chemoreceptor activation by lowered oxygen level, higher carbon dioxide level, and lower pH.

   B. *Conditions essential for maintaining an adequate oxygen supply:* removal of lung fluid, synchronous expansion of chest and abdomen, patent airway, and sufficient surfactant.

   C. *Expected newborn respiratory pattern:* shallow and irregular rate of 30 to 60 breaths/min, short periods of apnea less than 20 seconds, and loud and clear breath sounds.

   D. *Signs of respiratory distress:* see Signs of Respiratory Distress subsection; nasal flaring, retractions, and increased use of intercostal muscles, grunting with respirations, seesaw respirations, rate of less than 30 or more than 60 breaths/min at rest, apnea longer than 20 seconds, and adventitious breath sounds.

25. *Complete table related to closure of fetal circulatory shunts:* see Cardiovascular System subsection of Physiologic Adaptations section for method of closure and Table 16-2 for location and purpose.

26. *Newborn—cold stress:* see Temperature Regulation subsection of Thermogenic System section and Fig. 16-2:

   A. *Dangers of cold stress:*

   - Metabolic and physiologic demands on the newborn increase, leading to increased oxygen need and consumption.

   - Oxygen and energy are diverted from brain cells, cardiac function, and growth.

   - Decreased oxygen leads to vasoconstriction, respiratory distress, and reopening of the ductus arteriosus.

   - Acidosis, increased level of bilirubin, hypoglycemia.

   B. *Newborn behaviors associated with cold stress:* include increased respiratory rate; cyanosis;

decrease in oxygen level, pH, and glucose level; and signs of acidosis.

   C. *Measures to stabilize newborn temperature:* see Heat Loss subsection of Thermogenic System section; implement measures that reflect application of heat loss mechanisms of convection, radiation, evaporation, and conduction:

   - Dry infant and cover with warmed blankets or wrap with mother on her abdomen.

   - Cover head.

   - Use radiant heat shield or warmer to stabilize temperature initially; assess newborn and perform procedures.

   - Adjust environment.

27. *Table related to heat loss mechanisms and measures to prevent heat loss:* see Heat Loss subsection of Thermogenic System section.

28. *Characteristics of physiologic jaundice:* see Jaundice subsection of Hepatic System section; major characteristic is the appearance of jaundice after the first 24 hours of life. Jaundice should last less than 7 to 10 days.

29. Sleep-wake; deep, light; drowsy, quiet alert, active alert, crying; quiet alert, smile, vocalize, move in synchrony with speech, watch parents' faces, respond to voices.

30. Habituation; environmental stimuli; constant, repetitive, decreased

31. Temperament

32. Consolability; hand-to-mouth, voices, noises, visual

33. Cuddliness

34. *Complete table related to periods of a newborn's transition to extrauterine life:* see Transition to Extrauterine Life section for identification of each period, description of timing and duration, and typical newborn behaviors for each phase.

35. T, 36. F, 37. F, 38. T, 39. T, 40. F, 41. F, 42. T, 43. F, 44. F

45. K, 46. F, 47. B, 48. J, 49. D, 50. I, 51. H, 52. L, 53. A, 54. E, 55. G, 56. C

57. *Factors influencing infant behavior:* see subsection for each factor listed in Behavioral Characteristics section; each factor is described in terms of its influence on newborn behavior.

58. D is correct; the newborn at 5 hours old is in the second period of reactivity during which tachycardia, tachypnea, increased muscle tone, skin color changes, mucus production, and passage of meconium occur; although a newborn can have periods of apnea, these should not exceed 15 seconds; the average heart rate of a newborn when awake is 120 to 160 beats/min.

59. A is correct; the rash described is erythema toxicum; it is an inflammatory response that has no clinical significance and requires no treatment because it will disappear spontaneously.

60. D is correct; B and C are common newborn reflexes used to assess integrity of neuromuscular system; measurement of legs is not a method for determination of hip dysplasia.

61. C is correct; telangiectatic nevi are also known as stork bite marks and can also appear on the eyelids; milia are plugged sebaceous glands and appear like white pimples; nevus vasculosus or a strawberry mark is a raised, sharply demarcated bright or dark red swelling; nevus flammeus is a flat red-to-purple port wine lesion that does not blanch with pressure.

Critical Thinking Exercises

1. *Complete table related to physiologic functioning of newborn compared to that of an adult:* use specific subsection for each function in the Physiologic Adaptation section to complete the table.

2. *Parental concern regarding head variations:* see Caput Succedaneum and Cephalohematoma subsections of Integumentary System and Molding in Skeletal System sections; discuss each finding in terms of what it is, why it happens, its significance for the newborn's health status and adjustment, and how and when it will be resolved; Fig. 16-4 can be used to facilitate parental understanding.

3. *Parental concern regarding "bruises" on back and buttocks of their newborn:* discuss mongolian spots, what they are, and why they occur; see Mongolian Spots subsection of Integumentary System section.

4. *Parental interest in sensory capabilities of newborn:* see Sensory Behaviors subsection of Behavioral Characteristics section:

    A. *Specify what nurse should tell parents:* discuss newborn's capability with regard to vision, hearing, touch, taste, and smell.

    B. *List stimuli parents can provide to facilitate their newborn's development:* use face-to-face, eye-to-eye contact and objects to look at, especially those with bright or black and white patterns; talk to infant; play music; use heartbeat simulator; touch infant; and use infant massage.

5. *Parental concern regarding newborn weight loss:* determine percentage of weight loss, making sure it is not more than 10%; explain to the parents that their newborn's weight loss of 6% is well within the expected range, tell them why the loss occurs, discuss feeding measures, and inform them that the birth weight will be regained within 2 weeks.

CHAPTER 17: ASSESSMENT AND CARE OF THE NEWBORN AND FAMILY

Chapter Review Activities

1. F, 2. T, 3. F, 4. F, 5. T, 6. F, 7. F, 8. F, 9. F, 10. T, 11. F, 12. T, 13. F, 14. T, 15. F, 16. F,

17. T, 18. F, 19. T, 20. F, 21. T, 22. T, 23. T, 24. F, 25. F, 26. F, 27. T

28. Prepuce (foreskin); parents

29. Tetracycline, erythromycin; lower conjunctiva

30. Vitamin K; 0.5 to 1 mg, 25, 5/8

31. Edema, redness, purulent drainage; erythromycin solution, triple blue dye, alcohol

32. Preterm, premature

33. Term

34. Postterm, postdate

35. Postmature

36. Large for gestational age (LGA)

37. Appropriate for gestational age (AGA)

38. Small for gestational age (SGA)

39. *Assessment of gestational age:* see Gestational Age Assessment subsection of Care Management section and Fig. 17-5:

    A. *Signs for neuromuscular maturity:* assess such signs as posture, arm recoil, popliteal angle, scarf sign, heel to ear; note that the full-term newborn is more flexed and resists efforts to pull limbs in a certain direction (e.g., bringing heel to ear or elbow across sternum).

    B. *Signs for physical maturity:* assess such signs as skin condition, presence of lanugo, plantar creases, breast size, eye and ear formation, condition of genitalia.

    C. *Designation of AGA, LGA, and SGA:*
    - First, determine gestational age using the new Ballard scale.
    - Second, measure newborn's head circumference, length, and weight.
    - Third, plot estimated gestational age and measurements on graph to determine classification.

40. *Health teaching in preparation for discharge:* see Teaching Guidelines box—Sponge Bathing and specific subsection for each teaching topic in Care Management: Discharge Planning and Teaching section.

41. *Safety and medical aseptic principles when sponge bathing newborn:* see Teaching Guidelines box— Sponge Bathing:
    - **Safety:** prevent heat loss, gather all supplies before starting, never leave infant alone, check water temperature, and never hold infant under running water.
    - **Medical asepsis:** wash head to toe, inner to outer canthus, and genitalia from front to back; avoid use of soap, especially harsh soaps; promptly change diapers; do cord and circumcision care; and maintain personal cleanliness such as handwashing.

42. *Creation of a protective environment in terms of environment, infection control, and safety:* see Protective Environment subsection of Interventions section:

- **Environment:** check adequate lighting, ventilation, warmth, and humidity; eliminate fire hazards; promote safety with electrical appliances.
- **Infection control:** use Standard Precautions correctly, including handwashing and gloving as appropriate, adequate floor space to keep bassinets 60 cm apart, areas for cleaning and storing equipment and supplies, keeping persons with infection away or using appropriate precautions; instruct persons in contact with newborns.
- **Safety:** include security measures, identification measures, and instruction of parents.

43. D is correct; thinning of lanugo with bald spots is consistent with full-term status; pulse and weight are not part of the Ballard scale; the popliteal angle for a full-term newborn would be 100 degrees or less.

44. C is correct; the hemoglobin should be 14 to 24 g/dl; hematocrit should be 44% to 64%; glucose should be 40 to 60 mg/dl; bilirubin should be 0 to 1 mg/dl.

45. B is correct; signs of hypoglycemia include cyanosis along with apnea, jitteriness and twitching, irregular respirations, high-pitched cry, difficulty feeding, hunger, lethargy, eye rolling, and seizures; C and D are consistent with hypocalcemia.

46. A is correct; the control panel should be set at 36° to 37° C; the probe should be placed in the right upper quadrant of the abdomen below the intercostal margin, never over a rib; axillary, not rectal, temperature should be taken every hour.

47. B is correct; the infant should be NPO for up to 4 hours to prevent vomiting and aspiration; the site should be checked every hour for 12 hours; diaper wipes should not be used on the site because they contain alcohol, which would delay healing and cause discomfort; the yellow exudate is a protective film that forms in 24 hours and should not be removed.

Critical Thinking Exercises

1. *Apgar scoring:* see Table 17-1:

A. *Baby boy Smith:* heart rate, 160 beats/min (2); respiratory effort, good (2); muscle tone, active movement (2); reflex irritability, crying, with stimulus (2); color, acrocyanosis (1); score: 9; interpretation: score of 7 to 10 indicates that infant will have no difficulty adjusting to extrauterine life.

B. *Baby girl Doe:* heart rate, 102 beats/min (2); respiratory effort, slow and irregular (1); muscle tone, some flexion (1); reflex irritability, grimace response to stimulus (1); color pale (0); score: 5; interpretation: score of 4 to 6 indicates moderate difficulty adjusting to extrauterine life.

2. *Assessment of newborn girl:*

A. *Protocol for assessment during first 2 hours:* see Table 17-1, Box 17-1, and Initial Physical Assessment section.

B. *Legal responsibility for identification:* complete the identification process before the mother and newborn are separated; follow agency policy, which often requires that mother and newborn have matching identification bands; newborn's footprint and mother's fingerprints are placed on a footprint form.

C. *Two priority nursing diagnoses:* consider nursing diagnoses related to ineffective airway clearance, hypothermia, and ineffective thermoregulation.

D. *Priority nursing care measures:* discuss each of these areas:

- Stabilization of respiration and airway patency
- Maintenance of body temperature
- Immediate interventions in terms of identification, prophylactic medications, and promotion of bonding

3. *Care of circumcision site and cord:*

A. *Nursing diagnosis:* risk for infection related to removal of foreskin and healing of umbilical cord site.

B. *Expected outcome:* cord and circumcision sites will heal without infection.

C. *Teaching regarding care:* see Teaching Guidelines boxes—Care of the Circumcised Newborn at Home and Sponge Bathing—(Cord Care section); emphasize importance of assessing sites for progress of healing and signs of infection; educate about measures to keep the area clean and dry; list measures to enhance comfort; ensure that parents know how to assess circumcision site for bleeding and what to do if it occurs and how to assess urination and what to do if newborn has difficulty voiding.

4. *Newborn with hyperbilirubinemia:* see Therapy for Hyperbilirubinemia section to formulate the answer:

A. *Respond to parents' concern:* tell parents in simple terms that their newborn is exhibiting physiologic jaundice; explain why it happens and that it is an expected finding experienced by many newborns.

B. *Identify expected findings of physiologic hyperbilirubinemia:* mention jaundice, watery greenish stool, sleepiness, cephalocaudal progression, and elevated serum bilirubin level.

C. *Precautions and care measures during phototherapy:* increase fluids, feed frequently (at least every 3 hours), cover eyes (close eyes before covering and make sure that nose does not become covered; remove eye covering periodically to check eyes), monitor temperature for increase or decrease, perform skin care by cleansing stools promptly and not using lotions, place uncovered under lights and change position every 2 hours, cover genitalia, and remove from lights for feeding, cuddling, and eye contact.

5. *Newborn with mucus in airway:* see Stabilization and Relieving Airway Obstruction subsections:

   A. *Signs of abnormal breathing:* see Signs of Potential Complications box—Abnormal Newborn Breathing; include rate change, altered breath sounds, and signs of distress.

   B. *Nursing diagnosis:* impaired gas exchange related to upper airway obstruction with mucus.

   C. *Steps for using bulb syringe* (see Fig. 17-2 and Procedure box—Suctioning with a Bulb Syringe): perform gentle percussion over chest if indicated; suction mouth first and then each nare; compress bulb before insertions; insert tip along side of mouth, not over tongue, which could stimulate the gag reflex; continue until breathing sounds clear; be sure to teach parents how to use a bulb syringe.

   D. *Guidelines for use of mechanical suction:* see Procedure box—Suctioning with a Nasopharyngeal Catheter with Mechanical Suction Apparatus: suction for 5 seconds or less per insertion, use less than 80 mm Hg setting, lubricate catheter with sterile water, insert orally along base of tongue or up and back into nares, activate suction as catheter is removed, and repeat until breathing sounds clear.

6. *Maternal concerns regarding immunizations:* emphasize that breastfeeding provides only temporary immunity to some infections; immunizations must be given as recommended in terms of timing and number to achieve active immunity to what could be life-threatening infections; provide mother with written materials to read and a person to call to ask questions and discuss concerns; make referrals to address her financial concerns.

7. *Newborn scheduled for circumcision—pain concerns:* see Neonatal Pain section and Table 17-4:

   A. *Common behavioral responses to pain:* include body movements (withdrawal of upper and lower limbs); vocalization (cry); and cry face, fussy, irritable, and listless responses.

   B. *Changes in vital signs and integument:* include increase or decrease in heart rate and blood pressure; rapid, shallow respirations; and pale or flushed, moist integument.

   C. *Nursing diagnosis:* acute pain related to effects of circumcision.

   D. *Nonpharmacologic and pharmacologic relief measures:* see Management of Neonatal Pain:

      Nonpharmacologic: swaddle afterward, promote nonnutritive sucking, take to mother to be fed

and comforted, distract (older infant), apply protective Vaseline or other ointment to site, change diaper frequently, and position on side.

Pharmacologic: use local anesthesia and/or topical preparations.

CHAPTER 18: NEWBORN NUTRITION AND FEEDING

Chapter Review Activities

1. *Energy and fluid requirements of newborns:*

   A. *Fill in the blanks:*

      1. 110, 100, 95, 100

      2. 67, 20; 20

   B. *Calculate daily energy requirements:* Jim (440 kcal); Sue (600 kcal); Sam (712.5 kcal); Jean (1050 kcal)

2. *Location and function of lactation structures:*

   A. *Label illustration of lactation structures of the breast:* see Fig. 18-2. A. Alveolus; B. Ductule; C. Duct; D. Lactiferous duct; E. Lactiferous sinus; F. Nipple pore; G. Ampulla; H. Areola

   B. *Fill in the Blanks:* 1. Lobes; 2. Alveoli; 3. Glandular tissue; 4. Pores; 5. Milk ducts; 6. Myeloepithelial; 7. Areola

3. *Identification of advantages of breastfeeding for infant, mother, and families and society:* see Benefits of Breastfeeding section, which identifies several benefits for each category.

4. *Describe four breastfeeding positions:* see Positioning subsection of Care Management: The Breastfeeding Mother and Infant section and Fig. 18-6; describe football hold, cradle (traditional position), modified cradle (across the lap position), and side-lying.

5. *Feeding readiness cues:* see Feeding Readiness section:

   A. *Cues:* they include hand-to-mouth or hand-to-hand movements, sucking motions, strong rooting reflex, and mouthing.

   B. *Rationale for feeding according to these cues:* if cues are missed, baby may cry vigorously, become distraught, or withdraw into sleep; these behaviors will make feeding more difficult or impossible; feeding when the infant exhibits readiness enhances the chance of success and encourages the mother to continue breastfeeding.

6. *Differences between foremilk and hindmilk:* see Uniqueness of Human Milk section:

   • **Foremilk:** bluish-white, part skim and part whole milk, lactose, protein, and water-soluble vitamins

   • **Hindmilk:** cream "let-down" into the feeding, denser in calories from fat to ensure optimal growth and contentment between feedings

7. *Label illustrations of reflexes:* see Fig. 18-5:
   - **Milk production reflex:** A. Sucking stimulus; B. Hypothalamus; C. Anterior pituitary gland (prolactin); D. Milk production
   - **Let-down reflex:** A. Sucking stimulus; B. Hypothalamus; C. Posterior pituitary gland (oxytocin); D. Let-down reflex

8. *Stages of lactogenesis:* see Uniqueness of Human Milk section:
   - **Stage I:** begins in pregnancy when breasts are prepared for milk production and colostrum is formed in the breasts.
   - **Stage II:** colostrum changes to mature milk, with milk coming in on the third to fifth day after birth and onset of copious milk production.
   - **Stage III:** milk changes over about 10 days later, when the mature milk is established in stage III.

9. *Proper latch-on and removal:* see Latch subsection of Care Management: The Breastfeeding Mother and Infant section and Figs. 18-7 and 18-8.
   A. *Steps a woman should follow to ensure proper latch-on:* express a few drops of colostrum or milk onto the nipple; support breast; hold baby close to breast; touch baby's lower lip with nipple to simulate rooting reflex; with baby's mouth open and tongue down, pull baby onto nipple and areola of breast.
   B. *Signs of proper latch-on:* there is a firm tugging sensation on nipple, with no pinching or pain; baby's cheeks are rounded; jaw glides smoothly with sucking; swallow is audible; mouth covers nipple and 2 to 3 cm of areola around the nipple; and nose, chin, and cheeks touch the breast.
   C. *Removal from breast:* break suction by inserting finger into side of baby's mouth.

10. F, 11. F, 12. T, 13. F, 14. T, 15. F, 16. F, 17. F, 18. T, 19. T, 20. F, 21. T, 22. F, 23. T, 24. T, 25. T, 26. F, 27. F, 28. F

29. *Calming a fussy baby:* see Fussy Baby subsection of Special Considerations section and Box 18-3 for several measures such as swaddling, holding, and talking soothingly that can be used.

30. *Complete table related to assessment of infant and mother with regard to breastfeeding:* see Assessment—Infant and Mother subsections of Care Management section and Box 18-1.

31. B is correct; birth weight is regained in 10 to 14 days; six to eight wet diapers are expected at this time; baby should be fed every 2 to 3 hours, for a total of 8 to 12 times per day.

32. A is correct; swaddling is recommended; B, C, and D are all appropriate actions to calm a fussy baby.

33. D is correct; no soap should be used because it could dry the nipple and areola and increase the risk for irritation; vitamin E should not be used because it is a fat-soluble vitamin that the infant could ingest when breastfeeding; lanolin, colostrum, and milk are the preferred substances to be applied to the area; plastic liners can trap moisture and lead to sore nipples.

34. B is correct; a hormonal contraceptive could decrease the milk supply if given before lactation is well established during the first 6 weeks after birth; after 6 weeks a progestin-only contraceptive could be used because it is the hormonal contraceptive least likely to affect lactation; even complete breastfeeding is not considered to be a reliable method because ovulation can occur unexpectedly, even before the first menstrual period.

35. C is correct; the baby should be placed on the right side after feeding because this allows air bubbles to come up easily; tap water can be used unless the water supply is unsafe or unless otherwise instructed; formula should never be heated in the microwave because it could be overheated or heated unevenly.

Critical Thinking Exercises

1. *Analysis of a woman's breastfeeding technique:* + indicates competency and − indicates need for further instruction:

   A. −, B. +, C. −, D. −, E. +, F. −, G. +, H. +, I. −, J. −, K. +, L. −, M. −

2. *Infant feeding method decision making during prenatal period:* see Choosing an Infant Feeding Method section:

   A. *Nursing diagnosis and expected outcome:* decisional conflict related to lack of knowledge and experience regarding infant feeding methods; couple will choose method of infant feeding based on accurate information regarding the pros and cons of each feeding method.

   B. *Rationale for couple making the decision together:* both should learn about the pros and cons of feeding methods, with an emphasis on the benefits of breastfeeding and how the partner can help with the method chosen, because partner support is a major factor in a woman's choice to breast feed and in her breastfeeding success.

   C. *Why make the decision prenatally:* the prenatal period is a less stressful time, allowing for full consideration of options—feeding methods (including breastfeeding) that would be incorporated into life activities such as work outside the home, breastfeeding techniques and benefits by attending classes and reading.

   D. *How nurse can facilitate the decision-making process:* provide factual information about feeding methods in a nonjudgmental manner; dispel myths; address personal concerns of the couple; and make needed referrals to women, infants, and children (WIC), lactation consultant, breastfeeding classes, or La Leche League.

3. *Breastfeeding mother's questions and concerns:* see Anatomy and Physiology of Lactation section:

A. *Breast size:* discuss development of lactation structures in the breasts during pregnancy; emphasize that it is this development, not the size of the breasts, that is important.

B. *Let-down reflex:* explain what it is, why it happens (including physical and emotional triggers), what it will feel like, and why it is so important in terms of the hindmilk that the baby receives.

C. *Signs that breastfeeding is going well for mother and baby:* see Assessment of Infant and Mother subsections of Care Management-Breast Feeding section and Box 18-1, which identifies maternal and fetal indicators of effective breastfeeding.

D. *Nipple soreness:* see Sore Nipples subsection of Care of the Breastfeeding Mother section; discuss, demonstrate, and observe measures to prevent and treat sore nipples, including good breastfeeding techniques such as latch-on, removal, alternating of starting breasts and positions, and breast care measures such as air-drying nipples, avoiding use of soap, applying colostrum and then breast milk after feeding, and applying ice to nipples and areola 2 to 3 minutes before feeding.

E. *Engorgement:* see Engorgement section; prevention measures include frequency of feeding every 2 to 3 hours with 15 to 20 minutes on each breast; treatment measures include warm packs and massage before feeding, ice afterwards, cabbage leaves, and support.

F. *Afterpains and increased flow:* see Lactogenesis subsection of Anatomy and Physiology of Lactation section; explain that oxytocin is released during a feeding as a result of newborn sucking; this hormone triggers the let-down reflex but also stimulates the uterus to contract, causing afterpains in the first 3 to 5 days after birth; this hormone will reduce excessive bleeding.

G. *Breastfeeding as a birth control method:* see section on breastfeeding and contraception; emphasize that breastfeeding is not an effective contraceptive method because, even though ovulation might be delayed, its return is unpredictable and could occur before the first menstrual period; discuss contraceptive methods that are safe to use with breastfeeding.

H. *Weaning:* see Weaning subsection of Care Management-Breastfeeding section; emphasize that weaning needs to be a gradual process, eliminating one feeding at a time.

4. *Starting solid foods:* see Introducing Solid Foods section; emphasize importance of waiting to introduce solids at 4 to 6 months of age when the infant is physically and developmentally ready; early introduction of solid foods can lead to allergies, excessive caloric intake, and diminished interest in breastfeeding; dispel myth that solids encourage sleeping through the night.

5. *Infrequent feeding of sleeping baby:* see Frequency of Feedings, Duration of Feedings, and Special Considerations subsections of Care Management and Box 18-2:

A. *Nursing diagnosis and expected outcome:* risk for imbalanced nutrition: less than body requirements related to infrequent feeding patterns and deficient maternal knowledge; mother will breastfeed infant at least eight to ten times each day.

B. *Nursing approach:* describe feeding readiness cues to facilitate proper timing of feedings, which should occur every 3 hours during the day and every 4 hours at night, for a total of 8 to 12 feedings per day; discuss techniques to awaken sleeping baby.

6. *Bottle-feeding mother:* see Formula Feeding section and Teaching Guidelines box—Formula Preparation and Feeding:

A. *Nurse's response to mother's concern:* discuss how the mother can facilitate close contact during feeding and socialize with the infant; have her sit comfortably, touch, talk, sing, or read to baby to make the feeding time a close, intimate, and pleasant experience for both mother and baby.

B. *Guidelines for bottle-feeding:* include instruction related to such topics as how much formula and frequency of feedings; how to prepare formula, bottles, and nipples; principles of feeding such as using semiupright position, not propping bottle, making sure that fluid fills nipple, and looking for cues of satiety; burping; and choosing formula type.

CHAPTER 19: ASSESSMENT OF HIGH RISK PREGNANCY

Chapter Review Activities

1. T, 2. F, 3. T, 4. F, 5. F, 6. T, 7. F, 8. T, 9. F, 10. T

11. *Role of nurse when caring for high risk pregnant women undergoing antepartum testing:* see section on Assessment of the High Risk Pregnancy; answer should emphasize education, support measures, and assistance with or performance of the test.

12. *Woman scheduled for vaginal ultrasound:* see Ultrasonography section:

A. *Cite reason for the test for this woman:* to determine location of the gestational sac because pelvic inflammatory disease could have resulted in a narrowing of the fallopian tube, increasing the risk for ectopic pregnancy.

B. *Preparation for the test:* explain the purpose of the test, how it will be performed, and how it will feel; assist her into a lithotomy or supine position with hips elevated on a pillow; point out structures on the monitor as the test is performed; bladder does not have to be full for this type of ultrasound examination.

13. *Nurse's role related to ultrasound examination:* see Ultrasonography section; instruct woman to come with a full bladder if appropriate; explain purpose and method of examination; assist woman into a supine position with head and shoulders elevated and hip slightly tilted to the right or left; observe for supine hypotension during the test and orthostatic hypotension when rising to an upright position after the test; indicate how the fetus is being measured and point out fetus and his or her movements during the examination.

14. *State two risk factors for each pregnancy problem listed:* see Box 19-2, which lists several risk factors for each category (i.e., preterm labor, polyhydramnios, oligohydramnios, intrauterine growth restriction, postterm pregnancy, and chromosome abnormalities).

15. High risk pregnancy

16. Detection of fetal compromise, asphyxia, prevent, minimize

17. Daily fetal movement count, kick count; 12 hours; three movements within 1 hour, nonstress test, contraction stress test, biophysical profile (BPP); fetal sleep cycle, depressant medications, alcohol, smoking a cigarette, decrease

18. Ultrasonography; transabdominally, transvaginally; abdominal ultrasound, vaginal ultrasound, vagina, pelvic, pregnancy; ectopic, embryo, abnormalities, gestational age

19. Doppler blood flow analysis; hypertension, intrauterine growth restriction, diabetes mellitus, multiple fetuses, preterm labor

20. BPP, ultrasonography, fetal monitoring; fetal breathing movements, fetal movement, fetal tone, nonstress test, amniotic fluid volume; biophysical, central nervous system, hypoxemic

21. Magnetic resonance imaging; ionizing radiation

22. Amniocentesis; transabdominally, amniotic fluid; genetic disorders, pulmonary maturity, fetal hemolytic disease

23. Percutaneous umbilical cord sampling, cordocentesis, blood sampling, transfusion; umbilical blood vessel

24. Chorionic villus sampling; genetic makeup, 10, 12

25. Maternal serum alpha-fetoprotein (AFP); 16, 18

26. Triple marker test; 16, 18; maternal serum AFP, unconjugated estriol, human chorionic gonadotropin, age

27. Nonstress, accelerate

28. Contraction stress; late deceleration; nipple-stimulated contraction stress, oxytocin-stimulated contraction stress

29. D is correct; an amniocentesis with analysis of amniotic fluid for the lecithin/sphingomyelin ratio and presence of phosphatidylglycerol is used to determine pulmonary maturity; B refers to the contraction stress test; C refers to serial measurements of fetal growth using ultrasound examination.

30. C is correct; the woman should eat about 2 hours before the test to stimulate fetal movement; the test will evaluate the response of the FHR to fetal movement. Acceleration is expected; external, not internal, monitoring is used.

31. B is correct; the triple marker test is used to screen older pregnant women for the possibility that their fetus has Down syndrome; serum levels of AFP, unconjugated estriol, and hCG are measured; maternal serum AFP alone is the screening test for open neural tube defects such as spina bifida; a 1-hour 50-g glucose test is used to screen for gestational diabetes; an antibody titer (indirect Coombs' test) or amniocentesis would determine problems related to her Rh-negative status.

32. C is correct; at least three uterine contractions, lasting 40 to 60 seconds each, within a 10-minute period must occur to conduct the test; a suspicious test is recorded when late decelerations occur with less than 50% of the contractions; a negative test result is recorded when no late deceleration patterns occur; a positive test is recorded when there are persistent late decelerations with more than 50% of the contractions; unsatisfactory is the result recorded when there is a failure to achieve adequate uterine contractions.

33. A is correct; a supine position with hips elevated enhances the view of the uterus; a lithotomy position can also be used; a full bladder is not required for the vaginal ultrasound but would be needed for most abdominal ultrasounds; during the test the woman might experience some pressure, but medication for pain before the test is not required; contact gel is used with the abdominal ultrasound; water-soluble lubricant can be used to ease insertion of the vaginal probe.

Critical Thinking Exercises

1. *Woman having a BPP performed:* see BPP section and Table 19-3 for identification of the variables assessed as part of the test and how the test is scored:

A. *Nursing diagnosis:* anxiety related to the unexpected need to undergo a BPP.

B. *Nurse's response to woman's concern about the test:* describe how the test will be performed using ultrasonography and external electronic monitoring; explain that the purpose is to view the fetus within his or her environment, fetal movement, and heart rate response to activity.

C. *Meaning of a score of 8:* a score of 8 to 10 is a normal result indicating fetal well-being.

2. *Amniocentesis:* see Amniocentesis section and Nurse's Role in Antepartal Assessment for Risk section:

Preparing woman for the test: explain procedure, witness an informed consent, assess maternal vital signs and general health status, and get FHR before the test; ensure that ultrasound is performed to locate placenta and fetus before the test.

Supporting woman during the procedure: explain what is happening and why and what she will feel throughout, help her relax, and assess and observe her reactions during the test.

Providing postprocedure care and instructions: monitor maternal vital signs and status and FHR; determine when test results will be ready and whom to call; provide RhoGAM because she is Rh-negative and her husband is Rh-positive; teach her to check for signs of infection, bleeding, rupture of membranes, and contractions; make a follow-up phone call to check her status and discuss any concerns she might have regarding the test or the results.

3. *Nonstress test:* see Nonstress Test subsection of Electronic Fetal Monitoring section:

A. *Purpose of the test:* to determine adequacy of placental perfusion and fetal oxygenation by observing response of FHR to fetal movement.

B. *Preparation:* tell her that eating before the test can enhance fetal activity; schedule the test at a time of day that the fetus is usually active; assist the woman into a semirecumbent or seated position.

C. *Indicate how the test is conducted:* attach to-cotransducer to the fundus and ultrasound transducer to the site of the PMI; instruct the woman to indicate when the fetus moves; assess change, if any, in FHR as a result of movement.

D. *Analyze the tracing*

1. *Tracing indicates a nonreactive result:* no accelerations with fetal movement and limited variability.

2. *Tracing indicates a reactive result:* good variability and normal baseline range with accelerations as defined.

4. *Contraction stress test:* see Contraction Stress Test subsection of Electronic Fetal Monitoring section:

A. *Purpose of the test:* helps determine how her fetus will react to the stress of uterine contractions as they would occur during labor; uterine contractions decrease perfusion through the placenta, leading to fetal hypoxia; late decelerations during this test could be interpreted as an early warning of fetal compromise.

B. *Preparation for test:* assess woman's vital signs, general health status, and presence of contraindications for the test; attach external monitor for FHR assessment and uterine activity; assess FHR and activity; explain purpose of test, how it will be performed, and how long it will take; assist her into position as for NST.

C. *Indicate how the test is performed:* see Nipple Stimulation Contraction Stress Test section; stimulate nipples according to agency protocol until 3 uterine contractions of good quality occur within a 10-minute period, make sure that contractions subside after the test is completed, and assess maternal and fetal responses to the test.

D. *Indicate how oxytocin (Pitocin) contraction stress test would be performed:* see Oxytocin-Stimulated Contraction Stress Test section; administer oxytocin intravenously (similar to induction or augmentation of labor but with lower dosage) according to agency protocol; increase rate until uterine contractions meet the criteria for the test; monitor woman and fetus and contractions during the test and afterward until contractions subside.

E. *Analysis of results:*

1. *Negative result:* no late deceleration patterns.

2. *Positive result:* late decelerations with the appropriate number of contractions and limited variability.

CHAPTER 20: PREGNANCY AT RISK: PREEXISTING CONDITIONS

Chapter Review Activities

1. *Physiologic basis for clinical manifestations of diabetes mellitus:* see Diabetes Mellitus—Pathogenesis section for a concise explanation of each clinical manifestation listed in terms of cause and interrelationship.

2. Hyperglycemia, insulin secretion, insulin action

3. Polyuria; polydipsia, polyphagia; glycosuria

4. Pregestational diabetes mellitus; gestational diabetes

5. Glucose control, euglycemia (normoglycemia)

6. Hypoglycemia; hypoglycemic, nausea, vomiting, cravings, glucose

7. Hyperglycemia, ketoacidosis; insulin, 14 to 16 weeks

8. Phosphatidylglycerol, lecithin, sphingomyelin

9. Glycosylated hemoglobin (hemoglobin A_{1c}.)

10. Blood glucose; 25 to 30; 50% simple, complex,

11. Breakfast, lunch, dinner, bedtime, night; postprandial; insulin dosage or diet, nausea, vomiting, diarrhea, infection

12. Ketones; daily, first voided morning; meal, illness, 200 mg/dl

13. Two thirds, before breakfast, longer acting (NPH), short-acting (regular or lispro); one third, before dinner; hypoglycemia, short-acting, before dinner, longer acting, bedtime; short-acting, longer acting

14. *Complete table related to maternal risks/complications and fetal/neonatal risks/complications associated with pregestational diabetes:* see Maternal Risks/Complications subsection and Fetal and Newborn Risks/Complications subsection for a description of the risks/complications:

    • **Maternal:** miscarriage, childbirth complications related to macrosomia, pregnancy-induced hypertension, hydramnios, postpartum hemorrhage, premature rupture of membranes, infection, hypoglycemia, hyperglycemia, and ketoacidosis

    • **Fetal and neonatal:** congenital anomalies, macrosomia with related birth injuries, IUGR, intrauterine death, RDS, neonatal hypoglycemia, hypocalcemia, hypomagnesemia, hyperbilirubinemia

15. *Complete table related to metabolic changes of pregnancy and impact of these changes on pregnancy:* see Metabolic Changes Associated with Pregnancy subsection of Diabetes Mellitus section for full description related to each stage of pregnancy, including the antepartum trimesters and the postpartum period.

16. T, 17. F, 18. T, 19. T, 20. F, 21. F, 22. F, 23. T, 24. F, 25. F, 26. T, 27. F, 28. F, 29. F, 30. T

31. *State effect of thyroid disorders on reproduction and pregnancy:* see Thyroid Disorders section for a full description of hyperthyroidism and hypothyroidism; consider effects of these disorders on reproductive development, sexuality, fertility in terms of ability to conceive and sustain a pregnancy, and potential fetal-newborn complications related to maternal treatment of her thyroid disorder.

32. *Maternal and fetal complications related to maternal cardiovascular disease:* see Cardiovascular Disorders section; complications can include increase in miscarriage, incidence of preterm labor and birth, IUGR, maternal mortality, and stillbirth.

33. T, 34. F, 35. T, 36. T, 37. F, 38. F, 39. F, 40. F, 41. T, 42. T, 43. F, 44. T, 45. T, 46. F, 47. T, 48. T, 49. F, 50. T, 51. F, 52. T

53. D is correct; the woman is exhibiting signs of diabetic ketoacidosis; insulin is the required treatment, with the dosage dependent on blood glucose level; intravenous fluids might also be required; A is the treatment for hypoglycemia; although B and C might increase the woman's comfort, they are not the priority.

54. C is correct; a 2-hour postprandial blood glucose level should be lower than 120 mg/dl; A, B, and D all fall within the expected normal ranges.

55. B is correct; calories should be increased to 30 to 35 kcal/kg; a minimum intake of 250 mg of

carbohydrates is recommended daily; protein intake should range between 12% and 20%.

56. D is correct; washing hands is important, but gloves are not necessary for self-injection; vial should be gently rotated, not shaken; regular insulin should be drawn into the syringe first; because she is obese, a 90-degree angle with skin taut is recommended.

57. D is correct; other signs of cardiac compensation include moist, productive, frequent cough and crackles at base of lungs; supine hypotension, not cardiac decompensation, is a common finding during pregnancy related to compression of vena cava and aorta,.

58. A is correct; this woman is exhibiting signs of cardiac decompensation; further information regarding her cardiac status is required to determine what further action would be needed.

59. B is correct; bed rest is not required for a woman with a class II designation; she will need to avoid heavy exertion and stop activities that cause fatigue and dyspnea; actions in A, C, and D are all appropriate and recommended for class II.

Critical Thinking Exercises

1. *Preconception counseling for a woman with diabetes:* see Preconception Counseling subsection in Diabetes Mellitus section for full explanation.

    • Discuss purpose in terms of planning the optimum time for her pregnancy (when she has established glucose control within normal limits) because this will significantly decrease the incidence of congenital anomalies.

    • Diagnose any vascular problems.

    • Emphasize importance of her health and well-being before pregnancy for a healthy pregnancy outcome for herself.

    • Discuss how her diabetic management will need to be altered during pregnancy.

    • Include her husband because his health is important; he is her support during pregnancy.

2. *Pregnant woman with pregestational diabetes experiencing hypoglycemia:* see Table 20-2, Patient Instructions for Self-Management box—Treatment for Hypoglycemia, and Metabolic Changes Associated with Pregnancy and Pregestational Diabetes Mellitus subsections of the Diabetes Mellitus section:

    A. *Problem she is experiencing:* signs and symptoms she exhibits suggest hypoglycemia as a result of insufficient caloric intake with no adjustment in insulin dosage.

    B. *Action:* check blood glucose level if possible, eat or drink something that contains a simple carbohydrate, rest for 15 minutes and recheck blood glucose level, and repeat if glucose level remains low.

3. *Woman with pregestational diabetes—care management:*

   A. *Additional fetal assessment measures:* see Fetal Surveillance subsection for a discussion of a variety of antepartum tests for fetus; tests can include ultrasound examinations, maternal serum alpha-fetoprotein, fetal echocardiography, Doppler blood flow analysis through cord, maternal daily fetal movement counts, nonstress test, biophysical profile, and contraction stress test.

   B. *Stressors facing woman and her family:* list alterations in pattern of daily living, including usual management of diabetes; need for additional antepartum testing and prenatal visits; and financial implications.

   C. *Complete table related to care management during antepartum, intrapartum, and postpartum periods:* see specific subsections for diet, glucose monitoring, and insulin in Antepartum subsection of Care Management section to formulate answer; see Patient Instructions for Self-Management boxes in this section for additional suggestions for nursing interventions, including health teaching; plan of care for a woman with diabetes might also be helpful.

   D. *Activity and exercise recommendations:* see Exercise subsection of Antepartum subsection of Care Management section; recommend exercise according to her specific diabetic status, discuss when she should exercise and emphasize the importance of checking blood glucose level before, during, and after exercise and adjusting calorie intake and insulin administration accordingly.

4. *Hispanic-American woman with gestational diabetes:* see Gestational Diabetes section:

   A. *Complication being experienced with validating findings:* gestational diabetes; 50-g glucose screen result 152 mg/dl ($\geq$140 mg/dl); glucose tolerance test results reveal three values exceeding the normal range (fasting, 1-hour result, 3-hour result); see Fig. 20-4.

   B. *List risk factors in this situation:* older than 30 years of age, obese, mother has type 2 diabetes, and previous birth of baby more than 9 pounds.

   C. *Pathophysiology of gestational diabetes:* pancreas is unable to meet demands for increased insulin to compensate for the insulin resistance during the second and third trimesters and maintain normoglycemia.

   D. *Identify maternal and fetal-neonatal risks and complications:* see Maternal-Fetal Risks subsection of Gestational Diabetes section; similar to risks for pregestational diabetes, except for congenital disorders.

   E. *Outline the ongoing assessment required:* see Antepartum Care subsection; emphasize need for monitoring blood glucose level and urine for ketones, antepartum fetal surveillance, and increased frequency of prenatal visits.

   F. *State dietary changes:* see Diet subsection; woman is placed on a standard diabetic diet at 25 to 30 kcal/kg for a total 1500 to 2000 kcal/day.

   G. *Implications of gestational diabetes mellitus on her future health status:* see Postpartum subsection; more than 90% of women return to normal glucose levels, but gestational diabetes is likely to recur in subsequent pregnancies, and there is an increased risk for development of type 2 diabetes later in life; discuss lifestyle changes to lose weight and increase exercise; infant is also more likely to be obese and have diabetes mellitus in the future.

5. *Woman with type 2 diabetes unable to take oral hypoglycemic agents:* inform her that many of these agents have teratogenic potential and are less effective in regulating blood glucose levels; help her inject her own insulin through teaching, demonstration, practice, and support; see Patient Instructions for Self-Management box—Self-Administration of Insulin for preparing and injecting insulin; she will also need to learn how to check her own blood glucose level, which is another invasive technique.

6. *Pregnant women with mitral valve stenosis:* see Cardiovascular Disorders section:

   A. *Need to take heparin instead of warfarin:* see Antepartum subsection; explain why an anticoagulant is needed; inform her that warfarin (Coumadin) can cross the placenta and harm the fetus but that heparin, as a large molecule, will not.

   B. *Information to ensure safe use of heparin:* discuss her need to come for routine blood work to check clotting ability and to avoid foods high in vitamin K because vitamin K inhibits function; discuss alternative sources for folic acid; discuss side effects, including unusual bleeding and bruising.

   C. *Organic heart disease classification:* it is symptomatic with increased activity; for therapeutic plan see Antepartum subsection, focusing on specific measures for Class II:

   • **Rest, sleep, activity patterns:** use activity restriction in terms of avoiding heavy exertion; stop if signs of decompensation occur; and get 8 to 10 hours of sleep per night, with 30-minute naps after meals.

   • **Prevention of infection:** follow good hygiene and health habits to maintain resistance, identify infection early and treat promptly, and use prophylactic antibiotics.

   • **Nutrition:** follow well-balanced diet, high in iron and protein, with adequate calories and sodium restriction; stress need for potassium; and keep weight gain within limits.

- **Bowel elimination:** prevent constipation to avoid Valsalva maneuver.

D. *Factors that increase stress:* see Assessment and Nursing Diagnoses subsection of Care Management in Cardiovascular Disorder section:
- **Physiologic factors:** anemia, infection, edema, constipation.
- **Psychosocial factors:** depression, anxiety and fear, financial concerns, anger, impaired social interactions, feelings of inadequacy, cultural expectations, inadequate support system.

E/F. Symptoms and signs of cardiac decompensation: see Signs of Potential Complications box—Cardiac Decompensation, which identifies signs and symptoms for woman and health care provider.

G. 28, 32, hemodynamic changes reach their maximum

H. *These interventions to prevent cardiac decompensation:*
- Teach about rest; activity limitations; infection prevention; diet to prevent anemia and constipation; and stress reduction measures, including relaxation techniques.
- Ensure emotional and psychosocial support from health care provider and support system.
- Make referral as needed.

I. *Care during labor:* see Intrapartum subsection:
- Do comprehensive assessment for decompensation.
- Decrease fear and anxiety with one-on-one care and support in a calm atmosphere; keep her informed about what is occurring and how she and her fetus are doing.
- Provide pain relief (epidural is recommended); use comfort measures.
- Stress that vaginal birth is the best approach from a side-lying position, avoiding Valsalva maneuver and using open-glottis pushing with assistance of forceps or vacuum, oxygen via mask, and antibiotic prophylaxis.

J. 24, 48; see Nursing Alert in the Care Management section; problems occur as a result of hemodynamic changes associated with birth of baby and the circulatory and hormonal changes that occur with separation and expulsion of the placenta.

K. *Stress reduction measures during the postpartum period:* see Postpartum subsection; rest in side-lying position; assist with activities of daily living, progressive ambulation, pain relief, and measures to prevent infection and constipation; assist with newborn care.

L. *Breastfeeding:* yes, but she will need extra support as a result of the increased energy demands associated with breastfeeding.

M. *Discharge planning:* mobilize support system to help after discharge; make referrals for home care as needed; use time management techniques to plan specific times for activity, rest, and sleep; and discuss sexuality issues, contraception, and future pregnancies.

7. *Pregnant woman with epilepsy:* see Epilepsy subsection of Neurologic Disorders section; inform her that the effects of pregnancy on epilepsy are unpredictable; convulsions might injure her or fetus and lead to miscarriage, preterm labor, or separation of the placenta; she must take her medication to prevent convulsions; medications will be given in the lowest therapeutic dose; folic acid supplementation is important because anticonvulsants deplete stores of folic acid.

8. *Abuse of drugs and alcohol during pregnancy:* see Substance Abuse section:

A. *Approach of nurse during first health history interview:* incorporate questions into overall prenatal history; be matter of fact and nonjudgmental in approach used; start with questions about use of over-the-counter drugs, prescription and legal drugs (alcohol), and then illegal drugs; screen for sexually transmitted infections; use toxicology screens and questionnaires as appropriate.

B. *Factors to consider when planning care and setting outcomes:*
- Consider the characteristics of substance abusers such as depression related to previous negative life experiences; abuse might serve as a means of relieving loneliness and emptiness in their lives; abusers might have grown up in an environment where abuse is normal and they have had little opportunity to learn sober living skills.
- Remember that these characteristics can make change and recovery very difficult and interfere with their ability to be caring and nurturing parents; follow-up care is critical.

C. *Nursing measures:*
- Assist with decreasing and then stopping abuse of the substance; educate about the effects of the substance being abused on the pregnancy and the fetus—be clear and to the point and confront if necessary; use the receptivity to change during pregnancy; make referrals for treatment; assess progress; and perform toxicology screens as appropriate.

- Recognize that their ability to cope with childbirth might be limited; plan for toxicology screening of the newborn.
- Plan carefully for discharge, with safety of infant of utmost importance; make arrangements for home visit follow-up and services to help mother care for baby and continue treatment; notify child protective services if indicated.

CHAPTER 21: PREGNANCY AT RISK: GESTATIONAL CONDITIONS

Chapter Review Activities

1. Preeclampsia, 20 weeks, second, hypertension, proteinuria; mild, severe

2. Hypertension, 140/90; 2, 4-6

3. Proteinuria, 30, >1+, two, 6

4. Distribution, degree, pitting; Dependent edema, lowest

5. Severe preeclampsia, 160 mm Hg, 110 mm Hg, 5 grams, oliguria, cerebral, visual, thrombocytopenia, 100,000/mm^3, Pulmonary edema, impaired liver function

6. Eclampsia

7. HELLP, hemolysis (H), elevated liver (EL) enzymes, low platelets (LP)

8. Disruptions in placental perfusion, endothelial cell dysfunction

9. *Principles for ensuring accurate blood pressure measurement:* see Box 21-1; emphasize consistency in position of woman and her arm, the arm used, proper size of cuff, and provision of a rest period before the measurement; taking an average of two BP readings is recommended.

10. F, 11. F, 12. T, 13. F, 14. T, 15. F, 16. T, 17. F, 18. F, 19. F, 20. F, 21. T, 22. T, 23. T, 24. F, 25. F, 26. F

27. *Risk factors associated with gestational hypertension:* see Box 21-2 for a list of factors, including renal and hypertensive disease, family history of preeclampsia, multiple gestation, first pregnancy, maternal age, diabetes mellitus, Rh incompatibility, and obesity.

28. *Assessment techniques to determine findings associated with preeclampsia:*
   - **Hyperreflexia and ankle clonus:** see Table 21-4, which grades deep tendon reflex (DTR) responses; Physical Examination subsection and Fig. 21-4 provide further information and illustrations depicting performance of DTRs and ankle clonus.
   - **Proteinuria:** see Laboratory Tests subsection and Table 21-2; describe dipstick and 24-hour urine collection methods to determine level of protein in urine.

- **Pitting edema:** see Fig. 21-3, which illustrates assessment of pitting edema and classifications.

29. *Preeclampsia and eclampsia:* effect on fetal well-being:
   A. *Describe effect:* see Pathophysiology subsection of Hypertension in Pregnancy section; major effects on fetus relate to insufficient uteroplacental circulation leading to IUGR, intrauterine fetal death, or perinatal mortality (especially if abruptio placentae occurs); preterm labor and birth, acute hypoxia, and abruption can occur with a convulsion.
   B. *Fetal surveillance measures:* see Care Management subsection of Hypertension in Pregnancy; measures can include serial ultrasounds to evaluate fetal growth, nonstress test, and biophysical profile.

30. E, 31. C, 32. B, 33. A, 34. D, 35. F, 36. T, 37. T, 38. T, 39. F, 40. T, 41. T, 42. T, 43. T, 44. T, 45. F, 46. T

47. Miscarriage, premature dilation of the cervix (incompetent cervix), ectopic pregnancy, hydatidiform mole (molar pregnancy)

48. Placenta previa, premature separation of the placenta, abruptio placentae, cord insertion, placental

49. Miscarriage, 20, viable; 500 g; threatened, inevitable, incomplete, complete, missed

50. Human chorionic gonadotropin (B-hCG), 48; doubles, falling, inappropriately, pregnancy loss

51. Internal os, entirely, edge, internal os; low-lying placenta, lower uterine segment, contract

52. Premature separation of the placenta, detachment, part, all, uterus

53. *Disseminated intravascular coagulation (DIC):* see Disseminated Intravascular Coagulation subsection of Clotting Disorders during Pregnancy section:
   A. *Predisposing conditions:* include abruptio placentae, severe preeclampsia, HELLP syndrome, retained dead fetus, amniotic fluid embolism, gram-negative sepsis.
   B. *Clinical manifestations:* look for unusual and/or excessive bleeding, petechiae, oozing from injection sites, hematuria. See Box 21-6 for laboratory results present in DIC.
   C. *Priority nursing care measures:* use careful and thorough assessment, including renal function and fetal well-being, lateral position, administration of blood, blood products, and oxygen as ordered; education and emotional support of woman and family.

54. J, 55. E, 56. H, 57. I, 58. G, 59. A, 60. C 61. B, 62. D, 63. F

64. Trauma during pregnancy: see Trauma during Pregnancy section:
    A. *Significance:* see Significance subsection; statistical data, including incidence, when injuries usually occur, and types of injuries.
    B. *Effects of trauma on pregnancy:* include increased incidence of miscarriage, preterm labor and birth, hemorrhage, abruptio placentae, stillbirth, and fetal and maternal death.
    C. *Effects of trauma on fetus:* see Etiology subsection; impact can include death, skull fracture, and intracranial hemorrhage.
    D. *Observe for clinical signs of abruptio placentae:* see Clinical Manifestations subsection; deformation of the elastic myometrium around the placenta can cause the placenta to separate; when the mother survives, fetal death is usually the result of abruptio placentae in the first 24 hours; signs include uterine tenderness, pain, irritability, contractions, bleeding, leakage of amniotic fluid, and change in fetal heart rate (FHR) pattern.

65. Resuscitate the woman first, stabilize her condition; fetal, maternal; bleeding, irritability, tenderness, pain, cramps, hypovolemia; FHR, fetal activity, amniotic fluid, fetal cells; primary survey, establishment and maintenance of an airway, ensuring adequate breathing, maintenance of an adequate circulatory volume, defibrillation

66. *Complete table related to infections:* see Table 21-9 for information related to treatment measures and nursing considerations for each infection listed.

67. Hepatitis A

68. Rubella

69. Toxoplasmosis

70. Cytomegalovirus

71. Hepatitis B

72. Herpes simplex virus

73. C is correct; the woman should be seated or in a lateral position, she should rest for at least 5 minutes, and the cuff should cover 80% of the upper arm.

74. A is correct; with severe preeclampsia, the edema should be generalized, with noticeable puffiness of the eyes, face, and fingers; the DTRs should be more than or equal to 3 with possible ankle clonus; and the BP should be equal to or higher than 160/110 mm Hg.

75. D is correct; a respiratory rate of 12 breaths/min indicates dangerous central nervous system (CNS) depression by the magnesium sulfate; the solution should be 40 g in 1000 ml of Ringer's lactate, assessment should occur every 15 to 30 minutes, and the maintenance dosage should be 1 to 3 g/hour.

76. B is correct; magnesium sulfate is a CNS depressant given to prevent seizures.

77. A is correct; the woman is experiencing a threatened miscarriage; thus a conservative approach is attempted first; B and C reflect management of an inevitable and complete or incomplete miscarriage; cerclage or suturing of the cervix is done for recurrent miscarriage associated with premature dilation (incompetent) cervix.

78. C is correct; A, B, and D are appropriate nursing diagnoses, but deficient fluid is the most immediate concern, placing the woman's well-being at greatest risk.

79. B is correct; methotrexate destroys rapidly growing tissue, in this case the fetus and placenta, to avoid rupture of tube and need for surgery; follow-up with blood tests is needed for 2 to 8 weeks; vitamins (folic acid) and alcohol increase the risk for side effects with this medication.

80. C is correct; the clinical manifestations of placenta previa are described; dark red bleeding with pain is characteristic of abruptio placentae; massive bleeding from many sites is associated with DIC; bleeding is not a sign of preterm labor.

81. A is correct; hemorrhage is a major potential postpartum complication because the implantation site of the placenta is in the lower uterine segment, which has a limited capacity to contract after birth; infection is another major complication, but it is not the immediate focus of care; B and D are also important but not to the same degree as hemorrhage, which is life threatening.

Critical Thinking Exercises

1. *Woman with mild preeclampsia—home care:*
    A. *Signs and symptoms:* see Table 21-2, which differentiates between mild and severe preeclampsia in terms of maternal and fetal effects, and Table 21-3, which lists changes in laboratory values.
    B. *Three priority nursing diagnoses:* nursing diagnoses should consider physiologic effects of preeclampsia such as ineffective tissue perfusion—placenta and risk for injury to mother or fetus; psychosocial effects include anxiety, ineffective and/or compromised individual and family coping, powerlessness, ineffective role performance, interrupted family processes, and deficient knowledge; assessment findings should guide the choice and priority of nursing diagnoses, especially with regard to those that apply to psychosocial impact.
    C. *Organization of home care:* see Home Care subsection of Mild Gestational Hypertension and Mild Preeclampsia section; help couple mobilize their support system, make referrals to home care if needed, and discuss frequency of prenatal visits and antepartum testing.

D. *Teaching regarding assessment of status and signs of a worsening condition:* see Table 21-2 and Patient Instructions for Self-Management box—Assessing and Reporting Clinical Signs of Preeclampsia; discuss signs and put them in writing so couple can refer to them at home; have woman keep a daily diary of her findings, feelings, and concerns; teach woman and family to take BP, weigh accurately, and assess urine; and advise whom to call if problems or concerns arise.

E. *Instructions about nutrition and fluid intake:* see Diet subsection and Patient Instructions for Self-Management box—Diet for Severe Preeclampsia; emphasize the importance of protein, calcium, balance of roughage and fluids, and avoidance of foods that are high in salt or contain alcohol; explain rationale for dietary recommendations.

F. *Coping with activity restriction:* see Activity Restriction subsection, Patient Instructions for Self-Management box: Coping with Activity Restriction, and the Plan of Care section; explain rationale for bed rest and activity restrictions; clarify what this restriction means (e.g., how long she can be out of bed in a day and what type of activity is okay); discuss importance of lateral position when in bed, relaxation exercises, and calming diversional activities.

2. *Woman with severe preeclampsia—hospital care:*

A. *Signs and symptoms:* see Table 21-2, which differentiates between mild and severe preeclampsia in terms of maternal and fetal effects.

B. *Three priority nursing diagnoses:* ineffective tissue perfusion and risk for injury take on higher priority as the preeclampsia worsens and her condition in terms of maternal and fetal safety becomes more serious; anxiety or fear would be the priority psychosocial nursing diagnosis.

C. *Precautionary measures:* see Box 21-3, which lists hospital precautionary measures in terms of environmental modifications, seizure precautions, and readiness of emergency medications and equipment.

D. *Administration of magnesium sulfate:* see Box 21-4 and Nursing Alert in Magnesium Sulfate subsection:

- **Guidelines:** list the guidelines for preparing and administering the medication solution safely; include essential assessment measures that must be completed and documented before and during the infusion.

- **Explain expected therapeutic effect:** discuss that this medication is used for its CNS depressant effects to prevent convulsions; describe how it will be given, how she will feel,

and what will be done while she is receiving the infusion.

- **Maternal-fetal assessments:** include vital signs; FHR pattern; intake and output; urine for protein; DTRs and ankle clonus; and signs of improvement or worsening condition, including signs of an imminent seizure.

- **Signs of magnesium sulfate toxicity:** list hyporeflexia, respiratory depression, decreased blood pressure and pulse, oliguria, diminished loss of consciousness (LOC), high serum magnesium levels, and signs of fetal distress.

- **Immediate action:** discontinue magnesium sulfate infusion; administer 10% solution of calcium gluconate slowly by intravenous push.

E. *Seizure occurs:* see Eclampsia subsection and Emergency box—Eclampsia:

- **Emergency measures at onset of convulsion and immediately following:** emphasize importance of maintaining a patent airway, preventing injury, and calling for help; observe effects of seizure on mother and fetus; document the event and care measures implemented during and after seizure; provide comfort and reassurance after the convulsion; orient her to what happened; never leave her alone because another seizure could occur or signs of complications can begin; inform family.

- **List potential complications that can occur:** include rupture of membranes, preterm labor and birth, altered LOC, abruptio placentae, and fetal distress.

F. *Postpartum period recovering from eclampsia:* see Postpartum Nursing Care section:

- Close and comprehensive assessment with emphasis on signs of hemorrhage (low platelets, DIC, effect of magnesium sulfate), impending seizures, and status of preeclampsia.

- Continue hospital precautionary measures.

- Continue magnesium sulfate and antihypertensive medications; oxytocin (Pitocin) is oxytocic of choice because methylergonovine (Methergine) could elevate BP even further, especially if given parenterally.

- Provide emotional and psychosocial support for woman and her family; provide time for them to be together and with their baby but be careful to keep environmental stimuli at a low level until the danger of seizures passes.

- Discuss how her recovery is progressing and the prognosis for the rest of the postpartum period and for future pregnancies.

3. *Woman with hyperemesis gravidarum:* see Hyperemesis Gravidarum section:

A. *Predisposing and etiologic factors:* see Etiology subsection, which lists physiologic and psychologic factors, including the factors present in this situation: primigravida, maternal age younger than 20 years; additional factors include obesity, ambivalence about pregnancy, required lifestyle alterations, multifetal pregnancy, molar pregnancy, and body change concerns.

B. *Assessment of physiologic and psychosocial factors on admission:*

- **Physiologic:** include full description of nausea and vomiting; presence of other gastrointestinal symptoms; relief measures used; weight, including changes; vital signs; signs of fluid, electrolyte and acid-base imbalances; urine check for ketones and specific gravity; complete blood count; serum electrolyte, liver enzyme, and bilirubin levels.

- **Psychosocial:** discuss concerns regarding self and pregnancy; assess support system.

C. *Priority nursing diagnoses:* include deficient fluid volume, risk for fetal and maternal injury, anxiety, and powerlessness; woman's condition and circumstances will determine the priority, with physiologic diagnoses taking precedence in the acute phase.

D. *Care measures:* see Initial Care and Follow-up Care subsections:

- Discuss measures to restore fluid and electrolyte balance with intravenous administration of fluids, electrolytes, and nutrients and measures to restore ability to tolerate oral nutrition and gradual progression from NPO to full diet; monitor progress to determine effectiveness of therapeutic regimen, readiness for discharge, and need for continuing treatment with home care; provide comfort measures, including oral care and environmental modifications.

- Provide psychosocial support for woman and her family; make referrals as appropriate to home care and counseling.

- Teach woman and family about the disorder, how it is treated, its effect on pregnancy and fetus, and the importance of follow-up care.

- Discuss follow-up care requirements and types of foods and ways to eat (similar to recommendations for morning sickness).

- Include family in plan of care, especially with regard to meal preparation and support and encouragement of the woman.

- Teach woman how to assess herself in terms of weight; urine for ketones; and signs of developing problems that should be reported, including weight loss, return of nausea and vomiting, pain, and dehydration.

4. *Pregnant women requiring abdominal surgery:* see Surgery during Pregnancy section:

A. *Factors that complicate diagnosis and treatment for abdominal problems:* enlarged uterus and displaced internal organs interfere with palpation; alter position of the affected organ and change the usual clinical manifestations associated with a specific disorder; it might mimic signs and symptoms associated with pregnancy such as nausea, vomiting, and elevated white blood cell count.

B. *Common condition requiring abdominal surgery:* appendicitis; see Appendicitis subsection for clinical manifestations.

C. Fetus; FHR, uterine activity; lateral tilt, compression of vena cava; FHR, uterine activity.

D. *Discharge planning:* see Care Management subsection and Box 21-7; teach woman and family about what to watch for such as signs of infection or other complications, including onset of preterm labor, and care of incision; activity and rest considerations; and nutrition guidelines for healing; encourage performance of daily fetal movement counts; make referrals for home care as required.

5. *Woman with ruptured ectopic pregnancy:* see Ectopic Pregnancy section:

A. *Risk factors:* see Incidence and Etiology subsection; history of sexually transmitted infections, pelvic inflammatory disease, tubal sterilization, and surgical reversal of tubal sterilization.

B. *Assessment findings:* see Clinical Manifestations subsection; findings begin with signs of an unruptured tubal pregnancy (missed period, adnexal fullness and tenderness, dull or colicky pain); these signs are subtle and often missed; signs of rupture are more acute (abnormal bleeding, acute abdominal pain and referred shoulder pain, signs of hemorrhage and shock) and might be mistaken for other acute abdominal conditions.

C. *Differential diagnosis:* includes appendicitis, salpingitis, ruptured ovarian cyst, and miscarriage.

D. Hemorrhage, because much of the blood accumulates in the abdominal cavity.

E. Methotrexate; destruction/regression, unruptured, 3.5 cm

F. *Two priority nursing diagnoses:* deficient fluid volume, acute pain, and fear or anxiety and anticipatory grieving.

G. *Nursing measures for the preoperative and postoperative periods:* see Care Management subsection; measures include assessment; general preoperative and postoperative procedures; fluid replacement; emotional support to facilitate grieving; discussion of impact on future pregnancies; referral for counseling as appropriate; preparation for discharge with instructions for postoperative self-care, including self-assessment for complications such as infection; measures to enhance healing; and importance of follow-up appointment to assess progress of recovery.

6. *Woman with signs of miscarriage:*

    A. *Basis for signs and symptoms:* Table 21-6; signs indicate the woman is experiencing a threatened miscarriage.

    B. *Expected care management:* include bed rest, sedation, avoidance of stress and orgasm; follow progress with hCG levels and ultrasound to assess integrity of gestational sac; watch for signs of progress to inevitable miscarriage; caution her to save peri pads and tissue passed; provide emotional support.

7. *Woman with signs of miscarriage:* see Table 21-6:

    A. *Questions:* determine what she means by a lot of bleeding and if she is experiencing any other signs and symptoms related to miscarriage such as pain and cramping; determine the gestational age of her pregnancy and if there is anyone to bring her to the hospital if inevitable miscarriage is suspected.

    B. *Assessment findings indicative of an incomplete miscarriage:* heavy, profuse bleeding; severe cramping; and passage of tissue; cervix remains dilated.

    C. *Priority nursing diagnosis at this time:* deficient fluid volume related to continuing blood loss secondary to incomplete miscarriage.

    D. *Nursing measures:* see Medical Management subsection as basis for nursing measures identified; prompt termination of pregnancy: assess before and after procedure, explain what will occur, provide emotional support, refer for counseling if needed, prepare for discharge, and arrange for follow-up to assess physical and emotional status.

    E. *Discharge instructions:* see Home Care subsection and Teaching Guidelines box—Discharge Teaching for the Woman after Early Miscarriage; advise regarding signs and symptoms of complications (bleeding, infection), what to expect regarding progress of healing (pain, discharge), and measures to prevent complications (hygiene, nutrition, rest).

    F. *Nursing measures for anticipatory grieving:* see Home Care subsection and Teaching Guidelines box—Discharge Teaching for the Woman after Early Miscarriage; acknowledge her loss and provide time for her to express her feelings; inform her about how she might feel (mood swings, depression); refer her for grief counseling, support groups, clergy; make follow-up phone calls.

8. *Woman with complete hydatidiform mole:* see Gestational Trophoblastic Disease section:

    A. *Typical signs and symptoms:* see Clinical Manifestations subsection; signs include scant-to-profuse vaginal bleeding (dark brown to bright red), larger uterus for dates, anemia, hyperemesis gravidarum, and signs of preeclampsia before 20 weeks of gestation.

    B. *Posttreatment instructions:* see Care Management subsection; perform frequent physical and pelvic examinations; measure serum hCG levels for at least 1 year following established protocol for frequency; emphasize importance of follow-up assessments and strict birth control to prevent pregnancy until hCG levels have been normal for a specified period of time.

    C. Choriocarcinoma, hCG, uterus

9. *Comparison of a woman with marginal placenta previa to a woman with abruptio placentae, grade II:*

    A. *Comparison of findings:* see Placenta Previa and Abruptio Placentae subsections and Table 21-7 to compare findings for each disorder in terms of characteristics of bleeding, uterine tone, pain and tenderness, and ultrasound findings regarding location of placenta and fetal presentation or position.

    B. *Comparison of care management approaches:* consider home care vs. hopsital care for woman with placenta previa; hospital care is the safest approach for woman experiencing abruptio placentae; discuss active vs. expectant management for each disorder.

    C. *Postpartum considerations:* potential complications should be the basis for the special postpartum care requirements; hemorrhage (placenta previa related to limited contraction of lower portion of uterus; abruptio placentae related to Couvelaire uterus and DIC) and infection (lower implantation site, anemia from blood loss) are the major physiologic complications that need to be addressed; emotional and psychosocial support are important related to the high risk nature of the pregnanacy, especially if fetal loss was an outcome.

CHAPTER 22: LABOR AND BIRTH AT RISK

Chapter Review Activities

1. Preterm birth

2. Preterm labor

3. Length of gestation (<37 weeks of gestation), weight at the time of birth (≤2500 g)

4. Preterm birth, intrauterine growth restriction

5. Biochemical markers; fetal fibronectin

6. Fetal fibronectin; late second and early third, placental inflammation

7. Endocervical length

8. Premature rupture of membranes

9. Preterm premature rupture of membranes; infection; chorioamnionitis

10. Dysfunctional labor, dystocia, five factors affecting labor

11. Dysfunctional labor, cervical dilation, effacement, primary, descent, secondary

12. Hypertonic uterine dysfunction, painful, frequent, cervical dilation, effacement; latent; therapeutic rest

13. Hypotonic uterine dysfunction, weak, inefficient, stop

14. Soft-tissue dystocia, placenta previa, leiomyoma, ovarian tumors, bladder, rectum

15. Fetal dystocia; cephalopelvic disproportion; fetopelvic disproportion; occipitoposterior position; breech presentation

16. Multifetal pregnancy

17. Cervical dilation, fetal descent; prolonged latent phase, protracted active phase, secondary arrest, protracted descent, arrest of descent, failure of descent; precipitous labor; hypertonic uterine contractions, tetanic-like

18. External cephalic version

19. Trial of labor

20. Induction of labor

21. Bishop score; dilation, effacement, station, cervical consistency, cervical position; prostaglandins, ripen

22. Amniotomy; induce, augment

23. Augmentation of labor; oxytocin, amniotomy, nipple

24. Forceps-assisted birth

25. Vacuum-assisted birth, vacuum extraction

26. Cesarean birth

27. Postterm, postdate

28. Shoulder dystocia; fetopelvic disproportion related to excessive fetal size (macrosomia), maternal pelvic abnormalities

29. Prolapse of umbilical cord; long cord, malpresentation, transverse lie, unengaged presenting part, modified Sims, Trendelenburg, knee-chest; presenting part

30. Anaphylactoid syndrome of pregnancy, amniotic fluid embolism; Amniotic fluid

31. F, 32. T, 33. T, 34. F, 35. F, 36. T, 37. T, 38. F, 39. T, 40. T, 41. T, 42. F, 43. T, 44. T, 45. T, 46. F, 47. T, 48. T, 49. F, 50. T, 51. F

52. *Identify factors associated with risk categories for preterm labor and birth:* use Boxes 22-1 and 22-2 to complete this activity.

53. *Bed rest more harmful than helpful:* see Activity Restriction subsection of Lifestyle Modifications section and Box 22-4:

- Discuss the adverse effects of bed rest in terms of maternal physical and psychosocial effects and the effects on the woman's support system.

- Cite the fact that there is no research evidence to support the effectiveness of bed rest in preventing preterm birth or decreasing preterm birth rates.

54. C, 55. B, 56. D, 57. F, 58. A, 59. E, 60. G, 61. E, 62. F, 63. C, 64. D, 65. A, 66. B

67. *Five factors that cause dystocia:* see Dystocia section and specific subsections for each factor:

- **Powers:** dysfunctional labor (ineffective uterine contractions or bearing-down efforts).

- **Passage:** altered pelvic diameters and shape.

- **Passenger:** malpresentation or malposition, anomalies, size, number.

- **Psychologic status of mother:** past experiences, preparation, culture, support system, stress and anxiety level.

- **Position of mother:** ability and willingness to assume positions that facilitate uteroplacental perfusion and fetal descent.

68. *Therapeutic rest:* see Hypertonic Uterine Dysfunction section:

- **Purpose:** help woman experiencing hypertonic uterine dysfunction to rest and sleep so active labor can begin, usually after 4- to 6-hour rest period.

- **Methods:** use of shower or warm bath for relaxation; comfort measures; and administration of analgesics to inhibit contractions, reduce pain, and encourage rest, sleep, and relaxation.

69. *Complete table related to dysfunctional labor:* see Dysfunctional Labor section for information related to each dysfunctional labor pattern in terms of causes, maternal-fetal effects, changes in labor progress, and care management.

70. *Anaphylactoid syndrome of pregnancy:* see Anaphylactoid Syndrome of Pregnancy section.

A. *Risk factors:* include multiparity, tumultuous labor, abruptio placentae, oxytocin induction, macrosomia, and meconium passage.

B. *Signs of amniotic fluid embolism:* see Emergency box—Anaphylactoid Syndrome of Pregnancy (Amniotic Fluid Embolism) for a list of signs in terms of respiratory distress, circulatory collapse, and hemorrhage.

C. *Recommended care management for amniotic fluid embolism:* see Emergency box—Anaphylactoid Syndrome of Pregnancy (Amniotic Fluid Embolism); consider interventions related to promoting oxygenation, maintaining cardiac output, replacing fluid losses, observing for and correcting coagulation failure (disseminated intravascular coagulation), preparing for emergency birth, and providing emotional support.

71. *Indications and contraindications for oxytocin induction of labor:* see Oxytocin subsection of Care Management section; several indicators and contraindications are listed in Box 22-8.

72. D is correct; women younger than 17 or older than 35 years old represent a higher risk for preterm labor and birth, along with parity of zero or more than four; history of preterm birth, multiple abortions, or short interpregnancy interval; and infections of the genitourinary tract, including recurrent urinary tract infections, and the reproductive tract such as bacterial vaginosis.

73. A is correct; the woman should count contractions for 1 more hour and drink two to three glasses of water or juice after emptying bladder; conservative measures are tried before coming to the clinic for evaluation; she can resume light activity if contractions subside but should call for further instructions if they do not.

74. B is correct; weight loss, not gain, occurs; sleep disturbances lead to fatigue and emotional changes; lack of weight-bearing activity leads to bone demineralization.

75. C is correct; fluid intake should be limited to 2500 to 3000 ml/day; increase in heart rate is associated with beta-adrenergic agonist drugs such as ritodrine or terbutaline; magnesium sulfate is a central nervous system depressant; woman should alternate lateral positions to decrease pressure on cervix, which could stimulate uterine contractions.

76. C is correct; it is inserted into the posterior vaginal fornix; the woman should remain in bed for 2 hours; caution should be used if the woman has asthma so ensure that physician is aware; the insert is removed for severe side effects such as tachysystole or hyperstimulation of the uterus; dinoprostone often stimulates contractions and might even induce the onset of labor, eliminating or reducing the need for oxytocin.

77. D is correct; a Bishop score of 9 indicates that the cervix is already sufficiently ripe for successful induction; 10 U of oxytocin is usually mixed in 1000 ml of an electrolyte solution such as Ringer's lactate; the oxytocin solution is piggybacked at the proximal port (port nearest the insertion site).

78. A is correct; frequency of uterine contractions should be no less than every 2 minutes to allow for an adequate rest period between contractions; B, C, and D are all expected findings within the normal range.

79. C is correct; the presentation of this fetus is breech; the soft buttocks are a less efficient dilating wedge than the fetal head so labor might be slower; the ultrasound transducer should be placed to the left of the umbilicus at a level at or above it; passage of meconium is an expected finding as a result of pressure on the abdomen during descent; knee-chest position is most often used for occipitoposterior positions.

Critical Thinking Exercises

1. *Preterm labor and birth prevention program:* see Predicting Preterm Labor and Birth and Early Recognition and Diagnosis subsections:
   - Preterm birth is a major factor contributing to perinatal morbidity and mortality; early detection is critical for successful tocolysis and antenatal glucocorticoid therapy.
   - Many risk factors for preterm labor have been identified (Boxes 22-1 and 22-2), but risk scoring systems miss 50% of women who go into preterm labor.
   - All women should be taught signs of preterm labor and measures to prevent it based on identified risk factors that can be affected by changes in lifestyle behaviors (see Box 22-3).

2. *Woman with a history of preterm labor and birth:*
   A. *Identify signs of preterm labor:* see Box 22-3 as a guide for teaching woman about preterm labor; see if woman can retrospectively remember experiencing these vague signs with her first pregnancy.

   B. *Implementation of plan to prevent preterm labor:*
   - Evaluate woman's lifestyle for risky behaviors and health history for risk factors for preterm labor.
   - Discuss how certain identified factors could be changed to reduce her risk, especially those related to lifestyle (see Lifestyle Modifications subsection).
   - Consider modification of sexual activity, stress level, activity (work, home), and hygiene (prevent genitourinary tract infections).
   - Administer 17-alpha hydroxyprogesterone caproate weekly.

   C. *Woman begins to experience uterine contractions:* empty bladder, drink two to three glasses of water or juice, lie down on left side, and count contractions by palpating abdomen for 1 hour; call if contractions continue and progress; resume light activity if they do not.

   D. *Criteria for use of tocolysis:* assess woman to make sure that she is indeed in labor and that she does not exhibit contraindications to tocolysis (Box 22-6).

   E. *Nursing measures during magnesium sulfate infusion to suppress preterm labor:* see Suppression of Uterine Activity—Tocolytics section, including Medication Guide—Tocolytic Therapy for Preterm Labor, and Box 22-6.
   - Assess labor progress and maternal-fetal responses to magnesium sulfate, including adverse reactions.
   - Monitor and regulate infusion following protocol for increments in dosage of magnesium sulfate.
   - Measure intake and output.

- Provide support and encouragement.
- Maintain bed rest in lateral position.

F. *Administration of betamethasone:* see Promotion of Fetal Lung Maturity section:
- **Purpose:** stimulation of fetal surfactant production.
- **Protocol:** see Medication Guide—Antenatal Glucocorticoid Therapy with Betamethasone, Dexamethasone; explain action and indications for use, and administer intramuscularly deep into gluteal muscle, 12 mg, twice, 24 hours apart; observe for adverse effects.

3. *Woman experiencing preterm labor discharged to home care:* see Suppression of Uterine Activity and Home Care subsections of Preterm Labor Care Management section and Plan of Care for Preterm labor section:

A. *Nursing diagnoses:* risk for maternal-fetal injury related to effects of terbutaline therapy and activity restriction requirement for the suppression of preterm labor; interrupted family processes related to demands of labor suppression regimen.

B. *Instructions for maintaining terbutaline pump:* discuss use of pump, including signs of problems and site care; site change and adjustment of settings can be done by woman or home care nurse; identify side effects of terbutaline and whom to call if they should appear; teach her how to assess her vital signs, especially how to count her pulse and assess for changes in her respiratory status.

C. *Side effects of terbutaline:* see Medication Guide—Tocolytic Therapy for Preterm Labor, which lists signs that should be taught to the patient.

D. *Instructions regarding home uterine activity monitor:* discuss how often to monitor (twice daily while lying on side), how to transmit and check results, and what to do if contraction patterns indicate resumption of preterm labor; teach her how to palpate abdomen for uterine contractions.

E. *Coping with activity restriction:* identify members of her support system and include them in discussions of how activity restriction will be managed and how they can help; make referrals to home care agencies if needed.

4. *Woman with occipitoposterior position and difficulty bearing down:* see Dystocia—Secondary Powers and Fetal Causes—Malposition sections:

A. *Identified factors that have a negative effect on bearing-down efforts:* amount of analgesia and/or anesthesia used, exhaustion, maternal position, lack of knowledge about how to push effectively, lack of sleep, and inadequate food and fluid intake.

B. *Measures to facilitate bearing-down efforts:* coach her in bearing-down efforts, help her into an appropriate position, apply counterpressure to sacrum, demonstrate open-glottis pushing and coach her efforts with every contraction, and help her to begin pushing when Ferguson reflex is perceived.

C. *Recommended positions:* hands and knees or lateral position when the fetus is in an occipitoposterior position can be very effective in facilitating internal rotation and reducing back pain.

5. *Emergency cesarean birth:* see Cesarean Birth section and Care Path—Cesarean Birth:

A. *Preoperative measures:* implement typical preoperative care measures as for any major surgery in a calm and professional manner, explaining the purpose of each measure that must be performed; use a family-centered approach; discuss what will happen; witness an informed consent; assess fetal-maternal unit, insert Foley catheter, start or maintain intravenous infusion, and provide emotional support.

B. *Immediate postoperative measures:* see Immediate Postoperative Care subsection; assess for signs of hemorrhage, pain level, respiratory effort, renal function, circulatory status to extremities, emotional status, and attachment-reaction to newborn.

C. *Ongoing postoperative care measures:* see Postoperative or Postpartum Care subsection, Care Path, and Patient Instructions for Self-Management box—Signs of Postoperative Complications; measures include assessment of recovery, pain relief, coughing and deep breathing, leg exercises and assistance with ambulation, and nutrition and fluid intake (oral, intravenous); provide opportunities for interaction and care of newborn, assisting her as needed; provide emotional support to help her deal with her disappointment and feelings of failure; help her and her family prepare for discharge, making referrals as needed.

6. *Fetal position and presentation—RSA:* see Malpresentation subsection of Dystocia section; RSA indicates a breech presentation; consider that descent might be slower; meconium is often expelled, increasing danger of meconium aspiration; and risk for cord prolapse is increased; depending on progress of labor and maternal characteristics, cesarean or vaginal birth might occur.

7. *Induction of labor:* see Induction of Labor section and Box 22-8:

A. *Bishop score:* see Table 22-2 for factors assessed to determine degree of cervical ripening in preparation for labor process; used to determine if a cervical ripening method will need to be used to increase the chances of a successful labor induction.

B. *Score of 5 for a nulliparous woman:* her score should be greater than 9 to ensure a successful induction; cervical ripening will be needed before induction.

C. *Administration of dinoprostone:* see Cervical Ripening Methods subsection and Medication Guide—Prostaglandin E$_2$: Dinoprostone (Cervidil Insert; Prepidil Gel):

- Insert into posterior fornix of vagina.
- Side effects include headache, nausea and vomiting, fever, diarrhea, hypotension, and hyperstimulation of uterine contractions with or without fetal distress.
- After administration the woman should remain in bed in a lateral position for approximately 2 hours; she might then be allowed to ambulate and be discharged if stable, returning in morning for induction.
- Monitor vital signs, uterine activity, and FHR pattern.

D. *Amniotomy:* see Procedure box—Assisting with Amniotomy; explain what will happen, how it will feel, and why it is being done; assess maternal-fetal unit before and after the procedure; document findings; and support woman during procedure, telling her what is happening.

E. *Induction protocol:* 1. A, 2. A, 3. A, 4. A, 5. NA, 6. NA, 7. NA, 8. A, 9. NA, 10. A, 11. NA

F. *Major side effects of oxytocin induction:* include uterine tachysystole, abruptio placentae, uterine rupture, and abnormal (nonreassuring) FHR patterns.

8. *Postterm pregnancy:* see Postterm Pregnancy, Labor, and Birth section:

A. *Maternal-fetal risks related to postterm pregnancy:* see Maternal-Fetal Risks subsection; maternal risk relates to excessive size of fetus and hardness of fetal skull, which increase risk for dystocia; fetal risk relates to postmaturity syndrome as the placenta ages and a stressful labor and birth process resulting in increased risk for birth injury and neonatal hypoglycemia.

B. *Clinical manifestations:* maternal weight loss; decrease in uterine size; meconium in amniotic fluid; and advanced fetal bone maturation, including the skull.

C. *Nursing diagnosis:* risk for fetal injury related to placental aging and difficult birth associated with prolonged pregnancy.

D. *Care measures to ensure safety of maternal-fetal unit:* see Collaborative Care subsection:

- Continue prenatal care with more frequent visits.
- Antepartum assessments include daily fetal movement counts, nonstress test, amniotic fluid volume assessments, biophysical profile, contraction stress test, Doppler blood flow measurements, and cervical checks for ripening.
- Provide emotional support.
- Prepare for cervical ripening, induction of labor, monitoring for late and variable deceleration patterns, amnioinfusion, and forceps- or vacuum-assisted birth or cesarean birth.

E. *Instructions for self-care at home:* see Patient Instructions for Self-Management box—Postterm Pregnancy:

- Make sure that woman knows how to assess fetal movements and signs of labor.
- Emphasize importance of keeping all appointments for prenatal care and antepartum assessments.
- Identify whom to call with concerns, questions, and reports of changing status such as onset of labor or change in fetal movement pattern.

CHAPTER 23: POSTPARTUM COMPLICATIONS

Chapter Review Activities

1. Postpartum hemorrhage (PPH); hematocrit, erythrocyte infusion; uterine atony

2. Late PPH, secondary PPH

3. Early PPH, primary PPH, acute PPH

4. Uterine atony

5. Hematoma; vulvar hematomas; vaginal hematomas; perineal, rectal, vagina

6. Inversion of the uterus; hemorrhage, shock, pain; fundal implantation, malformation, short, placenta, atony, leiomyomas, placental tissue

7. Subinvolution

8. Hemorrhagic (hypovolemic) shock

9. Coagulopathy; idiopathic thrombocytopenia purpura; von Willebrand disease

10. Thrombosis, inflammation, obstruction; superficial venous thrombosis; deep vein thrombosis (DVT); pulmonary embolism

11. Postpartum, puerperal infection; fever, two successive, 10

12. Endometritis; placental

13. Mastitis, first-time mothers who are breastfeeding; unilateral, flow of milk

14. Uterine displacement, posterior displacement

15. Uterine prolapse

16. Cystocele

17. Rectocele

18. Urinary incontinence; stress incontinence

19. Fistula; vesicovaginal fistula, rectovaginal fistula

20. Pessary

21. Anterior colporrhaphy, posterior colporrhaphy

22. T, 23. T, 24. F, 25. F, 26. T, 27. F, 28. T, 29. F, 30. T, 31. T, 32. F, 33. F, 34. T, 35. F, 36. T, 37. T, 38. T, 39. F

40. *List factors increasing risk for complications of childbirth:* see specific subsection of each complication identified.

41. *Hemorrhagic shock:* see Emergency box—Hemorrhagic Shock and Hemorrhage Shock section.

42. *Twofold focus of management of hemorrhagic shock:* restore circulating blood volume and perfusion and treat the cause of the hemorrhage.

43. *Four priority nursing interventions for PPH:* see Nursing Interventions subsection of Hemorrhagic Shock section; cite interventions related to improving and monitoring tissue perfusion, treating the cause of the hemorrhage, supporting the woman and her family, and fostering maternal-infant attachment as appropriate.

44. *Standard of care for bleeding emergencies:* see Legal Tip—Standard of Care for Bleeding Emergencies; provision should be made for the nurse to implement actions independently. Policies, procedures, standing orders or protocols, and clinical guides should be established by the agency and agreed on by health care providers, including nurses; the nurse should never leave the patient alone.

45. T, 46. T, 47. T, 48. F, 49. T, 50. F, 51. F

52. Intense, pervasive sadness, severe, labile mood swings; 10%, 15%; irritability; rejection, jealousy

53. *Predisposing factors for postpartum depression:* see Assessment and Nursing Diagnoses subsection in Psychologic Complications section and Box 23-6 for a list of several factors, including prenatal or previous depression, stress, limited support, and anxiety.

54. *Clinical manifestations for postpartum depression:* see Postpartum Depression without Psychotic Features section; manifestations include depressed mood, insomnia-hypersomnia, weight changes, psychomotor retardation or agitation, fatigue, feelings of worthlessness or inappropriate guilt, diminished ability to concentrate, and suicidal ideation.

55. *Nursing diagnosis:* risk for impaired parenting: see In the Home and Community and Psychiatric Hospitalization subsections; discuss measures to keep the mother and her baby safe such as mobilizing home care resources, calls, or home visits; in the event that hospitalization is warranted, help the woman meet her baby's needs and respond to her baby's cues in a supervised setting; assess for progress in attachment.

56. *Measures to prevent postpartum depression:* see Patient Instructions for Self-Care—Activities for Prevention of Postpartum Depression section for several ideas for interventions and areas for teaching.

57. Depression, delusions, harming the infant or herself; days, 2 to 3; 8, fatigue, insomnia, restlessness, tearfulness, emotional lability, suspicion, confusion, incoherence, irrational, obsessive concerns; infant, kill the infant; bipolar disorder; manic, elevated, expansive, irritable

58. *Focuses for care management of woman with postpartum depression with psychotic features:* see Medical Management subsection; antidepressants and lithium can be given unless the mother is breastfeeding; hospitalization and psychotherapy are usually needed; supervised contact with the newborn needs to be arranged.

59. B is correct; although blood pressure should be taken before and after administration of methylergonovine, the woman's hypertensive status would be a contraindicating factor for its use; thus the order should be questioned.

60. A is correct; puerperal infections are infections of the genital tract after birth; pulse will increase, not decrease, in response to fever; B and C will also occur but are not the first signs exhibited.

61. C is correct; heparin and warfarin are safe for use by breastfeeding women; heparin, usually administered intravenously, is the anticoagulant of choice during the acute stage of DVT; woman should be fitted for elastic stockings after the acute stage is past and edema subsides.

62. C is correct; the woman needs to avoid being a "superwoman" and placing unrealistic expectations on herself; sharing feelings, resting, and having some time away from the baby are all adaptive coping mechanisms.

63. A is correct; although the other questions are appropriate, the potential for harming herself or her baby is the most serious and a very real concern.

Critical Thinking Exercises

1. *Postpartum woman at risk for PPH:*

   A. *Risk factors for early PPH:* see Box 23-1, include parity (5-1-0-7), vaginal full-term twin birth 1 hour ago, hypotonic uterine dysfunction treated with oxytocin, use of forceps for birth, and increased manipulation with birth of twins.

B. *Nursing diagnosis:* risk for deficient fluid volume related to moderate-to-heavy blood loss associated with vaginal birth of twins.

C. *Nurse's response to excessive blood loss:* most common cause of the excessive blood loss 1 hour after birth would be uterine atony, especially because woman exhibits several risk factors:

- Assess fundus for consistency, height, and location; massage if boggy.
- Express clots, if present, once uterus is firm.
- Check bladder for distention (distended bladder will reduce uterine contraction); check perineum for swelling and ask woman about experiencing perineal pressure (hematoma formation is possible related to use of forceps for birth).

D. *Guidelines for administering oxytocin intravenously:* use Medication Guide—Drugs Used to Manage Postpartum Hemorrhage for administration guidelines in terms of dosage and route, contraindications, and side effects; nursing considerations should include explanations and support for woman and her family.

E. *Signs of developing hemorrhagic shock:* see Emergency box—Hemorrhagic Shock, which identifies the priority assessment a nurse should perform and the findings that would indicate progress from hemorrhage to shock; assessment includes vital signs, skin, urinary output, level of consciousness, mental status, and central venous pressure; assessment should be frequent, and findings compared with one another to note changes.

F. *Nursing measures to support the woman and family:*

- Explain progress—meaning of findings and need for treatment measures being used, including their purpose and effectiveness.
- Use calm, professional, organized approach that incorporates periods of uninterrupted rest.
- Provide comfort measures.
- Provide opportunities for interaction with newborn and updates on newborn's status.

2. *Puerperal infection:*

A. *Risk factors:* see Box 23-4; consider preconception, antepartum, and intrapartum factors.

B. *Infection prevention measures:* emphasize measures to maintain resistance to infection (nutrition, rest, hygiene); use Standard Precautions, including handwashing, proper use of gloves, disposal of contaminated materials such as perineal pads, and care of equipment; teach woman about prevention measures, including handwashing, genital hygiene, and safer sex practices.

C. *Typical signs of endometritis:* see Endometritis subsection; signs include fever, tachycardia, chills, anorexia, nausea, fatigue and lethargy, pelvic pain and uterine tenderness, and foul-smelling profuse lochia.

D. *Nursing diagnoses:* acute pain related to effects of infection on uterine tissue; interrupted family process or anxiety related to unexpected postpartum complication (use assessment findings to determine priority psychosocial nursing diagnosis).

E. *Nursing measures:*

- Assess progress of healing.
- Administer antibiotics as prescribed; teach woman about correct use.
- Ensure adequate hydration, nutrition, and rest to enhance healing.
- Provide comfort measures and medications for pain relief.
- Arrange for newborn interaction and care.
- Use support measures and teaching to prepare woman for discharge.

3. *Woman with mastitis:* see Mastitis section:

A. *Assessment findings associated with mastitis:* unilateral findings are present well after milk comes in and include inflammation and edema with breast engorgement, chills, fever, malaise, localized tenderness, pain, swelling, redness and axillary adenopathy.

B. *Nursing diagnoses:* acute pain related to inflammation of right breast; ineffective breastfeeding or anxiety related to interruption of breastfeeding while taking antibiotics and concerns regarding transmission of infection to newborn.

C. *Treatment measures:* use antibiotics, breast support, local heat and cold applications, adequate hydration and nutrition, and analgesics; maintain lactation with continued breastfeeding, if permitted, or with breast pumping.

D. *Measures to prevent recurrence of mastitis:* focus on good breastfeeding technique (latch-on and removal, alternating positions and starting breast), frequent feedings (avoid missing feedings or abrupt weaning), breast care, early detection and treatment of cracks, and cleanliness practices.

4. *Woman with DVT:* see Thromboembolic Disease section:

A. *Risk factors:* see Incidence and Etiology subsection; in addition to venous stasis and hypercoagulability of pregnancy continuing into the postpartum period, other risk factors for this woman would be cesarean birth, obesity, age older than 35 years, and multiparity.

B. *Signs and symptoms indicative of DVT:* see Clinical Manifestations subsection; include unilateral leg pain and calf tenderness, swelling, redness and warmth, and positive Homans' sign; woman might also be asymptomatic with DVT, depending on degree of involvement.

C. *Nursing diagnosis:* anxiety related to unexpected development of a postpartum complication.

D. *Expected care management:* see Medical Management and Nursing Interventions subsections:

- Assess for unusual bleeding, signs of pulmonary embolism, and circulatory status of lower extremities.

- Administer anticoagulant (usually heparin during acute stage and then warfarin after the first few days), as ordered.

- Arrange for bed rest with elevation of affected leg; assist to change position; caution not to rub site.

- Fit with elastic stockings after acute phase when swelling has diminished and ambulation is permitted.

- Provide pain management using analgesics without aspirin and local application of warm, moist heat.

- Explain disorder and purpose and effectiveness of treatment measures used.

- Assist woman with care of self and newborn.

E. *Discharge instructions:*

- Teach how to assess leg and spot signs of unusual bleeding.

- Teach proper use of elastic or support stockings.

- Explain how to take anticoagulant safely and importance of follow-up to assess progress.

- Explain practices to prevent bleeding while taking an anticoagulant and importance of avoiding pregnancy because warfarin is teratogenic.

5. *Woman diagnosed with cystocele and rectocele:* see Cystocele and Rectocele and Care Management subsections of Sequelae of Childbirth Trauma section:

A. *Signs and symptoms most likely exhibited:* bearing down and pelvic pressure, urinary and bowel elimination changes, and bulging into the vagina noted during a vaginal examination.

B. *Management of cystocele and rectocele:* see Care Management section; focus on teaching woman about Kegel exercises, diet (fiber and fluids), stool softener, mild laxative, genital hygiene, including sitz baths, and proper use of commercial products; nursing approach should be caring and supportive.

C. *Instructions for use of a pessary:* tailor instructions for the type of pessary that is being used; include how to insert and remove, how to care for and cleanse the pessary, genital hygiene measures, and signs indicative of infection.

CHAPTER 24: THE NEWBORN AT RISK

Chapter Review Activities

1. F, 2. T, 3. T, 4. F, 5. F, 6. F, 7. F, 8. F, 9. F, 10. T, 11. T, 12. F, 13. F, 14. T, 15. T, 16. F, 17. F, 18. T, 19. F, 20. F, 21. T, 22. T, 23. F, 24. F, 25. F, 26. T, 27. F, 28. F, 29. T, 30. F, 31. T, 32. F, 33. T, 34. F, 35. T, 36. F

37. *Purpose of exogenous surfactant administration:* see Surfactant subsection of Oxygen Therapy section; preterm infants born before 32 weeks of gestation have difficulty producing enough surfactant to survive extrauterine life; exogenous surfactant will facilitate alveoli expansion and stability, easing respirations and enhancing gas exchange until the newborn can produce sufficient quantities on his or her own; administered via an endotracheal tube directly into the lungs.

38. *Kangaroo care:* see Kangaroo Care subsection in Developmental Care section and Fig. 24-6; it uses skin-to-skin holding to help preterm newborns interact with parents; it benefits newborn and parents by increasing feeling of being in control and allowing better temperature and oxygen stability with fewer episodes of crying, apnea, and periodic respirations; the newborn is in the quiet, alert state longer, thereby enhancing attachment and development.

39. *Complete the table related to physiologic problems of the preterm newborn:* each physiologic function with its potential problems is discussed in its own subsection of the Assessment section.

40. *Infections represented by TORCH:* see Table 24-7 for infections represented by each letter.

41. *Sepsis:* see the Sepsis subsection of Neonatal Infections section:

A. *Risk factors:* see Table 24-5, which identifies risk factors related to mother, intrapartum process, and neonate.

B. *Signs of neonatal sepsis:* see Table 24-6 for early signs of sepsis and signs according to body systems.

C. *Effective nursing measures:* see Nursing Intervention subsection of Care Management section; organize measures according to prevention, cure, and rehabilitation activities.

42. *Physiologic basis for ABO incompatibility:* see ABO subsection of Hemolytic Disease of the Newborn section; fetal blood is A, B, or AB; and mother's blood type is O; naturally occurring antibodies can cross the placenta, resulting in hemolysis of the fetus-newborn's red blood cells (RBCs); women with blood type O already have anti-A and anti-B antibodies in their blood.

43. B, 44. E, 45. C, 46. A, 47. D

48. *Respiratory distress syndrome:*
    A. Pulmonary surfactant, atelectasis, functional residual capacity, ventilation-perfusion, ventilation
    B. Tachypnea, grunting, nasal flaring, retractions, hypercapnia, respiratory (or) mixed, hypotension, shock; birth, 6 hours of birth; crackles, poor air exchange, pallor, apnea
    C. 72; surfactant
    D. Ventilation, oxygenation, exogenous surfactant, neutral thermal

49. Microcephaly

50. Hypospadias; epispadias; exstrophy of the bladder

51. Hydrocephalus

52. Congenital heart defect

53. Talipes equinovarus

54. Choanal atresia

55. Meningocele

56. Omphalocele; gastroschisis

57. Esophageal atresia; tracheoesophageal fistula

58. Anencephaly

59. Diaphragmatic hernia

60. Myelomeningocele

61. D is correct; retractions reflect increased effort and work to breathe; A, B, and C are all normal findings consistent with efficient respiratory effort in the preterm newborn.

62. B is correct; although A, C, and D are appropriate and important, respiration with adequate gas exchange takes precedence, especially because adequate surfactant is not produced before 34 weeks of gestation.

63. A is correct; sterile water is used to lubricate the tube; air, not sterile water, is used to check placement prior to feeding; because newborns are nose breathers, the mouth is the preferred route for insertion unless the infant is unable to tolerate it.

64. B is correct; isolation is not required, nor are gloves, for routine care measures; the nurse should be using Standard Precautions as would be used with all patients; zidovudine treatment begins after birth and continues for 6 weeks following delivery until human immunodeficiency virus (HIV) status has been determined.

65. D is correct; $Rh_o(D)$ immunoglobulin (RhoGAM) should be administered to the mother within 72 hours of birth; pathologic jaundice is unlikely because Coombs' test results indicate that antibodies have not been formed to destroy the newborn's RBCs; RhoGAM is given to prevent formation of antibodies; it would not be given if antibodies have already been formed as indicated by positive Coombs' test results.

66. A is correct; lateral or prone position prevents pressure on the sac that could cause damage; parents can hold newborn if they are supervised and instructed about how to hold infant without touching sac; sterile, moist, nonadherent dressings are used to protect the cord; Credé's method is used to ensure that all urine is emptied from the bladder to prevent stasis of urine as a result of incomplete emptying because retention is common.

Critical Thinking Exercises

1. *Weaning from oxygen process:*
    A. *Signs of readiness:* signs of respiratory distress are no longer exhibited; arterial blood gas levels and oxygen saturation are maintained within normal limits; newborn displays spontaneous adequate respiratory effort without difficulty and exhibits good color and improved muscle tone during increased activity.
    B. *Guidelines:* approach carefully in a gradual stepwise fashion from one method to another with close observation for signs of good or poor tolerance of the change; reassure and keep parents informed throughout the process of weaning, pointing out signs that their newborn is breathing effectively and is well oxygenated.

2. *Neonatal intensive care unit (NICU) environment:* see Environmental Concerns subsection of Care Management section:
    A. *Common stressors:*
       • **Infant stressors:** continuous exposure to light and noise, administration of sedatives and pain medications, and invasive procedures and medications required for treatment.
       • **Family stressors:** size and compromised, often fluctuating, health status of newborn; difficulty interacting with newborn and making eye contact; increased learning needs regarding status of newborn and care needs; concern regarding potential disabilities.
    B. *Cues related to overstimulation or relaxed state:* see Infant Communication subsection for a description of several cues for each state.
    C. *Measures to provide a balance of stimuli for the newborn:* see Infant Stimulation subsection; use water beds, kangaroo care, bundling, and coordinated plan of care to provide for period of interrupted rest and sleep; use pain medications and sedatives as needed; provide diurnal light patterns; decrease noise level; use stroking, talking, mobiles, decals, music, and wind-up toys for stimulation.
    D. *Guidelines for infant positioning:* see Developmental Care subsection; change position frequently, observing effect of position change on breathing and oxygenation and preventing aspiration; consider

boundaries, body alignment, sense of security, and comfort when positioning; teach parents.

E. *Nursing measures to support parents of an infant cared for in the NICU:* see Parental Tasks subsection; be with parents at first visit, helping them to see their infant rather than focusing on the equipment; explain characteristics of a preterm infant and purpose for procedures and equipment; encourage expression of feelings, concerns, and questions; assess their response to the newborn; make referrals to support group and arrange for home care.

3. *Postterm pregnancy:* see Postmature Infant section:

A. *Rationale for increased mortality:* increased oxygen demands are not met; and likelihood for impaired gas exchange occurs, leading to hypoxia, passage of meconium into amniotic fluid, and risk of aspiration of meconium into lungs.

B. *Typical assessment findings:* wasted appearance caused by loss of subcutaneous fat and muscle mass, peeling of skin, meconium staining, and wide-eyed appearance associated with chronic intrauterine hypoxia.

C. *Two major complications:* meconium aspiration syndrome and persistent pulmonary hypertension of the newborn; see separate subsection that describes each complication.

4. *Newborn whose mother is hepatitis B positive:* see Hepatitis B subsection of TORCH Infections section:

A. *Protocol for newborn care:* administer hepatitis B immunoglobulin 0.5 ml intramuscularly within 12 hours of birth; administer hepatitis B vaccine concurrently at a different site, repeating at 1 and 6 months of age.

B. *Safety of breastfeeding:* it is safe to breastfeed after the infant has been cleansed and the vaccine has been administered.

5. *Newborn whose mother has active herpes at the time of birth:* see Herpes Simplex Virus subsection of TORCH Infections section:

A. *Four modes of transmission:* transplacental, ascending infection by way of birth canal, direct contamination during passage through an infected birth canal (mode for this baby), and direct transmission to the newborn by an infected person.

B. *Clinical signs of active infection in the newborn:* include encephalitis (central nervous system [CNS] involvement); disseminated infection (involvement of virtually all organ systems, especially liver, adrenal glands, and lungs); or localized infection, including vesicles on skin, in oral cavity, and in eyes.

C. *Recommended nursing measures related to:*

- **Management after birth before discharge:** wear gloves when handling the newborn;

inspect for lesions and obtain cultures from mouth, eyes, and lesions as indicated; delay circumcision; discharge with mother if cultures are negative; breastfeeding is allowed if there are no lesions on the breasts; arrange for follow-up health care.

- **Vidarabine or acyclovir therapy:** provide general supportive care and treatment with acyclovir; vidarabine ointment can be used for 5 days to prevent keratoconjunctivitis.

6. *Newborn whose mother is HIV positive:* see HIV/AIDS subsection of TORCH Infections section:

A. *Potential for newborn infection:* there is a 13% to 39% risk for transmission unless zidovidine (AZT) was used during pregnancy, in which case the risk would be reduced to 8%.

B. *Modes of transmission:* prenatal (transplacental), perinatal (exposure to maternal blood and secretions during childbirth process), and postpartum (maternal secretions, including breast milk).

C. *Opportunistic and secondary infections:* common AIDS-defining secondary infections can include *Pneumocystis jiroveci* (formerly known as *Pneumocystis carinii*) pneumonia, candidiasis, cytomegalovirus infection, cryptosporidiosis, herpes simplex or herpes zoster, and disseminated varicella.

D. *Care measures:*

- Use Standard Precautions; protect infant from further exposure to maternal body fluids; gloves for routine care and isolation are not required.

- Cleanse skin with soap and water and alcohol before invasive procedures.

- Use antimicrobials as indicated for treatment and prevention of infection; give routine immunizations for children with symptomatic or asymptomatic infection; treat with combination therapy.

- Make arrangements for counseling, referrals, and follow-up for care and testing as indicated.

E. *Breastfeeding safety:* because breast milk can contain the virus, the newborn should not be breastfed; teach mother how to bottle-feed and demonstrate how she can have close contact with her newborn during feeding; in addition, discuss infection control measures that she can implement.

7. *Newborn with fetal alcohol syndrome (FAS):* see Table 24-8 in Substance Abuse section:

A. *Typical characteristics:* see substance abuse section for a full description of the newborn diagnosed with FAS.

B. *Long-term effects:* impaired visuomotor perception and performance; lowered IQ scores; delayed language development; reduced capacity to process and store factual data; motor, mental, and social delays; it is one of the leading causes of mental retardation in the United States.

C. *Nursing measures:* involve parents in care of newborn and teach them about expected effects of FAS, encourage attachment; help parents create a warm and caring home environment that enhances development; make appropriate referrals to community services for the newborn and treatment program for the mother to help her with her alcohol abuse problem (father might also need assistance).

8. *Effect of maternal substance abuse on the newborn:* see Substance Abuse section:

A. *Signs of withdrawal from heroin and methadone:* see Table 24-8.

B. *Effect of cocaine exposure:* see Table 24-8 for identification of neonatal effects in terms of physical and behavioral assessment findings.

9. *Newborn of mother suspected of abusing drugs during pregnancy:*

A. *Signs of neonatal abstinence syndrome:* see Table 24-9 for a list of signs in terms of gastrointestinal, CNS, metabolic, vasomotor, and respiratory functions and Fig. 24-11 for a scoring system.

B. *Nursing diagnoses:* deficient fluid volume related to inadequate fluid intake and increased fluid loss associated with effects of heroin withdrawal; disorganized infant behavior or disturbed sleep pattern related to withdrawal from heroin; risk for infection related to maternal risk behaviors associated with drug abuse.

C. *Care management:* see Teaching Guidelines box—Care of the Infant Experiencing Withdrawal; encourage parent participation in care of newborn, providing education and social support as needed; maintain nutrition, fluid, and electrolyte balance with careful management of feeding; practice infection control and respiratory care; use swaddling and pharmacologic treatment; carry out discharge planning and referral.

10. *Pregnant woman who is Rh negative:* see Hemolytic Disease section:

A. *Physiologic basis:* see Rh Incompatibility subsection; if an Rh-negative mother's blood comes in contact with the blood of her Rh-positive fetus, she will form antibodies against Rh-positive blood, which can then be transferred via the placenta to the fetus; if a fetus is Rh positive, the presence of these antibodies in the bloodstream will result in destruction of RBCs (hemolysis).

B. *Meaning of a positive indirect Coombs' test:* indicates that the woman has formed antibodies, probably as a result of her miscarriage and not receiving RhoGAM to prevent antibody formation.

C. *Candidate to receive RhoGAM:* woman is not a candidate because RhoGAM cannot be given once antibodies have formed or sensitization has occurred.

D. *RhoGAM purpose and use:* prevents sensitization; Rh-negative mothers who are indirect Coombs' negative should receive RhoGAM after an abortion, after specific invasive tests such as chorionic villi sampling and amniocentesis, during the third trimester, and within 72 hours after the birth of an Rh-positive direct Coombs'-negative newborn.

E. *Newborn complications:* see Rh Incompatibility subsection:
   - **Erythroblastosis fetalis:** fetus compensates for anemia caused by hemolysis by producing large numbers of immature erythrocytes to replace the destroyed RBCs.
   - **Hydrops fetalis:** marked anemia with cardiac decompensation, cardiomegaly, hepatosplenomegaly, hypoxia, and generalized edema and effusion of fluid into body spaces.

F. *Prevention of perinatal mortality:* administer intrauterine transfusions and promote early birth if the Rh antibody titer rises to dangerous levels and bilirubin level is increasing.

11. *Care management of newborn with myelomeningocele:* see Table 24-10:
   - Preoperative and postoperative measures include how to position newborn to protect the site; assess neurologic function; prevent trauma and infection of the site; facilitate bladder emptying.
   - Parental support includes facilitating attachment process; provide information and emotional care; prepare for surgical care, usually in the first 24 hours; and make referrals for long-term care for parents and child to help them adjust to and cope with the effects of the congenital anomaly.

12. *Newborn with a diaphragmatic hernia:* see Table 24-10:

A. *Clinical manifestations:* severe respiratory distress that worsens as intestine fills with air, diminished breath sounds, heart sounds in the right chest, flat or scaphoid abdomen, and bowel sounds auscultated in the chest.

B. *Nursing diagnosis:* impaired gas exchange related to inability to expand lungs fully associated with diaphragmatic hernia.

C. *Care measures in immediate postbirth period:*
- Position newborn with head and chest elevated and affected side down to allow normal lung to fully expand.
- Aspirate gastric contents to decompress gastrointestinal tract.
- Provide oxygen therapy and mechanical ventilation.

13. *Newborn with cleft lip and palate:* see Table 24-10:
A. *Nursing diagnoses:* imbalanced nutrition: less than body requirements, risk for ineffective airway clearance, and risk for impaired parent-infant attachment; all of these are related to defective and incomplete development of the lip and palate.
B. *Nursing measures:*
- Maintain airway patency while ensuring adequate hydration and nutrition using devices that prevent passage of milk into airway.
- Support and facilitate parental attachment to infant and skill with feeding; prepare parents for discharge.
- Explain the condition, how it occurs, what it entails, and how and when it will be repaired.
- Refer to support group.

14. *Birth of baby with anencephaly:*
A. *Making the decision to see the baby:*
- Tell them about the option to see the baby.
- Give them time to think about the option so that they can choose what is best for them.
- Come back and ask for their decision; if they are unsure or say no, ask again before discharge.
B. *Measures to help the couple when they see their baby:*
- Prepare baby, making him or her look as normal as possible: bathe, use powder, comb hair, put on identification bracelet, dress, wrap in a pretty blanket (get help from a funeral director if needed); give parents the opportunity to provide care.
- Explain to parents how baby will look so they will know what to expect.
- Treat baby as one would a live baby when bringing baby to parents: use name; touch baby's cheek; talk about baby's features, emphasizing those that are normal and any resemblances.
- Provide time alone with baby and adjust length of time with the baby to meet their needs; observe for cues that tell you that they need more time or that they are done; provide opportunity for family as well.
- Determine what else they would need to make a memory, such as a footprint, photograph, lock of hair.